W9-BNK-297

"As America and the healing professions have begun to embrace alternative approaches to health care, children have been left out. This splendid book helps correct this situation. Doctors Ditchek and Greenfield integrate the best of alternative and conventional medicine to help children not only survive but thrive. This is the pediatric medicine of the future because of a simple fact: It works."

—Larry Dossey, M.D., author of *Healing Beyond the Body* and *Healing Words*

"*Healthy Child, Whole Child* is a groundbreaking synthesis of the best in alternative and allopathic medicine for the very young. Ditchek, Greenfield, and Willeford have written a brilliant and supportive book for all parents. Don't leave the delivery room without it!"

—Rachel Naomi Remen, M.D., author of *Kitchen Table Wisdom*

". . . [T]he one book every family should have. Written by two conventionally trained physicians, who also have expertise in alternative medicine, *Healthy Child, Whole Child* lays the foundation for preventing illness and ensuring optimal health for your children. No parent should take chances with the health of a child: thanks to Dr. Stu and Dr. Russ, there is a safe and effective guide that would make Dr. Benjamin Spock proud."

—Kenneth R. Pelletier, Ph.D., M.D., clinical professor of medicine, Stanford University School of Medicine, and author of *The Best Alternative Medicine: What Works? What Does Not?*

"*Healthy Child, Whole Child* will revolutionize the way children perceive what it means to be healthy. . . . Not only every parent, but every member of our society should own this book and incorporate its message into our lives. Dr. Ditchek, Dr. Greenfield, and Lynn Willeford have defined an innovative and practical model for rearing healthy, whole children."

—Tracy W. Gaudet, M.D., director, Duke Center of Integrative Medicine, Duke University Medical Center

# Healthy Child, Whole Child

*Integrating the Best of Conventional*

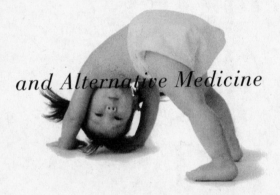

*and Alternative Medicine*

*to Keep Your Kids Healthy*

Quill

A HarperResource Book
*An Imprint of HarperCollinsPublishers*

# Healthy Child, Whole Child

Stuart H. Ditchek, M.D.
Russell H. Greenfield, M.D.

WITH LYNN MURRAY WILLEFORD

FOREWORD BY ANDREW WEIL, M.D.

Grateful acknowledgment is made to the following:
Clear Light Publishing for permission to reprint material from *Children's Book of Yoga* by Thia Luby. Copyright © 1998 by Thia Luby. Published by Clear Light Publishers; Just Imagine, Inc. for permission to reprint material from *Diaphragmatic Breathing* by Rebecca Kajander. Copyright © 1997 by Rebecca Kajander; Guilford Publications for permission to reprint material from *Hypnosis and Hypnotherapy with Children* by Karen Olness and Daniel Kohen. Copyright © 1996 by Karen Olness and Daniel Kohen; Houghton Mifflin Company for permission to reprint material from *Headache Help* by Lawrence Robbins and Susan Lang. Copyright © 2000 by Lawrence Robbins and Susan Lang.

First Quill/HarperResource edition published in 2002.

*Designed by Judith Stagnitto Abbate/Abbate Design*

*Line art by Alexis Seabrook*

Photo copyright © 2001 Julie Gang Photography

The Library of Congress has catalogued the hardcover edition as follows:

Ditchek, Stuart.
    Healthy child, Whole child : Integrating the Best of Conventional and Alternative Medicine to Keep Your Kids Healthy / Stuart Ditchek, Russell Greenfield, with Lynn Murray Willeford.—1st ed.
        p.  cm.
    Includes bibliographical references and index.
    ISBN 0-06-273745-7
    1. Children—Health and hygiene.  2. Children—Diseases—Alternative treatment.  3. Alternative medicine.
    I. Greenfield, Russell.  II. Title.

RJ47 .D55 2001
618.92—dc21
ISBN 0-06-273746-5  (pbk)                    00-054113

05 06 ❖/RRD 10 9 8 7 6 5 4 3

To my inspiration, Ruby, and to our children Teddy, Sammy, Yoni, Batsheva, and Leora. And to my mom and dad, who taught me hope and compassion.

—SHD—

To Julia, our children Abby and Jonathan, my mom, my brother, and the memory of my hero—my father, Alexander Greenfield.

—RHG—

To the family and friends who sustain me.

—LMW—

# Contents

# Foreword

## By Andrew Weil, M.D.

Writing forewords to books is not a high form of the literary art. When I do it, it is usually out of a sense of obligation to author-friends or publishers. That is not the case at present. *Healthy Child, Whole Child* is a really terrific work that embodies the spirit of the new medicine I have been trying to develop. It is a pleasure to introduce it to readers and help it find a place in the homes of parents who want to create healthy lifestyles for their children.

I know all three authors of this book, have taught them all, and worked with them. I am proud of their contributions to the growing field of Integrative Medicine and am delighted that they have taken on the tremendous task of applying it to the realm of children's health.

These are the basic principles of Integrative Medicine:

- A partnership must exist between patient and practitioner in the healing process
- Good treatment should include appropriate use of all available methods to facilitate the body's innate healing response
- Physicians must consider all factors that influence health, wellness, and disease, including mind, spirit, and community as well as body

- Doctors should neither reject conventional medicine nor accept alternative medicine uncritically
- Good medicine should be based on good science and open to new paradigms
- Doctors should use more natural, less invasive interventions whenever possible
- Medicine must address the broader concepts of health promotion and disease prevention as well as the treatment of illness
- Practitioners themselves must be models of health and healing, committed to the process of self-exploration and self-development.

Doctors Russell Greenfield and Stuart Ditchek and Lynn Murray Willeford observe all of these principles in *Healthy Child, Whole Child*. I can vouch, especially, for their adherence to the last one, because I know them all to be personally committed in their own lifestyles to health and healing and, as parents, to modeling healthy behavior for their children.

The field of pediatrics is ripe for Integrative Medicine. Pediatricians are open to it. They may lack knowledge and experience of other modalities of treatment because their training failed to provide them, but these doctors have no intellectual baggage in the way of learning. Most parents today want to make use of more natural methods of prevention and treatment for their kids. And the healing potential of young persons is greater than that of grown-ups. Give their bodies a chance and some support, and they will usually come back to the balance of health quickly, often dramatically.

At the University of Arizona Health Sciences Center, I codirect a national center for research in alternative medicine in pediatrics. Among other projects, my colleagues and I in the Department of Pediatrics and the Program in Integrative Medicine are studying the efficacy of cranial osteopathy and echinacea in managing recurrent ear infections and the usefulness of chamomile tea and hypnosis in improving recurrent abdominal pain. Both conditions are very common childhood ailments.

A great deal more of this kind of research needs to be done. But we do not have to wait for the results of studies to apply the basic principles of Integrative Medicine to raising healthy kids in the twenty-first century. That can be done right away, and Dr. Russ, Dr. Stu, and Lynn Willeford have done it. I think you will find, as I did, that they have produced a very readable, user-friendly guide that is rooted in common sense and in the same balanced approach to health and medicine that I advocate and teach. Raising healthy kids is one of the most important contributions we can make to the future. This book gives you the information and tools you need to do it.

— TUCSON, ARIZONA
JANUARY 2001

# Acknowledgments

**S***tuart:* The courage to conceptualize and write this book was supported and nurtured by my loving wife, Ruby. It was her belief in the importance of finding better ways to care for kids that inspired me to move forward. Without her patience and skill in supporting our children's needs I would not have been able to do this work—she is truly a master of stress management as it pertains to child care (especially our kids). I must acknowledge the complementary support meted out by my mom, Helen Ditchek; my sister, Karen Rosen; her husband, Jay Rosen; my mother-in-law, Susan Fishman; and my brother-in-law, David Fishman. Their emotional assistance was greatly appreciated. My dad, Teddy Ditchek, of blessed memory, whom we lost thirteen years ago, instilled in me the inner light that allowed me to dream and to care for people with compassion and without bias. His warmth continues to emanate from all those who knew him and loved him. I would like to thank Jane Friedman, who encouraged me to develop this book and opened my eyes to the privilege of educating the many rather than the few. It was Jane who introduced me to the important and groundbreaking works of Dr. Andrew Weil. Andy's warmth and loving logic have inspired me to a new level of compassionate care for my patients. Thanks also to Jeff Stone, who guided us through the book proposal process. His enthusiasm is unrivaled.

I would like to thank my mentor, Laurence Finberg, M.D., whose meticulous guidance throughout my training years at SUNY-Downstate, Kings County Medical Center, was a critical basis for my future work. Steve Shelov, M.D., chairman of Pediatrics at Maimonides Medical Center has been a great friend and teacher. His open-minded approach to pediatric care makes him a true leader in his field. Thanks to my associates at Integrative Pediatric Associates of New York—Shobha Michaels, M.D., and Zev Ash, M.D.—for being such wonderful partners and for providing unique care and warmth to our patients, to Paula Viespi D.C. for her gentle and conscientious care, to holistic dentist extraordinaire Robert Richter, D.D.S., and to Jeff Gruenglass for his constant technological and editorial assistance. A special thanks to Richard Pine, our agent, who had the vision to see the need for this book.

Most importantly I'd like to thank Russ Greenfield and Lynn Willeford for being such great friends and colleagues. Russ's unique career perspectives and warm insights and Lynn's keen writing, editorial skills, and understanding of the medical landscape made this book a robust reality. I consider them to be the closest of friends and look forward to many future endeavors together.

*Russell:* I must begin by recognizing the selfless support of my wife, Julia, who walks in beauty, and the stardust of our children, Abby and Jonathan. Their love makes anything possible, and everything beautiful. I count my blessings daily.

I reflect gratefully on my own childhood. I have my mom (Sophie), dad (Alexander), and brother (Michael) to thank for my growing up a Whole Child. They lovingly instilled in me a sense of family, the desire to learn, and a childlike appreciation for beauty and innocence. Individually and collectively, they are my role models for courage and dignity. I also offer gratitude and love to Jean and Julius Greenfield, Betty and James Stanley, and all the rest of my family.

I am grateful to my teacher and friend, Andrew Weil, M.D., who dreams of a better world and, not satisfied just to dream, works to make it so.

I owe a debt of gratitude to Tracy Gaudet, M.D., who supported my journey and enriched my life at great personal sacrifice. I thank my partners in the first class of the Program in Integrative Medicine at the University of Arizona Health Sciences Center for their support and camaraderie during our unique time together: Wendy Kohatsu, M.D., Roberta Lee, M.D., and Karen Koffler, M.D. Thank you to everyone at the Program in Integrative Medicine, who gave freely that I might learn, and to the faculty of the Department of Emergency Medicine at Harbor-UCLA Medical Center, for taking a wide-eyed boy and turning him into a doctor, and for instilling in me the love of teaching. I humbly thank all the people whom I've cared for as patients, who allowed me to witness their journeys, and have taught me so much about myself and about life.

To my friends, especially Keith Nelson and Colleen Grochowski, thank you for your enthusiastic belief in me.

A chance encounter in a gift shop led to the realization of shared dreams and this book. My coauthors, Stuart Ditchek, M.D. and Lynn Murray Willeford, are exceptionally kind human beings, gifted artists, and compassionate healers (even though Lynn has no initials after her name). The fact that we came together is evidence of there being order in this world, and I am grateful beyond measure for the time we have spent together.

*Lynn:* I want to thank my husband Blake; our son, Brook; my mother, Audrey Baston; and my sister Laurie Watts for their steadfast belief in my abilities and their unconditional love. I am also grateful to my South Whidbey support team; my writing mentors Peggy Taylor and Ann Medlock; the staff of *Dr. Andrew Weil's Self Healing* (for covering for me while I wrote the book); Andrew Weil, who opened my eyes all those years ago to a more expansive vision of health; and, of course, Russ and Stu.

We would all like to thank Andrew Weil, M.D. for his foreword, the late Michael Rothenberg, M.D., and Jo Rothenberg for their thoughts on our original outline, and Steven Shelov, M.D., for his invaluable input along the way. We want to thank Jo for lending us the electric pencil sharpener she and Michael used to edit the Spock and Rothenberg editions of *Baby and Child Care*. We want to take this opportunity to honor Andrew Weil, who through force of intellect, a belief in the indomitable human spirit, and the desire to do good in the world, is helping redefine the practice of medicine.

\* \* \*

We would also like to thank the following generous people for their information and feedback on specific chapters: nutritionist Cyndi Thomson Ph.D., R.D., assistant professor at the University of Arizona College of Public Health; Bob Lutz, M.D., medical editor for the Associate Fellowship of the Program in Integrative Medicine at the University of Arizona College of Medicine; physical-education teacher Amy Lutz, M.Ed.; Ken Bromberg, M.D., chief of pediatric infectious diseases at SUNY-Kings County Hospital Center; Susan Schacter, M.S., R.D. and Julia Schacter; Rosa Schnyer, L.Ac.; psychologist Steve Gurgevich, Ph.D., clinical faculty at the Program for Integrative Medicine at the University of Arizona College of Medicine; Francis Brinker, N.D.; Herbert Needleman, M.D., professor of psychiatry and pediatrics at the University of Pittsburgh School of Medicine; Judyth Reichenberg-Ullman, N.D., of the Northwest Center for Homeopathy; Ceci McCarten, M.D., chief developmental pediatrician at the McCarten Center in New York City; Larry Sugarman, M.D.; John Mark, M.D., and Sharon McDonough-Means, M.D., pediatric integrative medicine fellows at the University of Arizona Department of Pediatrics; Michael O'Connell, M.D.; Ilene M. Spector, D.O.; massage therapist Margaret Avery-Moon, N.C.T.M.B., president of Desert Institute of the Healing Arts in Tucson; aromatherapist, Andrea Morken and yoga instructor Susan Ferguson, R.N., B.S.N., R.Y.T. We thank Richard Pine, our agent, for the guidance he continues to offer a couple of upstart doctors.

Thanks also to the folks at HarperCollins who made publishing our first book such a pleasant experience: Ayesha Pande, Megan Newman, Nick Darrell, Miriam Sarzin, Diane Aronson, Jessica Putnam, Kate Stark, Chin-Yee Lai, Leah Carlson-Stanisic, designer Judith Abbate, and Shelby Meizlik.

Lastly, we offer thanks to the true leaders of integrative medicine, those who forged paths alone, believing not only in the medicine of the known, but also in the medicine of the possible.

We dedicate this book to parents and children around the world.

# Introduction

emily is concerned about the fact that umpteen ear infections kept her daughter on prescription antibiotics nearly all of last year, and she's decided it's time to start being proactive. Sleep-deprived Rick and Margarita are looking for an effective cure for their baby's colic. Ron would like to find some safe way to reduce his asthmatic son's reliance on steroid drugs without ending up in the ER more often. What do these parents have in common? They're all trying to make responsible health care decisions for their children while facing a bewildering array of options and an astounding lack of credible guidance. Maybe you have similar questions: How can I build up my child's immunity? What will help my child most when he's sick— a drug, an herbal extract, a homeopathic remedy, a chiropractic adjustment, a change in diet, a magnet in his shoe? Can I combine some of these therapies, and how? Which therapies are safe and effective for children and which are useless—or worse, dangerous?

So much has changed so fast in health care that we don't blame parents for feeling out of their depth. Where once there was just one kind of medicine, now there appear to be many, and few parents have the time or the knowledge to sift through and evaluate all the new information on therapies and remedies. Nor do many conventional pediatricians and family practitioners have the time to answer questions and respond to the medical and emotional concerns of the entire family. Now Dr. Welby works for an HMO and clearly cannot do much probing in the ten minutes of patient contact allotted him.

High technology and concern for the bottom line are fraying the ties between doctor and patient as medicine spins farther away from its roots in a personal healing relationship.

This soul-deep dissatisfaction with a system that doesn't seem to have the time or the inclination to treat whole beings has combined with concerns about the cost and safety of high-tech drugs to turn many adults toward less conventional health care. Americans are searching for safer, more natural, more effective, and more caring treatment, instinctively trying to create a system of health care that addresses the mind, body, and spirit in ways that conventional medicine rarely does. Homeopathy, naturopathy, mind/body medicine, herbal remedies, acupuncture, massage, body work—a myriad of modalities we never heard of as kids now offer new ways of caring for ourselves and our children.

In fact, according to a Harvard study, Americans now pay more visits to alternative practitioners in a year than they do to primary care physicians. They're visiting chiropractors for their aching backs, using biofeedback for their headaches, and seeing practitioners of Chinese medicine to relieve the side effects of chemotherapy. They're spending $250 million a year on homeopathic remedies, and close to $4 billion on nutritional supplements. Medical herbalism, once derided as "folk medicine," is now big business, with major pharmaceutical companies marketing St. John's wort for mood, ginkgo for memory and echinacea for everything else. And in a lot of cases, hype is outrunning research.

But is this stuff safe for kids? It's one thing to experiment with your own health, but as a parent you want to be more cautious with the health of your children. Yet with so many conventional and alternative therapies around—some with conflicting philosophies—how can you evaluate them and choose what's best for your children? You need expert help to sort through this information overload, tell you what works and what doesn't, and explain how to combine effective therapies into a well-integrated medical approach.

Consider us your guides through the thicket of pediatric health alternatives now available. We have been well educated and trained in conventional medicine, so we clearly understand its value, yet we are also knowledgeable about the uses of other healing therapies. As practitioners of the "integrative" medicine espoused by Harvard M.D. and best-selling author Andrew Weil, we are trained to draw the best preventive and therapeutic options from a variety of medical systems. Our goal is to facilitate the optimal functioning of your child's natural healing systems. This integrative approach respects and works along with other factors in health and wellness, such as nutrition, lifestyle, mind/body interactions, and even spiritual influences. We can give you authoritative, reliable information consistent with medical science, yet we remain open to possibilities beyond our current scientific understanding.

Who are we? Stuart Ditchek (hereafter Dr. Stu) is a practicing pediatrician and senior founding partner of Integrative Pediatric Associates of New York. Based in Brooklyn, Dr. Stu's practice carries a case load of 6,000, including children who come from other countries specifically to see him. A diplomate of the American Board of Pediatrics, an active fellow of the American Academy of Pediatrics, and a clinical assistant professor of Pediatrics at the New York University School of Medicine, Dr. Stu has all the conventional medical credentials one could wish for in a pediatrician. His style of practice—Integrative Pediatrics—is less conventional, however, drawing as it does on mind/body techniques, botanical remedies, and dietary and lifestyle changes as well as more "accepted" modalities. When it seems appropriate, he may refer a patient to a carefully chosen holistic dentist, chiropractor, acupuncturist, or therapist.

Russell Greenfield (Dr. Russ) is a specialist in emergency medicine who resigned a comfortable position as medical director of a hospital emergency department in North Carolina in order to become one of the first four physician-fellows to train with Dr. Andrew Weil at his Program in Integrative Medicine at the University of Arizona. Dr. Russ is now director of integrative medicine for the Carolinas Health Care System, and travels as a popular speaker, consultant, and instructor on integrative medicine; is a contributing editor to medical books and magazines; and serves as medical advisor to the newsletter *Dr. Andrew Weil's Self Healing*. He is a diplomate of the American Board of Emergency Medicine and an advisor to the federal and state medical boards, helping to design guidelines for the practice of integrative medicine.

In addition to being practicing physicians and researchers, Dr. Stu and Dr. Russ are dedicated fathers. Dr. Stu and his wife Ruby are raising five children from infant to preteen—Leora, Batsheva, Yoni, Teddy, and Sammy—in Brooklyn. Dr. Russ and his wife Julia and their children Jonathan and Abby have just left Tucson, Arizona, for Charlotte, North Carolina. East met West at a seminar put on by the Program for Integrative Medicine at Canyon Ranch Health Resort in Arizona, where Dr. Russ was an instructor and Dr. Stu distinguished himself as the rumpled attendee whose luggage had been lost by the airlines. We met in the gift shop there looking for presents for our kids, and began a conversation on the need for a guide to integrative pediatrics for parents. On the way from casual chat to printed page, we enlisted freelance health writer Lynn Willeford in our venture. Lynn has the necessary backgound in integrative medicine, as associate editor of the popular consumer newsletter *Dr. Andrew Weil's Self Healing* since its early days, and as a research assistant to Dr. Weil on his bestseller *Eight Weeks to Optimum Health*. In addition, as the proud mother of a college-age son, Lynn is able to provide the long view on raising kids integratively. The book in your hands is, in fact, the one she yearned for two decades ago.

We hope you will read *Healthy Child, Whole Child* from cover to cover, because we believe it is essential to have an understanding of the philosophy underlying integrative health care before trying to apply it to your children. We will introduce you to the basic concepts of integrative medicine in general and integrative pediatrics in particular. We offer a program to keep your young children healthy, and suggestions for what to do when they are not. To stress the importance to good health of optimizing the body's natural healing potential, we've put a discussion of the immune system right in the first section of the book, where we also tell you why we think your children should get vaccinations but shouldn't get so many prescriptions for antibiotics. We discuss the behaviors and attitudes that are the foundations of good health: good nutrition, regular exercise, time for relaxation, and protection from environmental and social pollutants. We'll answer such burning questions as: How can I get my kid to eat vegetables? How do we counter the "Big Mac attack"? Don't PE classes take care of my child's exercise requirement? Can kids really be stressed? and Is it safe to drink the water (or the milk)?

In Section II we introduce you to other healing approaches that can be included in good pediatric care. You'll learn what we think (and the research shows) about chiropractic, osteopathy, massage, botanical medicine, homeopathy, hypnosis, breathwork, meditation, biofeedback, energy medicine, acupuncture, and even the power of prayer. Then in the third section of the book we explain when and how these new healing modalities might be useful additions to or replacements for conventional care. We tell how to prevent or treat a sore throat, a cold, an ear infection, a gastrointestinal disorder, asthma, allergies, headache, attention deficit disorder, anxiety, and other conditions common in children. We wrap the book up with an introduction to our Healthy Child, Healthy Family Program, designed to help you and your family incorporate healthy behaviors and attitudes into your lives in a fun and participatory way.

There is a clear need for a book like *Healthy Child, Whole Child*. Parents of young children have been asking for such a guide, and older parents tell us how much they wish there had been something like this when their kids were growing up. As open-minded but conventionally trained physicians, we are uniquely qualified to write a book that honors and supports your child's natural healing potential, tells you what to do now to promote lifelong health for your children, and offers information on safe and effective treatment of common childhood conditions—all from a perspective that values both the art and the science of healing. We hope it will educate and empower you to work with your health-care professionals in achieving the goal dearest to our hearts as doctors and parents—wholly healthy kids.

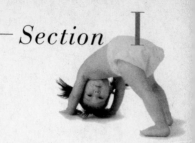

# Integrative Medicine for Children

# Chapter 1

# Read This First:

*What You Need to Know to Get the Most from This Book*

**b**efore we can talk about "integrative pediatrics" we need to explain the underlying concept of integrative medicine. "Integrative medicine" is a term popularized by the founder of the Program in Integrative Medicine at the University of Arizona, Harvard-trained physician and author Dr. Andrew Weil. It describes a model of healing that focuses on health rather than on disease, in which doctor and patient work in partnership, employing both conventional and less-established therapies to support the natural capacity for healing we all possess. Ideally, integrative medical care promotes well-being by addressing the mind, body, and spirit in a way that is effective, reasonably priced, and free of adverse side effects. Here are two examples from our practices to give you an idea of how these high-minded phrases translate into medical care in the real world.

Ten-month-old Michael (patient names have been changed throughout the book) came to Dr. Stu after his seventh ear infection. The previous infections had all been treated by antibiotics, but Michael's mom was concerned about the long-term effects of this treatment, which didn't seem to be very helpful, anyway. A purely conventional approach would have been to put the boy on preventive antibiotics for several months, and to consider surgical insertion of plastic tubes in his eardrums to relieve the fluid buildup in his inner ear if the condition did not resolve. But Dr. Stu thought he would see better results if he could uncover and address the *reason* the fluid was backing up in Michael's ears instead of just treating the boy's symptoms. Allergy or a case of gastroesophageal reflux (where the acidic stomach contents back up into the esophagus) can cause recurrent ear infections, so as an integrative pediatrician, Dr. Stu suggested dietary, lifestyle, and pharmaceutical approaches to address these possibilities. He eliminated cow's milk products from Michael's diet, changed his feeding positions, and tried a short course of acid-reducing medication. Within six weeks the fluids were gone from his middle ear, and Michael has not needed antibiotics for an ear infection since.

Dr. Russ integrated conventional and alternative therapies in a similar way when he treated Selena, a five-year-old liver-transplant recipient who was also diagnosed with a form of cancer. Since Selena's specialists were not confident she could be cured, her parents wanted Dr. Russ to do what he could to make her feel better. Dr. Russ worked in partnership with Selena's more conventional doctors to help her safely discontinue some of her medications. Among the interventions recommended were mind/body therapies and osteopathic manipulation to help ease her pain, and the herbal remedy milk thistle to help protect her transplanted liver. Selena's doctors voiced concern about her attending school because she could more easily pick up an infection, but her mom knew how important it was for her little girl "to be like every other kid," and allowed her to return to the classroom. Dr. Russ saw her a year later, and Selena looked great. Her cancer had not spread detectably, and she had not developed any infections. Although she had not been cured, her quality of life had been improved significantly.

# Defining Integrative Medicine

Integrative medicine is often confused with alternative medicine or complementary medicine, so we want to take a moment to explain the differences, with thanks to David Eisenberg M.D., who helped define these concepts. *Conventional,* or *allopathic, medicine* is the mainstream medicine taught in most American medical schools and practiced in most American hospitals. Its "don't just stand there, do something" attitude makes it excellent for medical and surgical emergencies, but it may be less useful for chronic conditions and unnecessarily aggressive in situations where time or a more gentle approach may be equally effective.

*Alternative medicine* includes therapies or philosophies not generally taught in American medical schools or offered in hospitals in this country and is used separately from or instead of conventional care. Some, such as Chinese medicine or ayurvedic (Indian) medicine, may be considered alternative here, but conventional in other countries. Alternative therapies run the gamut from the well researched to the hare-brained. Therapies considered alternative may, after further study or a change in perspective, eventually be incorporated to some degree into conventional medicine. This is what is happening now with herbal therapy.

*Complementary medicine* refers to therapies added to conventional treatment but not clinically integrated, so that practitioners may not even be aware of each other's involvement with a patient. An example of complementary medicine would be the use of herbal or nutritional therapies to alleviate the side effects of chemotherapy for cancer without the participation of the primary physician.

How does *integrative medicine* differ? Unlike conventional medicine, integrative medicine is not focused on fighting disease or suppressing symptoms, but on supporting the body's own natural healing processes. This principle is especially important in treating children, who have the potential to heal so much faster than adults. As most parents have witnessed, a child can bounce back from a fever or heal a cut virtually overnight.

With its emphasis on prevention, self-care, and the importance of trying gentle noninvasive therapies first, integrative medicine upsets the whole American paradigm of medicine as a war between doctors and invading diseases. Integrative practitioners work with the whole person—not just a collection of unconnected body parts—enlisting the patient's mind, body, and spirit in healing. They look for the underlying causes of health problems instead of only addressing the symptoms. An integrative practitioner offers a wider range of therapeutic options. We look at possible therapies—conventional and otherwise—with a cautious, scientific attitude, choosing those that are most likely to offer safe and effective treatment for a particular individual. This thoughtful integration of various modalities is in large part what distinguishes integrative medicine from alternative or complementary medicine.

There are many good physicians who are practicing integrative medicine and do not know it. They are the ones who understand the importance of an ounce of prevention. They really listen to their patients, and respect their values. They consider their patients to be partners, and are willing to learn about other therapeutic options and discuss them. The very presence of these "mindful doctors" is healing.

# Why We Practice Integrative Medicine

Although we are both conventionally trained physicians, the dawning realization that conventional medicine does not have all the answers caused both of us to change the way we practice over the past few years.

*Dr. Stu's story:* I was feeling pressed by the constraints of managed care to distance myself from my patients so I could get my work done in the required amount of time. I was losing the passion I had always had for my work because I just could not figure out how to treat the presenting problem, discuss preventive strategies for good health, and create the kind of close and caring relationship I wanted to have with my patients and their families in the ten to fifteen minutes that were allocated.

At the same time, I was also worried that my completely conventional attitude was no longer in sync with a number of my patients who were exploring alternative therapies. I was open to ways to avoid the heavy use of antibiotics and high-tech procedures so common in conventional medicine, but I have to admit I wasn't convinced that what I jokingly called "herbs and spices" was the way to go. I decided to use my scientific training to research and evaluate these alternatives, in hopes of protecting my patients from adverse side effects or money-hungry charlatans. I was delighted to come across the writings of Dr. Andrew Weil, a pioneer in the field of integrative medicine. I saw in Dr. Weil's approach a way to increase my focus on preventive medicine, augment my conventional armamentarium with a number of safe and effective alternative therapies more in line with the values of my patients' parents, and establish a more healing relationship with my patients. I've learned to look more for the root causes of health problems, such as stress or poor diet, and depend less on batteries of tests. My new openness has made the patient-doctor dialogue much more fruitful, and has allowed me to relax into enjoying my relationships with my patients.

*Dr. Russ's story:* I loved my work in the emergency department, but I was struck by how many of my patients were there because they felt their concerns had gone unheard during their ten-minute visit to their regular doctor. Few of my patients in the ED had any idea how to optimize their health or prevent disease. Although most of them had had their physical problems addressed, their gaping psychological and emotional wounds had been ignored for so long that they had finally reached a state of emergency. I became increasingly disillusioned by repeatedly treating people who had, to some extent, contributed to their ailment, whether it was the smoker's heart attack, the drinker's car accident, or the stressed-out executive's recurrent rash. These realizations stole some of the joy from the practice of medicine for me. As a hobby, I began exploring more holistic approaches to medicine. For instance, I was struck by the beauty, even the poetry, of Chinese Medicine, and could not understand Western medicine's arrogant stance that this ancient form of healing had nothing to offer American patients. In an ideal world, I thought, doctors would be able to use the best, safest, and least invasive therapies from all medical systems to prevent illness and enhance health. I wanted not only to be able to treat people in the most dire circumstances, but also to educate them, so that they might not have to return so often to the ED.

This dormant longing for a more holistic medical system was awakened when I came across an article in *Life* magazine about the new Program in Integrative Medicine that Dr. Andrew Weil had started at the University of Arizona. The very next day (after consulting my wife), I requested an application for one of the first two-year fellowships at the Program, and a week after I was accepted I quit my job in the emergency department and hauled my family from the rolling hills of North Carolina to the sagebrush and cactus of Tucson. At the time I had only the vaguest idea of what integrative medicine meant, but I hoped it would offer me tools to overcome what I saw as the limitations of conventional medicine. Naively, I thought I was just making a professional transition; I had no idea that it would require a personal transformation as well. In the first weeks and months of my training there, my skeptical mind was frequently forced to acknowledge that conventional medicine had a lot to learn about harnessing our own natural powers of healing. My training at PIM (and the birth of our children) also reawakened my previous interest in pediatric medicine, because I could see how children, with their inherently strong healing systems, could benefit greatly from an integrative approach to health.

# The Principles of Integrative Pediatric Medicine

Integrative pediatric medicine has eight basic principles in common with integrative medicine, as well as one additional principle specific to the care of children. The principles are:

*1. A belief in the innate healing powers of the body.* Your body was designed with an excellent system of defense, which we'll discuss in more detail in the next chapter. As physicians who practice integratively, we attempt to work with or support this natural healing capacity, because we believe that healing is going to come from within you, not from outside you. Our goal is always to use the best complementary and alternative therapies to strengthen and enhance the functioning of the child's innate healing capability, not take over for it.

The usual conventional medical approach, on the other hand, often ignores or tries to override the natural functions of the body's systems, attacking the symptoms of disease rather than dealing with the underlying causes of disease and not trusting that the body will often heal itself. In truth, many diseases do just run their course and go away. (As witness the old saying that a cold lasts seven days with medicine and a week without it.)

*2. Recognition of the interaction among body, mind, spirit, and environment.* The time-pressed conventional doctor generally focuses on what is called "the presenting problem," the symptom that brought you to his office that day. Yet no health problem exists in isolation. An integrative practitioner, or a good conventional one, knows the importance of not just looking at symptoms but also listening for deeper issues that might be contributing to the illness. We try to build a relationship with our patients that allows us to know the whole person—not just the medical and family history, but how the patient eats, exercises, and relates to his or her environment. We want to know what stressors are present and how the child's body reacts to them.

Conventional medicine has not been open to dealing with the mind or the spirit, although that is beginning to change. We have certainly seen for ourselves the healing possible when all parts of an individual are engaged. One example of this holistic approach to treatment is the case of Peter, a twelve-year-old boy with asthma, a constant cough, frequent upper respiratory tract infections, and migraine headaches, whose mother brought him to the clinic at the Program in Integrative Medicine when Dr. Russ was training there. Peter had seen some of the best doctors and specialists in the world, yet was still so sick he was missing one school day out of every three. Because the boy had a difficult home life, Dr. Russ believed his problems were not purely physical, but had a strong emotional/spiritual component. He offered Peter a sense of partnership; they swapped Kung Fu moves and video game secrets. Alternative measures such as lessons in self-hypnosis were recommended. When this very bright boy was given some control over his situation his symptoms improved dramatically. Within a month, Peter was feeling markedly better, and his attendance record at school had improved greatly. Integrative treatment that considered his situation and his feelings appeared to be more effective than treatment that only considered his physical self.

3. *A conviction that it is better to prevent disease than to have to treat it later.* There are innumerable studies illustrating the health-protective effects of good food, plenty of water, regular exercise, and reduction of stress. We think it is important to take the time to educate our patients about lifestyle measures such as these that will improve or maintain their health. Conventional providers are not as well versed in preventive care, because American medical schools have focused on treatment at the expense of prevention. The medical establishment, therefore, is poorly prepared to look at the deeper meaning of such things as the rising rate of some childhood cancers or the increase in asthma and allergy. In integrative medicine we believe it is safer, cheaper, and more effective to prevent disease before it starts than to have to treat it later. We think, for instance, that it makes more sense to teach your child to eat well and play often than to have to deal with a twelve-year-old with "adult-onset" diabetes brought on by obesity and sedentary ways.

4. *The belief that bodies respond uniquely, so treatment must always be customized.* Many conditions have different triggers in different people, so it makes sense that they may need different approaches to healing. Asthma is a good example: Dr. Russ has seen some people improve from osteopathic manipulation to the point where they can reduce their medications, some do better when they added acupuncture and breathing exercises to their conventional regimen, and others who find relief from a constitutional homeopathic remedy.

People vary in their biochemistry, digestion, hormonal levels, attitude, values, age and gender—all of which can influence what works and what doesn't. Since pharmaceutical drugs can vary in their effects four- to forty-fold, it is especially important to tailor the dose to the individual rather than vice versa. An integrative doctor strives to use the lowest possible dosage that is adequate to the job, recognizing that the effective dose of a prescription drug may well be less than the manufacturer's suggested dosage.

5. *A preference for gentle and inexpensive therapies over invasive or expensive ones.* In most cases nothing is lost by starting gently and becoming more aggressive if necessary. We have seen too many detrimental outcomes from overintervention, unnecessary drugs, and invasive procedures. For us the first choice for therapy is not the "big guns" but the "small sticks." For instance, why start steroid drug treatment for asthma if removing certain triggers in the environment could do the trick? Why surgically insert pediatric ear tubes if a change in diet might produce the same results?

As an example of the significant effects that even simple measures can have, we'll tell you about Isaac, a seventeen-year-old who had been battling the abdominal pain and bloody stools of Crohn's disease for four years. The immunosuppressive steroid drugs he'd been taking had significant side effects and seemed to work less well as time went on. He had become depressed and was losing so much weight that his mom did some research of her own and decided to try a dietary therapy. She took Isaac off cow's milk and most other dairy products and put him on a carbohydrate-restricted diet. She brought him to Dr. Stu to oversee this change in dietary regimen and help him taper off steroid drugs. To be truthful, Dr. Stu was still a very conventional doctor then and had no faith in this dietary approach. Yet he was forced to change his thinking when within two months Isaac was free of the pain and bloody stools and gaining weight. He was in remission for three years before his problems recurred. The now integrative Dr. Stu felt the setback might be due to the increased social and academic pressures Isaac was feeling, and added a stress-reduction component to the regimen. Isaac's newfound skills in mind/body techniques such as guided imagery and self-hypnosis have brought his condition back under control.

Dr. Russ remembers his constant surprise (and sometimes anger) during his training at the Program in Integrative Medicine when discovering gentle and effective therapies that were never mentioned in his medical school training. For instance, an older man who had been in constant pain for months from a narrowing of the spinal column called spinal stenosis came to the clinic looking for alternatives to the surgery that his doctors had told him offered the only chance to be free of pain. This was very early in his fellowship, so Dr. Russ had no faith that the osteopathic manipulation recommended by the clinic would work, because he had been taught that surgery was indeed the only option for such cases. Yet after the first osteopathic session the patient reported feeling much less pain. He returned a week later for another session. When he didn't come back to the clinic, Dr. Russ called to ask why. No need, said the man, I'm not in pain anymore. As the osteopath had predicted, the cause of the man's pain was not the spinal problem so clearly shown on the CT scans, but an easily treatable imbalance and inflammation in the surrounding musculature. That's when Dr. Russ realized that his conventional medical training had not necessarily taught him what works best, but just what works and fits within our current paradigm.

6. *A desire to integrate the best of conventional and "unconventional" medicine.* An integrative practitioner employs a wide-ranging set of tools—from conventional ones such as vaccines, antibiotics, pain medications, diagnostic tests, and surgery to mind/body techniques, homeopathy, massage, yoga, botanicals, nutritional intervention, and other alternatives. We want to stress that we do not turn our backs on the wondrous technological advances of the past few decades. Rather we embrace them, understand their limitations, and build on them.

But you have to know when to use what. There are times when only a prescription drug or invasive procedure will do, but there are just as clearly conditions for which conventional medicine has nothing very effective to offer. For instance, we have no satisfactory conventional treatments for viral illnesses, autoimmune disorders, and many forms of chronic headache or pain. In such cases alternative treatments might offer benefit. As a conventional doctor gone integrative, Dr. Stu has had great success with a first-line approach that emphasizes minimizing drug intake. For instance, very few of his patients with asthma use inhaled steroid drugs because of the effectiveness of the lifestyle, dietary, and behavioral approaches they have taken.

Yet, not every alternative therapy is effective, and people need someone with medical skills to help them evaluate these options intelligently. Considering that 83 million Americans spent $27 billion in 1997 on "unconventional" therapies, such as chiropractic, massage, herbal remedies, and dietary supplements, any doctor able to evaluate these options for safety and efficacy would surely be providing a public service. We are especially concerned that, according to a Yale University study, more than half of the people using alternative therapies did not tell their conventional doctors about them, leaving them unprotected from both harmful therapies and adverse interactions between otherwise useful therapies and conventional medications.

7. *A determination to forge a healing nonauthoritarian partnership with patients and parents.* Traditionally, the doctor has always known best, and patients who asked too many questions were treated as if they were challenging the doctor's credentials. Yet more healing actually goes on when the doctor and patient form a partnership in which the patient feels listened to and heard, and is accorded the right to make his or her own health decisions. We believe our role as doctors is to offer our findings and judgment, and be the patient's knowledgeable guide and advocate.

According to a study from Stanford University, one reason for the increased popularity of alternative therapies is that people see them as less authoritarian. Patients who use alternative therapies apparently feel a greater sense of control, a greater connection with their healer, and a better fit with their values about health. It is vital to create this sense of partnership in order to enlist all a patient's healing abilities. An integrative doctor—like any good doctor—knows that better results come not just from understanding the illness but also from understanding the person who *has* the illness. We realize that everyone who comes into our offices has underlying fears that may remain unspoken but need to be discerned and addressed. We encourage our patients and their parents to discuss these concerns. To find out how they perceive their illness and what treatment expectations they have, we listen actively and with empathy. We try to be very aware of subtle cues, leave room for any information to be offered that may require courage, and make sure that the parent and patient clearly understand what is to be done and why so they can "buy into" the program. We acknowledge that in health-care partnerships patients have the right to make the final decision, although they may choose to cede it to the doctor.

Of course, the concept of partnership implies equal responsibilities as well as equal rights. Ideally there should also be a partnership between parent and child, one that is based on love and encouragement. Along with the right to be an active and welcome participant in health care for your children, you must be willing to exert yourself as well. This may mean searching the library or the Internet for useful information to bring to your child's doctor, or changing your own unhealthy behaviors (Big Macs for lunch, too much TV, etc.) in order to be a better role model. It means taking the trouble to find a practitioner who meets your values and connects with and respects your child. Sometimes unconventional tactics may be used. Early in Dr. Stu's career he worked as a clinical consultant for a school with developmentally disabled kids. The children were frightened by the normal exam room paraphernalia, which made the exams difficult. It wasn't until a three-year-old boy with Down's syndrome pinned himself to the floor with fear that Dr. Stu tried a less orthodox approach, lying down next to the boy with his stethoscope, otoscope, and opthalmoscope on a cloth beside them. Once he got down to kid level, slowed the pace, gave the boy a chance to relax his fears of the strange instruments by trying to use them himself on his doctor, Dr. Stu was able to do the necessary exam. That's when he learned to meet his patients where they are.

8. *An acknowledgement that patients and parents have good instincts about their health.* An integrative physician expects to involve patients and their parents in the diagnosis and treatment of their problems. We almost always ask both parents and children what they think the cause or cure for their problem is, and we often find their instincts are right on target. By acknowledging their deeper knowledge of themselves or

their children, we empower our patients and their parents. Only they may know the deeper reasons for their condition. We have learned from experience that a stress-related disease is not going to go away for good until the child recognizes its cause, thus starting a process of acknowledgement, empowerment, and cure. For instance, Dr. Stu saw a fifth grader who had severe tics. Although her parents were sure she had Tourette's syndrome or some other neurological condition, Dr. Stu had his doubts. The child denied any problems at school, but knowing how much the family valued academic achievement, he sent the girl to a psychologist rather than a neurologist. Within two visits the child blurted out her belief (incorrect as it turned out) that her parents expected her to get at least a 95 on every assignment. Her tics went away as soon as she and her parents acknowledged and dealt with this underlying concern.

We also rely on the fact that most parents have a strong and pure instinct for their children's health and well-being. Parents know whether their baby's cries are from hunger or pain or fatigue, whether they mean "get this wet diaper offa me," or "I'm lonely, where is everyone?" They know if something's "off," and most of them have a true sense of when a *real* problem exists with their child. An "instinctive pediatrician" listens closely to parents and children, staying alert to the verbal and nonverbal cues that transmit this parental sense. It could be a persistent fever that just doesn't seem like other fevers the child has had, a cough or a cry that sounds different, a lack of energy in a kid who is usually running on all cylinders all day long. An observant parent makes a health practitioner's job that much easier.

There is also an additional principle that applies specifically to integrative pediatrics:

9. *The realization that children are not small adults.* When caring for a child we must never forget that we are caring for a complex developing system and must look at not just the short-term effects of a treatment but its long-term effects as well. We want to be cautious of any therapy that might interfere with the complicated processes that lead to growth and maturity. We must remember that drugs and herbal remedies that are appropriate for adults may not be equally safe for

children. Nor does Food and Drug Administration approval mean that a drug is necessarily safe for all ages and all conditions. In fact, nearly three quarters of pharmaceutical drugs prescribed for children have not been approved for this use because they have never been tested on children for optimal delivery method, dosage, and duration of therapy. We're pleased that the FDA has corrected this problem by now requiring age-specific safety profiles for new drugs. But most complementary and alternative therapies have not been tested on children either, a problem that still needs to be addressed.

As integrative practitioners, we also take the emotional effects of any medical procedure into account, especially with children. For example, even the simple, painless echocardiogram seems to upset children to the point that specialists ask us to prescribe sedatives to children undergoing this procedure. CT scan and MRI machines can be particularly scary, so we may use mind/body techniques, music, or aromatherapy to dispel children's fears. Children are also more easily traumatized by a bad experience, which colors how they react if the procedure must be repeated later.

# Visiting an Integrative Pediatrician

What can you expect from an integrative practitioner? Integrative pediatricians or primary care providers should be well versed in conventional medicine, and be knowledgeable or interested in learning about other therapies as well (they may practice them themselves or refer patients to alternative health providers they trust). They will offer advice regarding prevention of disease and optimization of health to all their patients, and offer inexpensive, gentle therapies that support the body's natural healing process as a first resort to those who are sick, moving up to more aggressive or more expensive modes only if necessary. They will look for ways to deal with the root causes of a problem and prevent its recurrence, using not only conventional interventions, but also changes in diet, behavior, environment, and attitude. Anything will be considered that may safely help the child. Mutual respect between provider, patient, and parent is a priority, so questions about or discussions of therapy are not only welcomed but also encouraged. The physician will use words carefully, providing hope and caring at every turn.

Your child's doctor may already provide such caring, informed, and empowering care, without using the label "integrative." We don't want to suggest that even completely conventional doctors cannot have caring relationships with their patients, because they clearly do. But there is a difference in perspective: An integrative doctor is more likely to provide preventive care or put greater emphasis on supporting the natural process of healing than suppressing symptoms.

# Getting More Integrative Care from a Conventional Physician

There is not yet a central service providing referrals to integrative pediatric care. You may be able to find an integrative practice in your area by asking friends for recommendations or asking respected alternative practitioners which M.D.s and D.O.s refer patients to them. But there are also ways you can get health care more in line with your values from a conventional physician or health maintenance organization. After all, our own patients had a lot to do with our switching from a purely conventional approach to one that is more integrative. So don't be afraid to tell your doctor about your health care needs and values, and about your expectations for the doctor-patient relationship. Patients and their parents have the potential to be a driving force in changing the way medicine is taught and practiced in this country.

- Keep a medical history file for each person in the family. Have copies of all tests or specialist reports faxed or mailed to you. Include doctor's visits, medications taken, side effects, and results. Include any supplements taken for the condition or other alternative therapy. Take the file to the doctor's office. If you belong to an HMO your primary care physician may change frequently, so you need to be familiar with your child's health history yourself.

- Write down the questions you want to ask, and hand the list to the doctor. Take notes when the doctor responds, or bring a friend or relative along to do so for you. Most people don't remember much after a doctor's visit.

- If your doctor has e-mail, send any further questions you have the next day.

- Educate yourself. You may need to be the one to find a qualified acupuncturist or a biofeedback trainer. Learn a little about your child's condition from reliable sources. Be prepared to send copies of pertinent studies or articles to the doctor before the next appointment, with a request for some feedback.

- Ask for any handouts or other printed materials available on subjects of interest to you.

- Ask if there are support or patient-education groups pertinent to your child's problem. Some practices or health management organizations realize there is not enough time in a typical office visit to provide all the education needed for people with chronic illnesses like asthma, and have set up after-hours classes or other programs.

- Be honest with your pediatrician about nontraditional approaches that have worked for your child, or which your child has tried. This is both educational for the physician and protective for your child, reducing the risk of drug/herb interactions, for example.

- Be prepared to change physicians if yours is not willing to be open-minded and consider alternative therapeutic options.

# Chapter 2

# Your Child's Invisible Shield:

*Immunity and How to Optimize It*

before the AIDS epidemic, the average person rarely talked about immunity. Oh, your mom might say you got a cold because you were "run-down" or that you needed to "build yourself back up" after a bout of flu, but there was no real awareness of the role and mechanisms of the immune system. We hadn't yet become as fluent in T-cell counts and natural-killer cells as we are today. But since AIDS taught all of us about the importance of a functioning immune system, parents now wonder whether they need to buy products that promise to boost immunity or create "superimmunity" in their kids. So let's talk about immunity—what it is, whether you can improve it, and whether it really needs to be "super" to do the job.

While everyone talks about "building immunity," few understand what's really involved in the day-to-day workings of the immune system. Our bodies are constantly exposed to potentially harmful bacteria, viruses, fungi, parasites, allergens, toxins, pollutants, pesticides, carcinogens, and radiation (even sunlight has its dark side). In fact, we are exposed to so many potential sources of illness that it's a wonder we're not sick all the time! Fortunately, our immune system is always on the job, whether repelling bacteria, silently erasing cuts and bruises, or restoring regular function to the body after a bout with the flu.

The primary function of this intricate and infinitely responsive system is to monitor activities throughout the body and protect the body from alien substances such as bacteria, viruses, allergens, and natural or chemical toxins, that carry immune-provoking substances on their surface called antigens. Through experience, the immune system becomes exquisitely sensitive to what is "me" and what is "not-me," and is able to target these foreign substances and either neutralize or destroy them before they can do harm.

We are rarely aware of the immune system when it is working efficiently. However, sometimes poor diet, stress, lack of exercise, environmental pollutants, or other causes weaken the immune system and allow infectious or inflammatory processes to set up shop. When that happens, the symptoms that make you think that your child is sick, such as fever or swollen glands, may actually be a sign that his immune system is mounting an appropriate response to infection. A moderate rise in body temperature slows the growth of invading organisms and speeds up your immune response, while the swelling of "the glands" (actually lymph nodes) indicates that increasing numbers of activated immune cells are gathering there to filter out and neutralize invaders. Problems also arise when the immune system does its job *too* well—attacking the body's own tissues as if they were invaders (as with autoimmune diseases) or overresponding to seemingly harmless substances like peanuts and cat dander (as with allergies and hypersensitivity).

# The Immune System

Integrative practitioners look at the immune system somewhat differently than conventional doctors do. Western medical practitioners generally view the immune system as a collection of individual organs, each of which has a specialized role to play in maintaining health. Integrative practitioners, on the other hand, define the immune system less by its various components than by the way that they work together as a functional system. That means proper immune function does not depend solely on how well any one particular organ works but on how well balanced the entire system is. A properly functioning immune system does not work only in the skin or only in the lymph nodes; it works all at once in an intricately coordinated dance of partners spread far and wide throughout the body.

The immune system is indeed everywhere. It includes specific glands, yes, but also the tiny hairs that line the tubes in your lungs, the mucous linings of your mouth and your gut, the physical and chemical barriers on your skin, the acid in your stomach, the protective enzymes in your tears and saliva, as well as the cells in your blood and your lymph (the clear fluid bathing all your tissues that transports immune cells and carries out debris). All the members of this vast defending army coordinate their activities and communicate back and forth with the brain and the endocrine glands by way of chemical messengers such as hormones, cytokines, histamine, and neurotransmitters. This intricate machinery (the ultimate in interactivity!) works to maintain that divine balance we call good health. Good health does not require "superimmunity," and we're not sure that products that claim to provide it can actually deliver. All you and your kids need is for the immune systems you were born with to function the way they are supposed to function.

A robust immune system protects not just from immediate illness, but from long-term disease as well. For instance, abnormal cells arise spontaneously in the body all the time, only to be repaired or destroyed by the immune system before they can lead to cancer. Your personal defense system is able to detect and eliminate many chemical carcinogens and natural toxins that enter the body through the air you breathe or the food you eat, and repair any damage they have caused. A strong defense against disease-causing agents (pathogens) becomes even more important now that research is suggesting a connection between bacteria and viruses and such long-term conditions as heart disease, stomach ulcers, and some cancers.

Where does immunity come from? We all have individual susceptibilities or resistance to disease that affect the operation of our immune systems. Some aspects of immunity are genetically determined. As a species we have protection against some diseases; we don't get feline (cat) leukemia, for instance. Within our own species, some of us are more or less susceptible to diseases or conditions by reason of our ethnic or racial heritage. Africans for example, have greater genetic resistance to malaria than Northern Europeans. In addition, your own familial inheritance may include susceptibility to conditions such as high cholesterol or diabetes.

Other forms of immunity are acquired either actively or passively, built up through natural exposure to various pathogens, through vaccinations, and even through your mother's milk, if you are breastfed. We'll talk more about them in a minute.

Immunity is also affected by how well the various parts of the immune system are functioning. The organs of the immune system include the skin, spleen, thymus, bone marrow, lymphatic system, tonsils and adenoids, appendix, and small intestine. Each of them plays a role in the production, storage, or transportation of the multitude of protective cells that are working round the clock to keep infection, chronic inflammation, or cancer from gaining a foothold in our bodies. A problem with one organ may affect others.

Although we tried to find one, there really is no better metaphor for the immune system than a military one—even for pacifists. The many elements of the immune system comprise a vast, interactive army with sentries, reconnaissance squads, regiments of warriors, "smart bombs," guerrilla bands, and even a Signal Corps of chemical and hormonal messengers. Control is shared amongst a junta of generals comprised of the brain and central nervous system, the endocrine (glandular) system, and the gastrointestinal system. Disorders in any one area can have significant impact upon the proper functioning of the immune system as a whole.

*(Although we are quite fascinated by how the immune system works at the cellular level, you may not share this fascination with us. In that case feel free to skip the following paragraph. Those of you interested in a brief overview of the role of immune cells in preventing disease should read on.)*

The foot soldiers of the immune system are the various white blood cells. Some respond nonspecifically to any particles that are "not-me," rushing in to attack and destroy them, and cleaning up the resulting mess. Other white blood cells called lymphocytes (T cells and B cells) are more specialized, responding only to specific antigens either by binding to their receptors and killing them or by producing antibodies (immunoglobulins) to do so. B-cells target bacteria and other foreign substances, produce antibodies, and activate the complement system—proteins that destroy the invaders and call for the pickup of any remains. T-cells destroy bacteria, cancer cells, and even cells harboring viruses. T-cells play many roles in the defense process: T-helper cells direct immune activity using chemical messengers like interferon and interleukin, T-killer cells target and kill specific invaders, and T-suppressor cells take the system off battlefield alert and return it to normal function. All these immune cells communicate with each other and with other parts of the body through chemical messengers. After an immune skirmish, memory cells that "remember" how to respond to this particular invader circulate, ready to produce the specific antibodies for it whenever it appears again. This is what we call "acquired" immunity.

How does a healthy immune system operate? Let's imagine your child has cut her hand. As bacteria penetrate the broken skin, sentry cells in the skin send out the alert. White blood cells in the front lines locate the foreign cells and jump into action, while sending chemical signals to other immune cells to bring in their more specific ammunition. The minor swelling and redness you may see around the cut indicate that blood vessels have become more porous in order to leak the liquids carrying more defensive cells onto the battlefield. As the battle rages, cellular debris is hauled away and filtered by the lymphatic system. Once the invading pathogens have been destroyed, memory cells retain the "signature" of the invader for a speedier response at the next encounter.

# Developing Immunity

Babies are born with the "hardware" of an immune system all in place: the organs, systems, and the immature cells (called stem cells) that will become immune cells. But they must develop their own "software" by teaching the components of the system how to work together. At first a baby operates with the antibodies transferred through the mother's bloodstream while the baby is in the womb and through the breast milk after birth. During birth, some microorganisms from the mother's vagina and perineum get into the baby's mouth. (Children born by Caesarean section pick up their first bacteria from the hospital and staff, instead.) These supply the "starter" bacteria for the infant's intestinal tract, where they help digest food, fight harmful bacteria, stimulate the immune system, and even produce vitamins.

The immunity borrowed from the mother wears off in a few months. Because the infant's own immune system has only just begun to develop, this is the time when your child is most vulnerable to serious infection. Slowly the immune system gains in strength as each encounter with a mild and otherwise unnoticed microorganism teaches the developing system how to recognize and deal with these "not-me" particles. With experience, the immune system becomes more skilled at defense, and accumulates more memory cells that can quickly produce antibodies. Memory cells from these encounters continue to circulate throughout the body so that the system can jump immediately into a correct response next time that particular virus or bacteria appears.

The immune system also has to learn which "not-me" bacteria are not only natural but beneficial, so that it doesn't destroy "good bugs" such as the *Lactobacilli* and *Bifidobacteria* in the digestive tract. All children carry both "good bugs" and "bad bugs" (pathogens) in and on their bodies. The pathogens cause no harm as long as they are kept in place and in balance with other microorganisms. For example, the bacterium *Clostridium dificile* normally lives in our colons, where it is kept in check by the rest of the organisms that compose normal intestinal flora. However, antibiotics may reduce the number of protective bacteria, upsetting the balance and allowing *Clostridium* to reproduce enough to cause an infection.

Children are not intended to be germ-free. In fact, young children need exposure to mild pathogens in order to become immune competent. That's why it is not necessary or even useful to fill children's rooms with antibacterial toys, bedding, and sprays in an effort to protect them from all contact with germs. Some medical researchers even theorize that this obsession with providing a germ-free environment may backfire over the long term, making children more vulnerable to developing allergies and asthma.

We are fascinated by this hotly debated "Hygiene Hypothesis." Its advocates believe that a germ-free environment deprives very young children of the exposure to innocuous bacteria that is necessary to balance the two arms of the developing immune system. One part of the system (Th1) fights infecting cells with an inflammatory response. The other (Th2) drives allergic response. A child is born with a stronger Th2 response. Normally, exposure to harmless microorganisms builds up the Th1 response. If all germs in the child's inner and outer environment are wiped out by antibiotic drugs and antimicrobial products, the Th1 response is not able to get stronger. The resulting imbalance in the two arms of the immune system, some say, is driving the increase in allergies and asthma that we are seeing today. If this proves to be the case, it might be better to let your children get a little dirty now and then.

# Influences on Immunity

The environment to which you are exposed, what you eat, and how much or how little you exercise all influence the quality of your immune response. Your brain also has tremendous influence on health and healing. There is, in fact, a whole new field of study called psychoneuroimmunology that looks at the connections between the brain and the endocrine and immune systems, and at how our thoughts and feelings affect the immune system's responses. One day we will probably take for granted the now-controversial idea that *every* major organ system and regulatory mechanism in the body is affected by outside events and their interpretation by the mind and emotions.

As evidence for the integration of these systems psychoneuroimmunologists point to the fact that white blood cells have receptors for chemical messengers from both the glands (hormones) and the brain (neurotransmitters). This chemical communication between the brain, the endocrine system, and the immune system seems to go in all directions—from the brain to the immune system, from the glands to the immune system, from the immune system to the brain, and so on.

Research in psychoneuroimmunology increasingly links factors such as stress and emotions to our susceptibility and response to infections, autoimmunity, and cancer. A number of studies have found that wounds heal more slowly in people under stress, and the late Norman Cousins wrote extensively from research and his own experience on the healing power of humor and a positive attitude. We'll talk more about this in the chapter on mind/body medicine.

# Optimizing Your Child's Immunity

Now that you understand a little about how the immune system operates, here's what you as parents can do to keep your children from catching every cold and flu that goes around. You can consider the sixteen steps that follow to be your blueprint for raising a healthy child. We will discuss each of them in greater detail in the chapters that follow. Please don't be intimidated by the length of this list. Just start with those steps that seem most achievable for your family and add additional strategies as you can.

- *Make sure your children get enough sleep.* Lack of sleep is a significant stress on the body. Haven't you noticed that you get more colds when you've been sleeping poorly?
- *Feed your kids a balanced, nutritious diet.* Breast-feed your babies, if possible, and give older kids lots of fruits, vegetables, and whole grains. Minimize the amount of highly processed foods they eat.
- *Protect children from environmental pollutants.* Ensure that their drinking water is pure. Wash your produce and buy organic foods when possible. Look for foods wrapped in nontoxic mate-

rials. Avoid the use of harmful household, lawn, and garden chemicals.

- *Teach your children how to reduce stress and how to cope with life's irritations in a healthy way.* As they get older, teach them to stay alert for the origins of some of their health problems in stress, anxiety, or other emotional states. Try to keep your own stress levels in check, as your kids will pick up on your anxieties.

- *Emphasize basic hygiene.* Teach your kids the proper way to wash their hands and brush their teeth.

- *Make physical activity a family goal.* Take frequent walks and bike rides together, or play hoops in the driveway after dinner. Limit your kids' sedentary activities, such as watching TV or playing video games. Exercise regularly yourself, and tell your children why you do.

- *Make sure your children drink plenty of water* to keep their organs functioning properly and their mucous membranes fat and happy. The mucous membranes that line your body passages are your prime defense against colds, flu, sinusitis, airborne toxins and even urinary tract infections.

- *Have fun.* Good times and lots of social ties reduce levels of stress hormones and improve immunity. And a sense of humor will get you and your children through many trying times.

- *Encourage optimism and the desire to be of use in the world.* It's never too early to instill a sense of meaning or spirituality in your children's lives so they feel part of something greater than themselves. Studies have linked positive attitude to faster healing.

- *Give your children massages, and teach them how to massage themselves and other family members.* We all long for some form of touch, and loving touch is very healing.

- *Get the recommended shots.* Immunization protects our children from diseases that once caused a great deal of pain and suffering.

- *Refrain from the urge to reach for antibiotics and antibacterial products* all the time to prevent your little ones from being "contaminated." Their immune systems need exposure to the common germs of everyday life to be able to fend off future infections.

- *Instill the attitude that the body has a natural desire to heal.* Teach your children to trust in the innate natural wisdom of the body, and its natural desire to be in healthy balance.

- *Do everything you can to keep your children from smoking* cigarettes, and make sure they are not exposed to the tobacco smoke of others. Tobacco use is an underlying risk factor for cancer, heart disease, emphysema, and other serious long-term conditions, and those who start smoking the youngest have the most trouble quitting. Even passive exposure to Mom or Dad's cigarette smoke contributes to allergies, ear infections, asthma, and other upper respiratory problems.

- *Offer your unconditional love.* Give each child your full and undivided attention at some point every day.

- *Be a good role model.* Be aware that the way you live your life is a lesson for your children. Do you really want them to be stressed-out, sedentary, caffeine-addicted, French-fry lovers when they grow up?

# Chapter 3

# A Shot in the Arm (or the Leg):

## *A Balanced Look at Vaccinations*

S hots! Now there's a word that can propel any child old enough to recognize it into a veritable cascade of activity designed to forestall the inevitable. Bribery, bargaining, pleading, empty promises—we've heard it all. Fortunately, immunization methods are getting less painful, and we have discovered through experience that children are incredibly forgiving. Not five minutes after having practically wrestled a kid to the ground to give him a shot, that same child will grab us around the knees and give us a big hug out in the waiting room. And that's a good thing, because immunization against deadly disease is one of the first steps parents can take to protect their children's health.

We know that vaccination is a controversial topic in alternative medical circles, and can be a source of tension between parents and the health professionals who care for their children. We think it's important for parents and pediatricians to be willing to engage in an honest dialogue on this contentious issue. Our fervent hope is that these discussions will strengthen the parent-doctor relationship and assuage parental fears about immunization. We think parents should recognize that pediatricians are devoted to the health and safety of the children in their care and would not knowingly act to endanger them. For their part, pediatricians should recognize that questions from parents do not imply a lack of trust, and that there *are* unanswered questions about vaccines that parents have a right—and a duty—to ask.

That said, we will declare our bias up front: We are strongly in favor of immunizing your child. (In fact Dr. Stu is so convinced that immunization is vital to the health and safety of a child that he doesn't accept into his practice families who will not allow their children to get their basic vaccinations.) As integrative practitioners we choose the safest, most effective treatments and protective practices from all the possibilities offered by conventional and alternative medicine. In this case we're going with conventional medical practice because we have seen the alternatives, and they are frightening to us as doctors and as fathers. We've been strongly motivated to vaccinate our own kids by those professional and personal experiences. As a young doctor training in the emergency room, Dr. Russ used to see many cases of bacterial meningitis, an inflammation of the brain and spinal cord, caused by *Haemophilus influenzae*. He was shocked by how quickly this form of meningitis attacked; it could lay previously healthy children so low so fast that they suffered terrible consequences if antibiotics were not administered immediately. Thanks to vaccines, it's now uncommon for an emergency-department doctor to see *H. influenzae* meningitis.

Similarly, Dr. Stu recalls the horror he experienced as a resident trying to ease the suffering of tiny patients with whooping cough (pertussis) as they struggled painfully for breath, choking and turning blue. As a result, he and his wife Ruby—a pediatric occupational therapist who has worked with kids suffering the neurological side effects of pertussis and other serious but preventable infections—enrolled their firstborn daughter in trials of an improved vaccine for whooping cough so that she would get maximal protection. All their kids have since participated in other vaccine studies, including *H. influenzae* and Lyme disease (which is endemic where they vacation).

Once you have watched children suffer and die of diseases that are now rare and preventable thanks to vaccines, you cannot imagine why parents would question the value of immunization. However, Americans rarely see these terrible diseases in action, thanks to the widespread availability of vaccines in this country and the mandatory requirements that many of them be given to children before they start school or day care. According to the Centers for Disease Control and Prevention (CDC), if we did not have vaccines we could expect 13,000 to 20,000 cases of paralytic polio a year, leaving thousands of children in braces, wheelchairs, or dependent on ventilators. Six hundred kids would die from meningitis caused by *Haemophilus influenzae*, and many of the survivors would be left deaf or mentally retarded. Another 7,500 or so would die from whooping cough, and close to 500 from measles. Pregnant women exposed to German measles (rubella) would suffer 2,100 stillbirths and deliver another 20,000 babies with heart defects, retardation, and/or deafness. Why wouldn't parents want to protect their children from so much suffering?

The number of vaccines required for your child will vary somewhat depending on your geographic location. We'd like to take a minute to acquaint you with the vaccines and the diseases they are designed to prevent:

**DTaP** is a combination vaccine that provides protection from diphtheria, tetanus, and pertussis (whopping cough), three common killers of children in the days before vaccines were available. Diphtheria is an aggressive bacterial infection that not only forms a choking membrane across the upper airway so a child cannot breathe, but also causes severe heart and nerve problems. Tetanus (lockjaw) is a muscular disorder caused by the poisons generated when spores from a common soil bacteria enter the body through a wound; the spasms of tetanus are very painful and can become deadly if the muscles associated with breathing are affected. Pertussis generally just causes a mild cough in adults, but can send a child into painful paroxysms of coughing that deprive the brain of oxygen and cause damage to the young infant's central nervous system.

The **MMR** shot is also a combination vaccine. It protects against measles, mumps, and rubella (German measles). Although these were once common childhood diseases—almost a childhood rite of passage—they can be quite severe in adults, the immune-compromised, or the very young. Measles can cause fatal encephalitis; mumps can lead to sterility in males; and rubella can be devastating to developing fetuses, killing some in the womb and causing deafness, mental retardation, and heart problems in others. As an example of the effectiveness of vaccination, there were one and a half million cases of measles in 1961 and 100 cases in 1999, 20,000 cases of congenital (passed from mother to fetus) rubella in 1964 and 7 in 1983.

The **polio** vaccine provides protection from a muscle-weakening virus, which, as late as the 1950s, was sentencing children and adults to wheelchairs and iron lungs. The oral vaccines containing weakened live virus protected the Baby Boomers, but in rare cases (six to seven cases a year in the United States and Canada) caused polio. Thanks to the effective American vaccine-monitoring program, our children today receive a safer, injectable vaccine made with inactivated poliovirus.

The ***Haemophilus influenzae*** type b (Hib), vaccine protects against the bacteria that most commonly causes meningitis in infants. During the 1980s there were about 7,000 cases of Hib-related meningitis a year in children; in 1998, thanks to a widespread vaccination campaign, only 54 cases were reported. Most of today's young doctors have never even seen this devastating illness, once a staple of pediatric emergency care.

The **hepatitis B** vaccine is required for children in only forty-two states, but absolutely necessary for any baby born of a woman who is hepatitis B-positive. Most other children are not at great risk for this disease, but this insidious, incurable, liver-damaging virus is very easily transmissible (100 times more transmissible than HIV). The younger the disease is acquired, the more likely it is to be chronic and cause cirrhosis and liver cancer. Immunization at birth is a safety net that protects against both infection during childhood and infection later in life from such risky behavior as unprotected sexual contact, piercing, injected drugs, etc. Because hepatitis B is a risk factor for liver cancer, you can think of this shot as the first vaccine for cancer.

There are two more vaccines sometimes required by schools or day-care centers:

**Hepatitis A**. The CDC recommends inoculation against this liver-damaging virus to children in those communities and states where the disease is endemic. Children over the age of two are immunized to protect themselves, but mostly to protect the adults in their lives, who generally develop more severe cases of the disease. Kids shoulder the responsibility for getting the vaccine because they are the greatest single source of hepatitis A infection for adults, and because our current health system does not foster the kind of environment where adults will readily seek out protection through vaccination and screening.

**Varicella**. Currently twenty-three states require immunization against varicella to enter school or day care. While this disease, more commonly known as chicken pox, is generally quite mild in children, it can be much more severe in immunocompromised children or in adults. In addition, there are several cases per year in the United States of absolutely healthy children who become critically ill when open lesions from scratched chicken pox become infected with a bacterium that's resistant to antibiotics. We will discuss this vaccine in more detail later when we give our recommendations.

In addition, there is a new vaccine called the **pneumococcal conjugate** vaccine (Prevnar) which has just been added to the list of routine vaccinations in children under five. Prevnar is strongly recommended for all babies and for children at high risk for infections of the blood and brain caused by *Streptococcus pneumoniae*, such as kids with compromised immune systems, sickle-cell disease, or HIV infection. The vaccine can also prevent the most resistant recurrent ear infections, therefore reducing the need for antibiotics.

And finally, you might consider an annual **flu shot** for children with asthma and other chronic respiratory infections, underlying heart or lung disease, or other chronic conditions that leave them at a greater risk of complications such as pneumonia from influenza. We don't normally recommend an annual flu shot for healthy children.

# The Case for Vaccinations

The most compelling reason to immunize your child is that it works. The development of vaccines is one of the greatest public health advances in history. Before there were appropriate vaccines available, we used to see whooping cough and Hib meningitis on a regular basis. Now we rarely see them at all. Nor does each summer bring the polio epidemics of the 1940s and 1950s, or every dirty cut raise the specter of tetanus. The effectiveness of vaccines as a tool for improving public health is the reason why all states in this country require certain immunizations before a child can enter the public school system. Because of this widespread use of vaccines, American parents can just assume that their children will survive the infectious diseases of childhood. Parents in the developing world, where vaccines are not readily available, don't have this luxury.

How do vaccines work? A vaccine, or immunization, is traditionally a weakened or killed form of a disease-causing virus or bacteria. Some of the newest vaccines are cloned from portions of a virus's genetic code that will provoke a similar immune response with fewer side effects. When a vaccine is injected or swallowed or inhaled (a method used with some newer vaccines), it stimulates the formation of antibodies to the disease. These antibodies will target and attack the particular pathogen when they come across it later, preventing you from actually getting sick from the disease. In some cases a vaccine protects you completely, in other cases it protects you partially (you get only a mild form of the disease) or for only a certain length of time (which is why we have booster shots for diseases like tetanus). The first primitive vaccine was developed in 1798 by Edward Jenner to prevent smallpox, a then-devastating disease that was finally eliminated in the world nearly two-hundred years later after a heroic global immunization campaign waged by the World Health Organization (WHO). In the years since Jenner's primitive vaccine, vaccines have been developed to protect us from such life-threatening diseases as whooping cough, diphtheria, typhoid, yellow fever, polio, and tetanus as well as more minor but still occasionally deadly ones such as measles, mumps, German measles, chicken pox, and pneumococcal infections.

In addition to our concerns that each individual child be immunized, we both feel strongly that there is an important "common good" argument to be made for vaccinations. Immunization protects not just the person at the sharp end of the needle, but also all the people with whom he or she comes in contact. Some people cannot be vaccinated themselves because of allergy, immune compromise, or fetal status, but when everyone else is vaccinated, the nonvaccinated benefit from the "herd immunity" created. The campaign to wipe out German measles is a case in point. Its major goal was the protection of pregnant women from exposure to rubella. As a society we all get vaccinated against rubella because that drastically reduces exposure of pregnant women to the disease and insures that females carry some vaccine-induced antibodies to rubella in their system to protect future pregnancies.

National vaccine programs like this only work if there is a high level of participation. It is not enough to say that your kids don't have to be immunized because everyone else will be. This strategy can backfire. A few years ago, a young child died of diphtheria in California—the only student in the class who had not been immunized.

We understand the importance of parents being able to make personal choices for their children's health. However, we think that the socially responsible parent will also consider all the children who are too young or too ill to be immunized and act to protect them as well. Unfortunately, if enough people decide not to have their children immunized, a pool large enough to sustain an epidemic is created. A temporary lapse in immunization practice from 1989 to 1991 led to pocket epidemics of measles in the United States that caused the preventable deaths of at least 120 people. Similar outbreaks have occurred in Japan (pertussis) and Ireland and The Netherlands (measles) following antivaccine scare campaigns.

We will need to continue vaccination programs even after some of these diseases become rare or are eradicated in the United States because of our porous borders. Millions of people from other countries—many of them not fully immunized—come into the United States as either visitors or immigrants. Likewise, millions of Americans travel every year to countries where these diseases are more prevalent; some of them return bearing pathogenic souvenirs.

# Concerns About Vaccinations

Many diligent parents have concerns about vaccines; some are legitimate, and some are based on misinformation. If you have concerns, your pediatrician or family-practice doctor should be willing to listen and respond to them thoughtfully and nonjudgmentally. In addition, you can get a great deal of excellent current information on vaccine safety from the National Immunization Program of the Centers for Disease Prevention and Control (CDC) (see Resources section). Don't let anyone make you feel bad for asking questions about vaccines. In the past such questions from doctors and parents have led to changes in some vaccine formulations and immunization schedules. For instance, the old inactivated whole-cell vaccine for diphtheria, tetanus, and pertussis (DTP) has now been replaced by an acellular version (DTaP) that does not cause as many systemic side effects. (Although it may cause progressively worse local reactions with each shot, these are not long-lasting effects.) Similarly, when experience showed that the first children to get MMR vaccine appeared to lose their immunity around age twenty-five, a booster shot was added between age four and six to maintain protection.

Currently the CDC, the National Institutes of Health (NIH), the American Committee for Immunization Practices (ACIP), the American Academy of Pediatrics (AAP), the National Vaccine Datalink Project, and the Food and Drug Administration (FDA) all oversee vaccine safety. New vaccines must be approved by the FDA after clinical trials like the ones that Dr. Stu's children participated in. Once the vaccine is approved and distributed, its effects are monitored closely, because side effects that may have escaped notice during clinical trials might become more obvious as larger groups of people experience them. This surveillance by several levels of government, pediatric associations, health maintenance organizations, and vaccine manufacturers is unceasing—a vaccine is monitored throughout its entire term of use. This system of multiple safeguards means that no single entity or organization has the power to impose the kind of cover-ups described by what we call "vaccine conspiracy theorists."

If you doubt that vaccines are under greater scrutiny than ever before, consider the case of the rotavirus vaccine. Rotavirus causes a devastating diarrhea that leads to dehydration and is a leading cause of death in children under five in the nonindustrialized world. Although good nutrition and sanitary conditions generally put American children at less risk, rotavirus still strikes a million kids in this country each year. A vaccine developed by Wyeth-Ayerst Laboratories (RotaShield) was approved by the FDA in 1998. As a few cases of a potentially serious bowel obstruction had turned up during the vaccine trials, the Advisory Committee in Immunization Practices called for close monitoring for that condition on the federal Vaccine Adverse Event Reporting System (VAERS) to see if the condition was vaccine-related. When data from a large California HMO and from the State of Minnesota suggested an increased risk for the bowel disorder in the weeks immediately following vaccination, the American Academy of Pediatrics and the American Academy of Family Physicians expressed concerns, and the CDC asked that distribution of RotaShield be halted. The company complied with the request, and the vaccine is no longer used in this country.

This is not to say that this particular vaccine might not be of great benefit in other situations. To our mind, Rotashield is not safe enough for widespread use in the United States given the low incidence here of serious cases of the disease and the gravity of the potential side effects. But it is a viable option for use in infants in developing countries where the risk of death from the infection is so high that the potential side effects dwindle in significance. Fortunately a safer version of the vaccine may be on the horizon as we go to press.

As vaccines improve, we would expect parental resistance to them to decline. However, more and more parents are requesting exemption from the vaccinations required by their states for entry into school. All states provide medical exemption for children with allergies to components of some vaccines or with a compromised immune system. Forty-eight states now allow exemption for religious reasons as well, and another fifteen allow exemption for philosophical reasons.

Ironically the decision to avoid vaccination is gaining popularity largely because of the very effectiveness of vaccines. It is certainly more difficult for parents to make an informed decision about the risks versus the benefits of vaccines if they have never seen the horrible effects of the diseases in question. In addition, there's a public relations imbalance—while the rare adverse effects of vaccines make the news, the many deaths and impairments *prevented* by the vaccines are invisible. Here's one example: Despite headlines reporting that former Miss America Heather Whitestone's hearing impairment was a side effect of the whole-cell pertussis vaccine she'd been given as a child, her hearing loss was actually caused by a meningitis infection that today would have been prevented by the Hib vaccination.

There are also difficulties with the way most of us look at statistics. A one in a million chance that your child might suffer a serious side effect from immunization tends to loom larger than the much higher risks of side effects from the disease itself if the disease is only an abstraction. And finally, psychology weights the scales unfairly as well. According to a recent study, parents say they would feel much worse about any adverse effect of vaccinations (in which they had an active role in a medical intervention) than any adverse effects from catching the preventable disease (in which they see themselves as having but a passive role in a natural event).

Parents carry a tremendous burden of responsibility when making decisions regarding their children's health. They long for reassurances from the health professionals caring for their children that nothing will go wrong. While we can rarely provide such complete reassurance, we can listen conscientiously and offer open, rational, and emotional support while discussing options.

# Six Myths (and One True Statement) About Vaccines

We'll now address the major concerns about vaccination one by one, looking at the claims in the light of current research and our own medical experience. (In the interests of full disclosure we will tell you that Dr. Stu is a member of the Vaccine Study Group of the State University of New York Downstate School of Medicine, and that his practice participates in FDA-supervised multicenter vaccine trials.) We don't have room to discuss any of these concerns in depth, so we will refer you to the Resources section at the back of this book. But briefly, here are some of the common reasons given to withhold vaccination:

*The adverse effects of vaccines are worse than the disease themselves.* Clearly false. We've seen antivaccine materials that refer to pertussis as "a mild cough and respiratory infection," (as it is in adults) but no one who's ever seen a child in the throes of whooping cough would use such a description. Most of the immunizable diseases are really quite scary, and we are fortunate that we see them so infrequently in this country that we have the luxury of worrying more about the possible risks of immunization. Actually, the risk of serious adverse effects from a vaccine is extraordinarily low compared to the risks of the disease itself. According to the data collected by the Vaccine Adverse Effects Reporting System (VAERS) of the FDA, only one death was even possibly associated with the millions of shots given between 1990 and 1992. Even one death from vaccines is tragic, but many, many more children would have died of these diseases or their complications without immunization. That makes the risk-to-benefit ratio very favorable.

We have seen thousands of children so far in our careers, and have never seen a child with permanent seizure or neurological side effects directly related to vaccination. The vast majority of children suffer only mild side effects: soreness at the site of the injection, rash, low-grade fever, and irritability. However, rarely, seizures from high fever have been associated with measles vaccination, and a serious muscular weakness called Guillain-Barré syndrome with a tetanus shot. We cannot guarantee that immunization is a 100 percent risk-free procedure. All children cannot be expected to respond in the same way to *any* treatment, given their individual exposures and genetic susceptibilities. There will always be some subgroups that may be adversely affected by any particular vaccine, which is why, for instance, we do not give pertussis shots to children with progressive neurological disorders unless we have a note from a neurologist that the condition has stabilized. However, the scientific literature overwhelmingly agrees that vaccines are safe for most children.

In order to assess claims of damage from vaccines, parents need to understand the difference between "association" and "causality." We can rarely prove that a vaccine *caused* an individual condition. We can say that the condition has been *associated* with a vaccine—that they both occurred about the same time—but this is not proof that the vaccine is to blame. For instance, some problems, such as sudden infant death syndrome (SIDS) and autism, typically occur or first become apparent at the age when most shots are scheduled and given. Their occurrence then does not mean that vaccines cause SIDS or autism; in fact, studies suggest that neither disease occurs more often in those given immunizations. It appears to be merely an accident of timing that links the vaccine with the disease.

The claim has been made that the rise in allergies and immune disorders is due to multiple vaccinations given at a very young age, but this has not been proven. Nor is juvenile diabetes associated with the Hib or hepatitis B vaccines, according to the CDC, which analyzed data from three large health maintenance organizations.

*Too many vaccines too early in life damage the immune system.* False. The first few months of life are when children are most at risk for these diseases because of their lack of natural immunity and inability to mount a strong immune response. For instance, pertussis may just cause a persistent cough in an adult, but it can cause brain damage if experienced before the age of six months. Giving the vaccine at a later age when the greatest risk for the disease has passed makes no sense.

The young immune system learns and becomes stronger by exposure to milder forms of pathogens, such as are found in vaccines. Shots given in the first few months of life (80 percent of them are given before the age of two) generally provide protection longer. **Varicella** vaccine, for example, does not "take" as well in children over twelve as it does in younger kids. With rare exceptions, we are not in favor of delaying or prolonging the vaccination series, because as children get older, they are less likely to be taken to the doctor or clinic for follow-up care.

*We don't need all these vaccines anymore because the diseases are nearly eradicated in this country.* False. As we discussed above, borders that look solid on the map are woefully inadequate to contain disease. Many of the diseases we consider nearly extinct are still alive and well in the developing world where lack of funds and lack of political will cripple attempts at general immunization. These diseases lurk at our own doorstep, ready to be tracked in by the next traveler.

*Measles/mumps/rubella (MMR) vaccine causes autism and inflammatory bowel disease.* False. In 1998 a researcher in Great Britain reported a link between MMR inoculation and these two disorders, and vaccine antagonists there immediately began demanding the withdrawal of the vaccine. Later, larger studies by others found no difference in the rate of autism before and after the introduction of the MMR vaccine in the country. The CDC has studied this question extensively in the United States and found no association.

*Vaccines contain toxic mercury.* Now false. In 1999 it was discovered that infants could possibly accumulate more than the FDA-approved safe level of mercury if all the vaccines they were given in their first year contained the mercury-based preservative thimerosal. Although thimerosal has been used for decades to prevent bacterial contamination of vaccines with no apparent ill effects, the AAP and the Public Health Service pushed to have manufacturers start removing it from all vaccines given to children as a safety measure. Thimerosal exposure has been cut 60 percent since then, and soon all vaccines for children in the United States will be mercury-free.

*Combination vaccines are more dangerous than single vaccines.* False. Fewer shots obviously means fewer tears and less trauma for the child and less cost to the parent. As you can see from the chart on page 42–43, most children are getting several shots containing four to six vaccines at each visit anyway. The primary problem with the "super-combination" vaccines being developed to administer four or more vaccines at once is not safety so much as effectiveness. The various vaccine strains could compete for dominance in the immune system, inhibiting a complete response to the antigen and complete protection from the micro-organism. This in fact is what happened during testing of a proposed combination shot for hepatitis A and B. It may become more difficult in the future to get vaccines singly as more and more of them are packaged in combination.

*Vaccines do not completely protect you from disease*. This is *true*. No vaccine offers 100 percent protection, because individual responses to vaccines vary. Vaccine protection typically varies from 79 percent for Lyme disease to 99 percent for measles (with the booster). Nor do all vaccines protect you forever. For instance, 5 percent of children vaccinated for chicken pox will develop a mild case of the disease if exposed to the virus later. However, most vaccines protect you during the time period when you are most at risk and almost all vaccines lessen the severity of the disease should you happen to contract it despite immunization.

# Our Vaccine Recommendations

We generally suggest that parents follow the recommendations of the American Academy of Pediatrics regarding immunizations. The AAP has taken a very activist approach to vaccines and vaccine safety in the past few years—witness their stance regarding the rotavirus vaccine—and we trust them to consider the safety of our children as a group and as individuals.

The following chart gives a simplified version of the current AAP recommendations as of the date of publication of this book:

| Year One | Year Two | Year Four and After |
|---|---|---|
| **DTaP** (diphtheria/tetanus/ pertussis) at 2 months, 4 months, and 6 months | **DTaP** at 15 to 18 months | **DTaP** at 4 to 6 years 1 **DT** at 11 to 12 years, and **tetanus** boosters every 10 years thereafter |
| **Polio** at 2 months, 4 months, and 6 to 18 months | | **Polio** at 4 to 6 years |

| Year One | Year Two | Year Four and After |
|---|---|---|
| **MMR** (measles/mumps/ rubella) at 12 to 15 months | | **MMR** at 4 to 6 years |
| **Hepatitis B**: three doses in first year (schedule depends on whether or not mother had Hepatitis B at time of child's birth) | | |
| **Varicella** (chicken pox) at 12 months | **Varicella** at 18 months | |
| **Hib** (*Haemophilus influenzae*) and 6 months | **Hib** at 12 to 18 months | |
| **Pneumococcal conjugate** vaccine at 2 months, 4 months, and 6 months | **Pneumococcal conjugate** vaccine at 12 to 15 months if child did not receive it as an infant | |

We sometimes modify these standards. Some parents are concerned about giving too many shots at so young an age, so if a mother insists (and is hepatitis B-negative), we are open to delaying the first hepatitis B shot until a child is six to twelve months of age or until entry into day care. However, the reason this immunization is now required is that children in certain areas of the country are at great risk for the disease at a very young age. You will need to talk with your child's doctor about conditions where you live to determine if it is safe to delay administration of this vaccine.

With the exception of immunocompromised kids, we are also willing to allow parents to decide about varicella vaccine in those areas where this vaccine is not yet legally required. Even pediatricians are not fully united in their opinions about the need for chicken pox immunization, so we think it is appropriate for parents and doctors to make this decision together on an individual basis. While the two of us vary in the strength of our support for varicella vaccination, we generally recommend it both to protect adults without immunity and to protect children from increasingly virulent infections that might arise from scratched pox. While any child with a lot of scratches or insect bites is at a slightly greater risk of contracting such a severe infection, some experts believe that the varicella virus weakens the immune system and makes it easier for such skin infections to develop from scratched pox.

Our own misgivings about the vaccine are becoming moot as more states require that children entering school or day care be vaccinated against chicken pox, a movement we do not applaud because we favor parental education and choice in this instance. We were initially put off by a marketing campaign by vaccine manufacturers that is clearly built on fear, and by the pressure to require immunization for its economic advantages. (Productivity is lowered by workers who have to stay home for a week with their itchy children.) Although we are not yet fully convinced that the immunization will last long enough to be protective into the adult years, when a case of chicken pox can be a lot more severe, evidence for long-term immunity is growing. We know that many parents, remembering their own bouts with chicken pox, would like to save their children from a week to ten days of discomfort through vaccination. Others cannot understand why they have to immunize their healthy children against a mild childhood infection. They tell us they prefer their children to acquire the disease naturally for longer-lasting protection. We can sympathize with this attitude, as we have taken this approach with some of our own children. However, as immunization is increasingly required, there may be fewer chances for our children to be exposed to chickenpox naturally, leaving them at greater risk from the disease as adults.

We are sometimes faced with parents whose concerns over the safety of the combination MMR vaccine cannot be assuaged. In those few cases where parents absolutely refuse to have their children immunized with the MMR vaccine for fear of developmental side effects (especially if there are already developmental problems in the family) we may offer this compromise: We will give the child the three (measles, mumps, and rubella) vaccines separately if the parent guarantees to bring the child in for the extra visits required to give the complete series of shots. We cannot advise such split dosing for the general population as the extra effort involved on the part of parents practically guarantees that some children will miss shots and not be completely immunized.

In addition, we recommend two other vaccines in certain situations. Hepatitis A is a liver disease endemic in some parts of the country, including the areas where we practice. It is well worth giving this protection to a child older than two who is living or traveling in places where the disease is common. Lyme disease is a tick-borne illness that in some people can cause chronic muscle or joint pains and fatigue. A Lyme vaccine is currently approved only for older teens and adults, with approval for children in the offing. If your family spends a great deal of time outdoors in the Northeast or other woodsy places where Lyme disease is endemic, you might consider this vaccine for your older children. Be aware, however, that there are concerns that this immunization can cause joint pain, and it is not yet approved for those under fifteen years of age.

# Easing the Aftereffects of Immunization

We rarely hold off giving a vaccine just because a child has a cold. If we did we could fall behind on the immunization schedule, because kids have so many colds. We do hold off on giving the MMR vaccine to a child with the sniffles, because viral infections may reduce the immune response to a live, attenuated-virus vaccine. We do not give a scheduled shot if a child has a fever over 101 degrees; we may delay a shot in children with milder fevers if the parent seems especially worried about it.

Some vaccines will cause slight side effects—swelling, itching, or redness at the site of the injection, a mild fever, or irritability. If your child displays a more serious response—high fever, persistent screaming, seizure—call the doctor, or, if unable to reach the doctor, consider a trip to the emergency department of your hospital.

There are a few ways to reduce the mild side effects of inoculations. First you might ask your doctor to massage the site of the injection for thirty seconds before giving the injection; children tend to find this soothing. You can calm your child yourself in a number of ways, such as rocking, stroking, speaking in a soothing voice, or giving a pacifier or a favorite toy. Such distractions reduce infant distress with the injections. A brief session of hypnotherapy beforehand can also make the experience more pleasant. You should take care to lower your own levels of anxiety so your child does not pick up on your tension and become tense, too. Treat vaccination matter-of-factly and your kids will, too. You can give a little children's acetaminophen for postinjection soreness. You can also toss a clean wet washcloth in the freezer; an hour later you'll have an easy-to-use cold compress to reduce any inflammation or pain at the injection site.

# Chapter 4

# Drugs and Bugs:

## *The Proper Use of Antibiotics*

t he development of antibiotic drugs may be the single greatest medical achievement of the twentieth century, curing a host of previously deadly bacterial infections. Injections of penicillin saved the lives and limbs of tens of thousands of soldiers during World War II. After the war, the number of deaths from infectious diseases dropped so precipitously that few today now realize how dangerous many infections—even strep throat and pneumonia—once were. Unfortunately, these "miracle drugs" were so effective that they soon became not just the weapons of choice against bacterial diseases, but an absolute cure-all for almost any condition. By now we have so abused antibiotic drugs that the "miracle" has turned into something of a mixed blessing.

When and how to prescribe antibiotic drugs has become a huge issue in the past few years, especially in the field of pediatrics. By misusing and overusing these drugs we have weakened their effectiveness, creating new strains of "superbugs" that are highly resistant to the antibiotics in our current arsenal. In our practices we are beginning to see untreatable diseases caused by these highly aggressive bacteria, diseases we have never seen before. We find this development so worrisome, and the need to educate parents so great, that we are devoting an entire chapter to antibiotics. (We encourage you to read this whole section, but if you're short on time, you can find our bottom line in "What Parents Can Do" at the end of the chapter.

Before we get any further in this discussion, let's talk a little about what an antibiotic is and what it can and cannot do. *Antibiotic* (from the Greek words for "against" and "life") commonly refers to a drug that kills or inhibits bacteria. It does not kill viruses, so antibiotics are useless against such viral diseases as colds, influenza, and most other viral upper-respiratory infections. The first of the widely available antibiotics were sulfonamide and penicillin. There are now more than a hundred antibiotics available, including tetracyclines, cephalosporins, quinolones, and more. Some are considered narrow-spectrum antibiotics, because they work only against certain categories of organisms. Others are so-called broad-spectrum drugs that affect a wider variety of microbes.

Even in the early days of antibiotic use, there were hints of a dark side to antibiotics. Alexander Fleming, the man who discovered penicillin, observed that greater exposure to the drug caused the targeted bacteria to mutate, and become harder to kill. He predicted even more problems once an oral form of penicillin made the drug more widely available. The inevitable process of natural selection insures that the most susceptible strains of targeted bacteria will be destroyed, leaving the hardier ones to survive and evolve new defenses against the drug's next attack. The mutated bacteria pass their resistance on to their progeny and to unrelated bacteria as well. These resistant bacteria cause more severe, less treatable infectious disease that requires higher doses of drugs, combinations of drugs, or new drugs altogether, to which—inevitably—the bacteria also adapt.

When antibiotics are used properly, the progression of antibiotic attack and bacterial adaptation goes more slowly, so it takes a while to build up complete bacterial resistance to a drug. But we have sped up the course of events by our overuse of the drugs. It took five years for the first strains of bacteria resistant to penicillin to show up; resistance to the newest antibiotic drug was seen in 10 percent of the subjects in the drug's pre-approval trials. In 1954 manufacturers produced two million pounds of antibiotic drugs; less than fifty years later they produce (and we use) more than twenty-five times that amount. We go through more than 160 million outpatient prescriptions for antibiotics a year (23 million of them for ear infections alone), about three times the number per person prescribed in more antibiotic-wary European countries like The Netherlands. The Centers for Disease Control and Prevention (CDC) estimates that almost half of all outpatient prescriptions for antibiotics are given for viral diseases not affected by antibiotics and are therefore useless.

Our overexposure to antibiotics—through prescription medicines and veterinary drugs in our food—and our overuse of antibacterial products are causing a frightening increase in the number of strains of bacteria resistant to all but one or two antibiotic drugs. Until recently, medical science dealt with the increased resistance of bacteria and reduced effectiveness of drugs by building bigger and stronger antibiotics (a microbial version of the arms race). Of course, as these second- and third-generation drugs were used more frequently, bacteria become wise to them as well. Unfortunately, we may be running out of antibiotic options. Essentially, modern pharmaceutical technology has created a "cure" for disease that ensures the survival of a more-evolved disease-causing organism. Or as a 1997 study put it, "Technology is losing the arms race with evolution."

It's ironic that improper use of the greatest medical discovery of the twentieth century has put the children and adults of the twenty-first century at risk. We have inadvertently created so many strains of bacteria that are invulnerable to drugs that some say we are facing an era when there will be few, if any, effective drugs to combat infectious disease. (And similar resistance is developing to antifungal and antiviral drugs.) Surprisingly, this gloomy prediction is coming not from critics of conventional medicine but from the medical establishment itself. Major campaigns for reducing antibiotic resistance have been launched by the National Academy of the Sciences, the CDC, the American Academy of Pediatrics, and the American Medical Association.

In a 1998 editorial in the *New England Journal of Medicine*, Dr. Stuart Levy of Tufts University, founder of the Alliance for the Prudent Use of Antibiotics, pointed out five underlying principles of bacterial resistance that are cause for concern:

1. Antibiotic resistance is inevitable, given enough time and enough drugs used.
2. Bacteria evolve to become progressively more resistant to a drug.
3. Bacteria that are resistant to one drug are likely to become resistant to others.
4. Bacteria lose this resistance slowly, if at all.
5. Resistant bacteria are easily transmitted from one person to another.

Here's an example of how bacterial resistance works. Several years ago, there was a community-wide outbreak in Brooklyn of a common intestinal infection caused by the bacterium *Shigella*. Children with this form of dysentery have bloody stools, high fever, and abdominal cramping. When necessary, they are treated with a sulfa-based drug. Because of the size of the outbreak, the New York City Health Department monitored the spread of this highly contagious infection, and soon determined that the effectiveness of the drug was decreasing as more and more children took it. By the third week of the outbreak, the *Shigella* organism was completely resistant to sulfa drugs, forcing a switch to a drug with a broader spectrum of activity (and the risk of causing resistance in greater numbers of bacteria). Knowing that most cases of childhood shigella in this country resolve on their own, the Health Department advised local pediatricians to stop using antibiotics unless a child's symptoms of fever and dehydration were worsening. Although some community pediatricians did not comply with this plan, Dr. Stu's office did hold back on antibiotics. A week's wait allowed more susceptible strains of *Shigella* to be restored in his young patients, making the bacteria sensitive to sulfa-based medications once again.

The resistant *Shigella* in this example may just have been endemic to Brooklyn, as researchers have found that the strains of bacteria that develop resistance vary geographically, depending on the particular prescribing and practice habits of doctors and hospitals in the area. What is resistant in one geographic area may be easily treated in another, although there is evidence that some of the resistant strains are spreading to far-flung corners of the globe. Most of the nastier strains of resistant bacteria are more commonly found in institutions such as hospitals and nursing homes, where there are large numbers of people with lowered immunity getting multiple drugs. However, some of these new bacteria are now showing up in healthy people, causing serious bacterial infections. It is no longer rare to hear of healthy young adults succumbing to a bacterial infection, the most well known example being Muppet creator Jim Henson, who died of streptococcal pneumonia in 1989 after a short illness. More aggressively virulent strains of bacteria like this are responsible for the sorts of situations that lead to tabloid headlines ("Flesh-eating strep devours boy's left arm").

Resistant strains of bacteria are arising more rapidly because increased day care attendance promotes more infectious disease, more people have access to antibiotics, and antibiotics are overprescribed. Many of the prescriptions written each year are therapeutically worthless—for instance, the millions of doses of antibiotics issued for colds, influenza, and other conditions caused by viruses. Other prescriptions turn out not to be effective in the long term; treating ear infections with antibiotics is obviously not reducing the overall incidence of recurrent ear infections, as prescriptions for ear infections have increased sevenfold over the past two decades.

Fortunately antibiotic practice is changing. We've moved past the days when some doctors prescribed a daily penicillin tablet as a preventive measure and others routinely passed them out "just in case," to a time when such wholesale dissemination of the drug is discouraged. National campaigns to reduce antibiotic use are focusing not just on educating physicians, but on educating consumers as well. Too often patients with a viral disease like a cold or flu demand antibiotics—the assumed "quick fix"—not understanding that antibiotics work only against bacteria. Unfortunately, since these colds and flus are generally self-limiting—that is, they run their course and clear up on their own—people who take antibiotics for them will attribute their recovery to the drug and insist on a prescription next time they start to sniffle. Doctors react to this actual or perceived pressure by prescribing antibiotics even when they know there will be no medical benefit, especially if they have free samples from the pharmaceutical companies to eliminate cost from the equation. This kind of thinking has got to change.

Ironically, *under*use of antibiotics can also promote the creation of supergerms. We all know people who stop taking a prescription as soon as they start to feel better, despite the doctor's orders to continue for a week to ten days. Not taking the complete dose of an antimicrobial has the unfortunate effect of killing off those bacteria most susceptible to the drug and leaving the strongest to survive, thrive, and possibly mutate to a form that does not respond to the drug. This is happening right now in this country with tuberculosis, and in other parts of the world with most of the major infectious diseases (travelers, beware). The same result comes when someone later uses saved-up pills to inadequately self-medicate another condition.

Antibiotics can also be *mis*used, as, for instance, when a broad-spectrum antibiotic is used when a narrow-spectrum one would do. As you might suspect from the name, broad-spectrum drugs are effective against a wide variety of bacteria, and therefore can promote resistance in many varieties at once. Using a narrow-spectrum antibiotic that just attacks certain bacteria reduces the amount of bacterial resistance engendered. We advocate starting with the simplest and least expensive forms of antibiotics and switching to more complex broader-spectrum drugs only if there is no clinical improvement over the first 48 to 72 hours.

Reducing the unnecessary use of antibiotics is especially important in young children. Antibiotics are referred to as "societal" or "environmental" drugs, because one person's use or misuse can affect everyone else in his or her family or community. Bacteria grow in and are shed by every human being, so we pass on our own resistant germs to others, affecting the bacterial culture of the entire community, and putting the weak and the immune-compromised at greater risk. Children who play together eventually share all the coexisting bacteria inherent to their own bodies. This is the reason why children in day care and nursery programs acquire new infections all the time and why some parents of school-age children wryly refer to them as "living incubators." If children within those small groups develop resistant bacteria, they are shared by every member of the group, and eventually with everyone with whom they come in contact.

Antibiotics affect society in another way as well, because they are present in so much of our food and possibly our water. Antibiotics are used, for instance, by fruit farmers to prevent or treat plant diseases. Even worse, the farm animals in this country are dosed with millions of pounds of antibiotics each year; in fact, almost half the antibiotics produced in this country are used to speed the growth of animals intended for food. These antibiotics, many of them the same as are used in humans, are given at what is called subtherapeutic levels— that is, at dosages insufficient to wipe the bacteria out, a virtual recipe for creating bacterial resistance. Use of antibiotics to promote animal growth has been restricted in Europe for decades for that very reason. Many of the antibiotics fed to farm animals to promote growth or—in higher doses—to treat infections, can be passed on to us in food, and are considered an important factor in the creation of drug-resistant bacteria in people. According to new studies, antibiotics excreted by both farm animals and humans are now turning up in our lakes, rivers, and other supplies of drinking water, giving them a second shot at our bacterial flora.

# Our Antibiotic Practices

Standards of treatment for antibiotic drugs have changed greatly in the past few years as the adverse effects of using these drugs improperly have become more obvious. It is clear that we need to treat infections in very young infants and immune-compromised children, and severe infections in otherwise healthy kids. We also intervene more frequently with antibiotics in children with problems such as muscular dystrophy who are at higher risk of respiratory infections because they are unable to get rid of bacteria-prone secretions from their airways.

These exceptions aside, pediatricians have not yet reached complete consensus on exactly which infections to treat with antibiotics and for what duration. However, you should expect your pediatrician to work with you in taking practical and safe steps to reduce your child's exposure to antibiotics. A cautious approach to antibiotics will not leave your children at the mercy of every bacterium that crosses their path, but rather supports their natural healing ability. Children are remarkably resilient creatures. They are less likely than adults to have chronic medical problems and more likely to bounce back quickly from the transient stress of an infection. With certain exceptions, well-fed, healthy children have the ability to mobilize an adequate defense on their own, if given a little time. Whenever possible, we try to wait and give our patients' little bodies a chance to muster their own defenses before charging in with the big antibiotic guns.

As integrative practitioners, we are committed to supporting natural efforts to heal. We know that invading organisms can slip through natural defenses and set off a bacterial infection. When this happens, the immune system usually just goes to work and clears up the problem with no need for drugs. But sometimes—because the bacteria are particularly strong or reproducing especially fast, or because the immune system is not functioning at peak efficiency—natural defenses are overwhelmed. This is when we turn to antibiotics, because these drugs can reduce the numbers of the bacteria enough for the immune system to be able to take over and heal the infection. We look at antibiotics not as a cure *per se*, but as an aid to the immune response. This is a very different philosophical perspective from that of conventional doctors.

Although antibiotics can be very useful, they are not completely benign drugs. The main side effect of antibiotics in children is diarrhea and gastrointestinal upset, as the drug alters the natural balance of flora in the bowel. This side effect can be countered with probiotics such as those that can be found in yogurt with live cultures. These drugs also carry the potential for allergic reactions, both mild and severe. Parents also report to us that some kids taking antibiotics act "very weird," with greater irritability, more crying, and more misbehavior.

There is currently a major push in this country to educate patients and parents about appropriate use of antibiotics. Physicians like us who take a measured approach to antibiotics already spend a lot of time educating parents about the reasons for this practice. When we don't recommend antibiotics immediately for what appears to be a low-grade bacterial infection, some parents act as if we had refused to call in a surgeon for acute appendicitis. Others demand the broadest-spectrum antibiotics available for the simplest of infections: "My child does not respond to amoxicillin," they say, "It never works for him." What these parents fail to realize is that the lack of response to antibiotics is not a function of the child's immune system, but rather a function of the bacterial strain, or the fact that the cause is a virus against which antibiotics have no activity. The important thing to remember is that children are not resistant to antibiotics—bacteria are!

The cultural paradigm of relying heavily on antibiotics is not going to change quickly. That inherent American desire for a quick fix makes our more cautious way of addressing childhood infections a tough sell at first, but our good results speak for themselves. We take the time to explain the reasons for not immediately prescribing antibiotics, and decide—together with the parents—which tactic to follow. We may decide on a period of watchful waiting if the parents are willing to monitor their child's progress, call in if the child's symptoms worsen, and schedule a follow-up visit seven to ten days later to check that the infection has resolved. We may respond more conservatively (with a prescription for an antibiotic) when careful follow-up is not likely to occur.

Sometimes parents are determined to get an antibiotic for their child because they have come to think of the word "antibiotic" as a synonym for "strong, effective medicine." In those cases we might give them a prescription, but ask that they wait a day or two to see if the condition worsens before filling it. With a prescription reassuringly in hand, most parents are more willing to wait to see if the problem clears up on its own. In fact, a study of this kind of prescribing found that nearly a third of those prescriptions were never filled. In general, we tend to prescribe the older antibiotic drugs like amoxicillin because they are more narrowly targeted, rather than the hotly marketed new drugs, which we save for more serious infections. Narrow-spectrum drugs engender resistance in fewer types of bacteria.

Here are a few examples to give you an idea of times when we feel antibiotics are necessary and when they are not. (Turn to Section III for more detailed discussion of treatment for the first four conditions described below.)

*Enrique comes to see us with a low-grade fever, a runny nose, and a cough. Although he feels a little under par, he has been busily stacking blocks in the waiting room. His mother asks for antibiotics for him.* It is most likely that Enrique just has a cold, or a mild case of influenza, and antibiotics are not needed. Twenty-one percent of all antibiotic prescriptions for children are written for colds and other viral upper respiratory infections, so it is essential that parents remember that antibiotics do not kill viruses. We would focus instead on relieving his symptoms and shortening the duration of the cold.

*Six-year-old Nathan has a fever, nausea, bloody diarrhea, and abdominal pain.* These and other symptoms could indicate a *Shigella* infection. Because of our experience, we now assume that children with mild shigella dysentery who are otherwise healthy will be able to mobilize an adequate immune response on their own. We monitor Nathan closely for signs of clinical deterioration, and keep antibiotics on the "hold" shelf unless needed.

*Monique has a fever of 101, and a sore throat.* Monique's symptoms could be caused by a virus or, of more concern, by the bacteria *Streptococcus*. If it's a virus, she has no need for antibiotic drugs. Not treating a childhood strep throat, however, is the equivalent of playing medical Russian roulette. While it is true that many strep throats will resolve without treatment, a small but not insignificant number will go on to such serious complications as valvular heart disease, post-strep reactive arthritis, or rheumatic kidney disease (glomerulonephritis). Because studies have shown that starting antibiotic treatment too soon increases the chance of recurrence of the infection, it makes sense to us to take the time to do a throat culture when possible. We prefer to do this standard 24-hour strep test rather than a rapid strep test because it allows time for the child to make natural antibodies to streptococcal bacteria on the infected tonsil and throat that will serve her well in the future. If the symptoms persist and she tests positive for *Streptococcus* (strep), we would then start her on antibiotics.

*Alan is a little fussy and has been tugging at his ear, leading his dad to think his son has another ear infection.* The treatment of middle ear infections (otitis media) remains an area of controversy (for more on this topic, see chapter 18). The standard of care in the United States has been to treat all ear infections in children with antibiotics. In some European countries, physicians restrict the use of antibiotics for ear infections, having found that "watchful waiting" is safe and appropriate as 70 to 80 percent of children's ear infections clear up on their own without treatment. Studies in this country are now reinforcing that finding, and antibiotics are generally saved for those with acute ear infections who do not improve over the waiting period. Our treatment of Alan would focus on pain relief, with a phone follow-up or a second visit in several days if his symptoms haven't cleared up.

*Sophie fell and cut her leg on a camping trip last week. The wound is now red and inflamed, with red streaks emanating from it.* Sophie clearly has a serious infection that requires oral, and perhaps injected, antibiotics.

*Kayla comes in with a tummy ache, a high fever, and burning with urination.* Upon examination we diagnose a urinary tract infection, which must always be treated with antibiotics in young children to prevent spread to the kidneys.

Parents who are monitoring their children during a "wait and see" period should watch for these signs that antibiotic treatment should begin or another medical evaluation should be made: worsening pain, fussiness or other atypical behavior, decreased intake of solids and especially liquids, reduced urine output, and difficulties with breathing. A good relationship between parents and physician is essential here, as the physician must be able to trust the parents' oversight of the situation and the parent must be able to trust that the physician will respond quickly if needed.

When we do prescribe systemic or oral *anti*biotics we also prescribe a complementary course of what are called *pro*biotics (or "good bacteria") to help maintain a healthy balance of bacteria in the large intestine. The bowel normally contains hundreds of strains of bacteria, which help digest our food, produce vitamins, and protect us from illness. Some of these bacteria can cause disease themselves, but other bacteria normally keep them in check. Unfortunately, antibiotics cannot tell a good bug from a bad one in the dark, and may upset the healthy balance of flora in a way that causes diarrhea in 20 to 40 percent of all children prescribed antibiotics (or vaginal yeast infections in some girls).

Probiotics are foods or supplements that contain one or more of the beneficial intestinal bacteria that would normally be killed by an antibiotic. Probiotic foods include yogurt with active cultures, kefir, naturally fermented pickles, kim chee, and dairy products fortified with various kinds of bacteria, including *Lactobacilli*. Probiotic supplements are also available, but unfortunately many have been tested and found unworthy of the claims made for them. You can increase your odds of getting an effective product that will still be viable when it gets to the large intestine by looking for an enteric-coated supplement that contains at least a billion active units of the named probiotic. Supplements containing the patented *Lactobacillus* GG (named for the two university scientists who developed it) have been proven in recent studies to greatly reduce both the incidence and the duration of diarrhea caused by antibiotics.

Our usual probiotic prescription is one cup of yogurt with active cultures a day throughout the course of antibiotics and for a week thereafter. If you prefer supplements, there are powdered and chewable forms available for children.

# What Parents Can Do

Doctors and parents share the blame for overuse of antibiotics, as do pharmaceutical companies who spend millions on ads pushing antibiotics. This partnership in overuse goes on daily in nearly every pediatric and family medicine practice throughout the country, and is a major factor in the creation of antibiotic-resistant bacteria. But we believe the concerted efforts at patient and physician education now taking place in this country will help preserve the usefulness of antibiotics. Here are ten ways you can do your part:

1. Don't pressure your doctor for antibiotic drugs. Do not request antibiotics for viral infections like colds and flu or suspected viral infections. Give mild conditions a few days to heal on their own. Even if antibiotics have appeared to be helpful in the past, keep in mind that your child might have healed just as quickly without them.

2. If your child's doctor prescribes antibiotics, make sure you understand his rationale for the prescription. Studies have found that pediatricians often think a parent wants a child to get an antibiotic when in fact the parent just wants the child to feel better.

3. Indicate your openness to a "wait and see" policy when appropriate.

4. Use antibiotics as prescribed. Don't stop taking them before you should, and don't use leftover antibiotics or someone else's prescription.

5. Keep track of your family's usage of antibiotics so you know what drugs have been used and to what effect.

6. If finances allow, consider buying organic meats and dairy products that are free of antibiotics. Milk can contain traces of dozens of different antibiotics used to treat dairy cattle or increase their milk production.

7. Train your children to wash their hands frequently (see box at the end of this chapter). Make sure that their preschools and schools allow/encourage hand-washing as well. In a Canadian study, day care centers instituting strict hygiene policies for students and staff were able to reduce diarrhea 27 percent, respiratory infections 20 percent, and urinary tract infections 25 percent. During outbreaks of infectious disease we even suggest that parents check the restrooms at their children's schools to make sure they are adequately stocked with soap and paper towels.

8. Avoid the use of antibacterial soaps, toys, blankets, etc. According to the CDC, plain soap and water are just as effective as the heavily advertised antibacterial soaps and do not encourage the growth of resistant bacteria. There have been

reports that bacteria are developing resistance to triclosan, a common antibacterial agent in soaps, although these findings are controversial. Proponents of the "hygiene hypothesis" postulate that early exposure to antibacterials and antibiotics may backfire because it does not permit the natural exposure to common bacteria that prevents later development of allergy and asthma.

9. Make sure your children get the recommended vaccinations. It's a lot better to prevent certain infections than to have to treat them with antibiotics.

10. Support your children's natural immunity.

# Hand Washing 101

Chores that are fun are more likely to get done, so we would like to recommend two diverting methods of washing hands.

● *THE MUSICAL METHOD.* Hygiene experts tell us we need soap, water, and at least 20 seconds to get hands clean. The "Happy Birthday" song is just about the right length. Teach your kids to sing and scrub at the same time: "*Happy birthday to you* (rub soapy palms together briskly), *Happy birthday to you* (interlace fingers and rub them quickly together up and down their length), *Happy birthday, dear me-ee* (rub along backs of hands), *Happy birthday to you* (scrub under nails as best as possible).

● *THE ARTISTIC METHOD.* If your child prefers the visual, show how much fun you can have when you work up a good bunch of soapy foam. In this case, the brisk rubbing of all the surfaces of the hands can be interrupted occasionally to blow bubbles. Just make the "OK" sign with your fingers, make sure there's a film of soap in the circle formed, and blow gently.

# Chapter 5

# The Joy of Eating:

## *It's a Family Affair*

Once upon a time the dining room table was the heart of the home, a place where friends and family gathered together to enjoy a home-cooked meal, share stories, and express gratitude for the gifts of life. Dinner was a time of connection and relaxation, not a forced refueling stop in a busy day, a time to watch the news, or a place to play out various food obsessions. Other cultures still stress this social aspect of dining, but the ability to savor food and family seems to have been lost—or perhaps just mislaid—in our own country.

Think we're exaggerating? Let's look at a few facts:

- Only a third of American families typically eat dinner together, according to a 1995 survey.
- Two thirds of American families have the TV on during dinner at least some of the time, and 40 percent have it on often or all the time.
- On average, elementary school-age kids get a quarter of their daily calories from food obtained outside the home.
- In 1999 the average American household spent almost as much on fast food as they did on health care.

Despite our best intentions, our own experiences tend to back up these statistics. We know too well how often mealtimes can be rushed occasions squeezed in between school, work, Scouts, sports, dance class, and all our other activities. We know that our eyes have sometimes been glued to the TV or our ears to the telephone during meals. We know that the plates at the table have sometimes been filled with take-out food or a processed meal tossed in the microwave. We know how often pleasant family meals deteriorate into arguments over how much and what types of food our kids are willing to eat. We know how difficult it is to serve healthy food that our kids will eat with pleasure when every day it seems there is a new "food villain" for us to worry about. We know, we know. We've got eight kids among us, and we've been there.

We would like to help you bring the pleasure back to eating. We are going to explain the basics of a healthy diet without creating categories of irredeemably "bad" foods or making every "good" food sound like a medical prescription. We are going to give you the information that will allow you to counter the unhealthy commercial and cultural messages about food that assault your children day in and day out.

Let's start by looking at the reality of how today's children eat. With fast food and take-out such a big part of their lives, only 1 percent of our kids between the ages of one and nine fully meet the federal guidelines for a healthy diet: 6 to 11 daily servings of grains, 3 to 5 servings of vegetables, 2 to 4 servings of fruit, and 2 to 3 servings of dairy products. How can that be?

- Three quarters of our kids eat only one serving of vegetables a day instead of the recommended three to five. And that vegetable is usually the potato—French fries count for a quarter of all the vegetables eaten by children—although tomato (from the sauce on pizzas and tacos) comes in second.

- Only 10 percent of girls and 25 percent of boys get the current RDA for calcium each day to help them build strong bones and teeth for life.

- American kids are eating more calories than ever, 40 percent of them from fat and excess sugar.

- Kids are eating more salty snack foods, more fatty baked goods, and more sugar-based fruity and carbonated drinks.

- Half of all six- to twelve-year-olds drink about 15 ounces of soda a day, and amazingly, a fifth of all toddlers drink seven ounces of soda a day.

With all this emphasis on fat, starch, and sugar, is it any wonder that the number of children who are overweight has *doubled* in the past thirty years?

The good news is that in 1995 most children under twelve *were* getting what were then called the Recommended Daily Amounts of most of their vitamins and minerals—thanks largely to fortified breakfast cereals, fruit drinks, and baked goods, which function as high-calorie vitamin supplements. (The term RDA will soon be replaced by DRI or Dietary Recommended Intake.) Although our kids are still eating more fat than they should be, fat consumption has been decreasing since the 1970s as more children switch to lower-fat milk. (The exception is preschool-age kids, who actually increased their daily fat intake from 1989 to 1995.) Our kids are eating leaner meats, and a little less visible fat, but they have increased their intake of fats hidden in grain products such as baked goods, pizzas, enchiladas, and tacos. Although hunger still exists, the nutritional spotlight has shifted from preventing diseases of deficiency to preventing health problems caused by *excess*.

Like their parents, our children are eating too much and exercising too little, causing an epidemic of obesity in America. We will discuss obesity in children at greater length in the next chapter, but we want to make sure that you understand that diet in the formative years can have long-term effects—good or ill—on your child's health as an adult. The seeds of such serious medical problems as adult obesity, cardiovascular disease, adult-onset diabetes, osteoporosis, stroke, and probably some cancers are sown during childhood. That's why it is essential for you to encourage good nutritional habits now that will serve your child for a lifetime.

On the flip side of this obesity epidemic is the issue of hunger in America. About 8 percent of our children suffer from what is euphemistically called "food insecurity"—they do not know where their next meal is coming from, and they often do not have enough to eat. This malnourishment has long-term implications as well, because deficiencies in important nutrients can affect both health and educational attainments. Poor children have a much greater risk of, for instance, iron deficiency, which can stunt intellect and slow learning. Lack of protein can slow growth; reliance on the high-fat, high-salt foods often found in inner-city markets can predispose toward diabetes and hypertension; and inadequate levels of antioxidant vitamins can impair immune function. It is important that we all work to ensure that the breakfasts and lunches provided for free at public schools be as nutritious as possible, especially since they may be the only meals that many children eat all day.

There is no way that we can cover nutrition from birth to age twelve in one chapter and be anywhere near as thorough as we'd like to be. If you are interested in a fuller discussion of nutrition, we list a few very good books on the topic in our Resources section at the back of this book. In the meantime, here's our overview.

> *Our children are eating too much high-calorie, low-quality food. Because they are also not getting enough exercise, they are gaining weight.*
>
> *Children who are overweight are at risk for long-term health problems.*

# Prenatal Nutrition

By now, everyone knows the importance of good prenatal nutrition. The poor dietary habits of an expectant mother clearly lead to low birth weight, birth defects, and potential intellectual deficits in her child, as well as health problems such as anemia in the woman herself. It's even possible that a pregnant woman's diet can affect her child's health into adulthood; some research suggests that the stage is set in the womb for hypertension, diabetes, high cholesterol, and other adult conditions.

The developing fetus is especially open to damage during the first trimester of pregnancy. In those first three months—during part of which the woman does not even realize she is pregnant—the spinal cord and central nervous system take form. Because it is particularly important to have an adequate supply of folic acid during this period to prevent neural tube birth defects such as spina bifida, we recommend that all women of child-bearing age get at least 400 *micro*grams (mcg) of the B-vitamin folic acid every day through fortified foods or a multivitamin.

Later in the pregnancy, other nutrients become important. For instance, a pregnant woman must get enough calcium—1,200 to 1,500 milligrams (mg)—and iron (30 mg) a day for two, so that her own stocks of these nutrients won't become depleted as her fetus builds bones, teeth, and the iron stores that will help tide the baby over the first four to six months of life (breast milk is low in iron).

Throughout your pregnancy it's important to eat a varied diet with enough calories—about 300 more a day than usual. You want to gain 25 to 35 pounds with your pregnancy, to increase the chances that your baby will be born at a healthy weight. Focus on high-quality foods like whole grains, produce of all types, lean meats, beans, and low-fat dairy foods. Moderate amounts of soy foods are healthy, but we do not recommend soy supplements; there is just not enough research on the fetal effects of high doses of the plant estrogens contained in these products. Do include more foods high in omega-3 fatty acids, such as salmon, herring, walnuts, and flaxseeds. Skip alcohol and tobacco, and ask your doctor if any of the herbs, dietary supplements, or medications you're currently taking can affect your unborn child. We don't recommend adding any new supplements except prenatal vitamins. Stick to no more than one or two cups of coffee a day, since a higher daily intake (five or more cups) has been found to double the rate of miscarriage and may leach calcium stores from the bones.

We encourage pregnant women to drink purified drinking water, wash their produce, and eat organic food (when available and affordable). We are concerned about the potential for subtle nervous system and hormonal disturbances in children born to mothers exposed to environmental pollutants called hormonally active agents, such as pesticides, polychlorinated biphenyls (PCBs), and dioxins. (See chapter 8 for a more detailed discussion of this topic.) Studies in wildlife and in humans suggest changes in neurological and sexual development can occur when a developing fetus is exposed to environmental estrogens such as these at the wrong time. Currently a lot of national and international research is focused on hormonally active agents, and until the results of this research are in, we do recommend that pregnant women take precautions to avoid unnecessary exposure to these pollutants. In addition, pregnant women should avoid eating too much fish caught in polluted waters (call your state health department for advice), as it may be high in dioxin, PCBs, or toxic metals.

> *Make sure you get 400 mcg of folic acid a day from the time you decide to get pregnant.*
> *Do not drink alcohol at all while you are pregnant or trying to conceive.*
> *Eat a varied, healthy diet throughout your pregnancy.*
> *Don't gain more than 25 to 35 pounds, but do gain enough so your baby has a better chance of being normal weight at birth.*

# Feeding Your Child to Age Two

We believe strongly that children should be breast-fed until they are at least one year of age, but we understand that this is not possible for all women. For instance, women with HIV and those taking certain medications cannot breast-feed without putting their children at risk for potential harm. If you cannot breast-feed your child, don't feel guilty, and don't worry that it will ruin your relationship with your baby. The one complaint we have about some organized advocates for breast-feeding is their dogmatic insistence that the only way to form a close bond with a new child is through breast-feeding. This is absolutely not true.

On the other hand, the makers of commercial baby formulas press their case too strongly as well, to the point where many pregnant women are routinely given educational materials on breast-feeding sponsored by formula makers. This practice, which is forbidden by the World Health Organization, was found in a recent study to significantly decrease the amount of time women nursed their children.

Breast-feeding does offer substantial benefits to both mother and child, so we urge you to consider it carefully. For baby, breast milk

- provides maternal antibodies while the baby's own immune system is developing
- reduces the incidence of diarrhea, upper-respiratory infections, ear infections, and other bacterial and viral illnesses
- lowers the chances of developing allergies, asthma, chronic digestive disorders, and some childhood cancers
- protects against obesity and type-1 diabetes in childhood
- protects against cardiovascular problems and type-2 diabetes in adulthood
- may increase intelligence
- provides a stronger response to immunization
- is more digestible than formula, more efficient a source of energy, and provides hundreds of compounds such as growth factors, hormones, and essential fatty acids not found in infant formulas.

And for mother, breast-feeding

- may reduce the risk of breast cancer in premenopausal women
- saves money and time on formula
- speeds postpartum healing of the uterus
- promotes fat loss.

Even with all these pluses, only 62 percent of American women try nursing at all, and only 15 percent nurse their babies for a full year—one of the lowest rates for breast-feeding in the world. Perhaps this is because we do not provide enough support for nursing mothers. New mothers are generally discharged from the hospital within 24 hours of giving birth, so few of them have a chance to learn how to breast-feed in a relaxed and comforting atmosphere. In addition, few employers provide private space for breast pumping, and most Americans stare aghast at any woman who, even discreetly, raises her blouse to feed her infant. Despite promotion of breast-feeding by the federal government and the American Academy of Pediatrics, we do not yet view nursing as a natural activity in this country. So we applaud those women who do choose to breast-feed their babies, and may there be more and more of them as the years go on.

Breast-feeding is both natural and optimal, but nursing mothers still need education and support. (Check the back of the book for some resources.) Above all, they need good nutrition, good hydration, plenty of rest, and the support of family and friends to help them achieve these goals. Getting enough calories (about 2,500) and enough water (eight glasses) each day is clearly essential, as mothers who eat and drink too little while they are nursing make less milk, and it is lower in the high-quality fatty acids needed for growth and development. *What* you eat is as important as *how much* you eat, as it may also affect a baby's digestion and mood. Colic and fussiness can sometimes be traced to foods eaten by the mother. If you suspect your diet is affecting your child, try eliminating a suspect food for a few days to see if it makes a difference. In our experience, dairy is often the culprit. If this turns out to be true for you, start taking a calcium supplement as soon as you give up dairy products to make sure you get enough of this essential mineral for nursing mothers. At three to four months of age, breast-fed infants should be started on an infant vitamin/mineral supplement like TriViSol or PolyViSol drops to provide additional amounts of iron and vitamins A, C, and D. This is especially important for dark-skinned infants who do not absorb vitamin D as well from the sun.

In addition to good nutrition, nursing mothers require rest. A fatigued or anxious mother may produce less milk, and her baby may develop poor nursing patterns—such as a weak suck or spitting up—that lead to low weight gain. We realize that it can be difficult to find the time to take care of yourself when you have a new baby. But we subscribe to the "in-flight oxygen mask" rule cited by every flight attendant we've ever encountered: Take care of yourself first, so you can care for your children. A nursing mother must get the meals and rest she needs so that she can best provide for her baby. Our advice is to ignore the dusty tabletops, cut back on work or volunteer responsibilities if you can, and ask for help from friends and family. You're not being selfish—you're being a good mother.

If you will not be breast-feeding your child, you will need to choose an infant formula. Regular cow's milk can cause gastrointestinal bleeding and iron deficiency in infants, so it is not an option for children under a year of age. There are basically three categories of formula: milk (casein)-based, soy-based, and specialized "predigested" formulas for children with allergies or significant gastroesophageal reflux (vomiting and spitting up). All have been developed to match human breast milk as closely as possible. We generally recommend milk-based formulas such as Similac or Enfamil, which are well tolerated by most babies. Soy formulas are a second choice because of our concerns that the phytates in soy formulas can bind iron and calcium so they are not as available to the developing child. Look for formula with added DHA (docosahexanoic acid) or other forms of omega-3 fatty acids, which appear to help with brain development. We do not know of any organic infant formulas at this time.

You may begin to introduce solid foods to formula-fed infants at about four months of age. You'll want to wait longer with breast-fed babies—until about six or seven months—as they may suck less strongly and take in less breast milk once they start eating solids. Our advice is to start with a simple bland food like iron-fortified rice cereal, and slowly add other foods, one at a time, so you can tease out any potential food allergies, which might show up in the form of skin disorders, recurrent respiratory tract infections, or gastrointestinal problems. You can buy pureed foods or make them yourself with a portable food grinder or food mill. Dr. Stu's wife used to prepare several meals' worth at once by pureeing the foods into ice cube trays and defrosting as needed. However, babies younger than seven months should not be fed homemade pureed carrots, beets, turnips, spinach, or collard greens because in some parts of the country (generally agricultural areas) these vegetables are too high in nitrates for a very young child. Commercial manufacturers screen for nitrates, so their products are safe at any age. If you do buy commercial baby foods, make sure they contain low levels of added salt, sugar, and other fillers, and look for the organic products offered by several manufacturers.

We recommend that you move to vegetables after rice cereal, starting with red/orange ones like squash and sweet potatoes, then moving to green ones like peas and string beans. Fruits would come next. We hold off on introducing berries, peanuts, egg whites (yolks are okay), and other frequently allergenic foods until a child is older. Yogurt, cottage cheese, and pureed meats can be added after seven months. As far as first beverages go, when your child is old enough for regular soy or cow's milk (over twelve months), give her pasteurized organic full-fat milks until eighteen months, when you can switch to 1% milks. In contrast to adults, babies need plenty of fat in their first two years, as fat fuels the creation of brain tissue. We hope you will not introduce sweet things at all during a child's first year. Be cautious with the amount of fruit juice you allow your child thereafter. Excessive intake of fruit juice can cause gastrointestinal problems and tooth decay or be a contributing factor in failure to gain weight in the second year of life.

---

*Breast-feed your child for a full year if at all possible.*

*If you use formula, try a milk-based (casein) one first.*

*Regular cow's milk is not an option for children under a year.*

*At three or four months, start breast-fed babies on an infant supplement that provides vitamins A, C, and D and iron.*

*Introduce solid foods to formula-fed infants at about four months of age, and to breast-fed babies at six to seven months of age or later.*

*Hold off on introducing sweet foods other than pureed fruits until a child is at least a year old and limit them thereafter.*

# Feeding Your Child from Two to Twelve

When you take away aroma, flavor, and the social aspects of food, you are left with food's rock-bottom purpose—fuel. The food we eat provides the energy we need to keep us going and growing. The energy-producing value of a food is expressed in calories. The federal Recommended Daily Allowances of energy for children are: about 1,300 calories a day for children aged one to three, 1,800 calories a day for kids four to six, and 2,000 calories a day for children seven to ten; after age ten, recommendations vary by gender. Foods high in fat or sugar provide a lot of calories per ounce, but they may be low in nutrients. Nutrient-dense foods like fruits and vegetables are generally lower in calories by comparison, so you can eat more of them and reach the same caloric goal. Although the three macronutrients—fats, carbohydrates, and protein—can all be used as fuel by the body, each has different qualities. Simple sugars provide quick energy and the more concentrated fats provide sustained energy. Proteins are used as last-ditch fuels only. While they provide the raw materials to build muscle and tissue, they are complex molecules that burn less easily.

Over the course of a week, 50 to 60 percent of your child's intake of calories should come from carbohydrates, 20 to 30 percent from fats, and 10 to 20 percent from proteins. Don't obsess about these numbers—just use them as a rough guideline to help in planning nutritionally balanced meals and snacks. Concentrate on high-quality sources of these macronutrients. This is clearly an area for improvement nationally. It's sad but true that the top ten sources of energy for American children aged two to eleven are (in order): milk, bread, cakes/cookies/donuts, beef, ready-to-eat cereal, soft drinks, cheese, salty snacks, sugars/syrups/jams, and chicken.

Fortunately, it is easy to get all the healthy foods you need with plenty of room for a few treats. The United States Department of Agriculture (USDA) has developed a Food Guide Pyramid for Children, which we have adapted just a little by adding a base of water to highlight our belief in the importance of staying well hydrated (see page 73).

Base your child's diet on the foods and fluids at the bottom of the pyramid. Save the foods at the top for occasional treats. Specific foods listed in each category are intended as examples of healthy choices in that food group.

*Water.* Your body may feel quite solid, but more than half of it is water. Water is absolutely essential for good health. Without enough water, your heart, blood, and kidneys are unable to filter out and excrete the waste products of the body efficiently. Water moisturizes the mucous membranes so they can perform their immune duties, lubricates the joints, and keeps the digestive system working smoothly. Yet according to one recent study, 70 percent of preschoolers did not drink *any* water in the course of a day. Children are more vulnerable to dehydration—which can cause dizziness, weakness, constipation, and headaches—because of their smaller size. Children who do not drink enough water through the day tend to be tired and somewhat wacky by late afternoon.

Water remains our beverage of choice for children, so we are appalled by the exponential increase in the amount of soda and fruity sugar-based drinks that kids glug down. Children under 80 pounds should drink a cup of water a day for every 10 pounds, which means a 60-pound child needs to drink 48 ounces of water a day. Save soft drinks for special occasions. If your kids get bored with plain water, mix sparkling water with a little fruit juice (or thawed frozen concentrate) for a change of pace. We had no trouble convincing our own little athletes of the importance of always carrying a 25-ounce sports bottle filled with water and emptying at least two of them a day. When tucking their kids in at night, Dr. Russ and his wife always leave a glass of water on their bedside tables.

*Grains.* It's generally accepted that about 55 percent of the calories in a healthy diet should come from carbohydrates, a broad category that encompasses grains, fruits, vegetables, and sugars. Carbohydrates

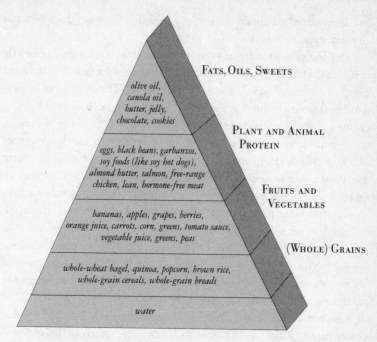

FATS, OILS, SWEETS

*olive oil,
canola oil,
butter, jelly,
chocolate, cookies*

PLANT AND ANIMAL
PROTEIN

*eggs, black beans, garbanzos,
soy foods (like soy hot dogs),
almond butter, salmon, free-range
chicken, lean, hormone-free meat*

FRUITS AND
VEGETABLES

*bananas, apples, grapes, berries,
orange juice, carrots, corn, greens, tomato sauce,
vegetable juice, greens, peas*

(WHOLE) GRAINS

*whole-wheat bagel, quinoa, popcorn, brown rice,
whole-grain cereals, whole-grain breads*

*water*

The Healthy Child Food Pyramid

provide us with the most easily accessible energy to fuel both our bodies and our minds. While carbohydrates are essential to good health, we are learning the hard way that not just any carbohydrate will do. The type of carbohydrate you choose makes a big difference.

The most vitamins, minerals, and fiber are found in the less-processed carbohydrates: whole-grain products, dried beans, fruits, and vegetables. Refined carbohydrates like white breads, cookies, candies, pasta, most children's cereals, and white rice have fewer of these nutrients and cause greater variation in your levels of blood sugar (glucose). Unfortunately, refined carbohydrates are what most people eat in this country. And they are eating more of them, ironically, because they are trying to cut back on fat. While many fat-free baked goods and other products lack calories from fat, they are actually full of calories from sugar and other simple carbohydrates. (Didn't you wonder why they tasted so good? And why you didn't lose weight when you ate them even though they had no fat?)

The increased intake of carbohydrates in this country, especially refined carbohydrates with added fat, is considered a factor in the worrisome increase in type-2 diabetes in children. That's why we recommend that your children get as many as possible of their six to eleven servings a day of carbohydrates from foods like bran flakes, oatmeal, whole-grain breads, produce, and whole-grain entrees and side dishes such as barley soup or bean burritos in whole wheat tortillas. Croissant sandwiches, high-sugar cereals, giant cinnamon rolls, and cookies as big as their head should be reserved for special treats rather than everyday fare. In our experience, both personal and professional, the worst evangelizers for sweet foods are grandparents, who seem to feel it is their obligation to introduce very young children to candy and ice cream despite parental wishes to the contrary. Our message to your children's grandparents: Spoil 'em some other way. You cannot get too much love, but you can get too much sugar.

Less refined carbohydrates contain healthy insoluble and soluble dietary fibers, which benefit your kids both immediately (by preventing constipation) and in the long-term (by preventing cardiovascular disease and diabetes). After the age of two, fiber intake in grams from grains and produce should equal your child's age in years plus five (for instance, 11 grams a day for a six-year-old). Unfortunately, only a third to a half of kids between the ages of four and ten meet this standard. Those who do eat a lot more cereals, produce, legumes, and nuts and a lot less fat that those who fall short.

You can help kids meet their fiber needs by keeping ready-to-eat servings of fruits and vegetables in the refrigerator, and little bags of almonds or walnuts on the snack shelf. Learn to cook and enjoy dishes based on legumes like pinto or red beans. Look for breakfast cereals like bran flakes or oat circles that offer whole-grain goodness. Avoid those highly refined cereals marketed to kids—we're floored that manufacturers can take a grain product basically stripped of its naturally healthful components, drench it in several forms of sugar, add artificial flavorings and some very vivid artificial colorings, and merely by tossing in a few vitamins and minerals, maintain that the product is good for your child. Make sure that the breads you buy are firm and not squishy, and that they feature "whole-wheat flour" or "cracked wheat" as the first ingredient. (Don't be fooled by the term "wheat flour"—it's just white flour.) Once you look, you'll see all sorts of whole-grain breadstuffs on the shelf, from bagels and muffins to pancake mixes and frozen waffles. We encourage you to experiment with whole grains beyond whole wheat, oatmeal, and brown rice. Your family might also like quinoa as a side dish, barley in a thick soup, or bulgur (cracked wheat) as the basis of a hot-weather salad. We recommend a few cookbooks to get you started in the Resource section at the back of the book.

*Fruits and Vegetables.* Children should eat three to five servings of vegetables a day and two to four servings of fruit. Study after study has shown the powerful effects of a diet that contains this level of produce. Eating fruits and vegetables can help prevent diabetes, obesity, cardiovascular problems, osteoporosis, many cancers, and even some vision problems. These benefits seem to come from the wide variety of antioxidant vitamins and minerals and phytochemicals (plant compounds) found in fruits and vegetables. These phytochemicals, in addition to being antioxidants that neutralize cell-damaging free radicals, also have their own specific effects on our metabolism. The quercetin in citrus fruits, for instance, can reduce the symptoms of allergy, and the lutein in corn and spinach is good for your eyes.

Because there are so many beneficial compounds spread throughout the fruit and vegetable kingdom, our advice is to "eat the rainbow." Eating five or more servings of variously colored fruits and vegetables a day assures you of getting a full range of vitamins, minerals, fiber, and phytochemicals. Different colors of fruits and vegetables indicate the presence of different phytochemicals in the plant pigments—orange foods like squash and carrots tend be higher in alpha and beta carotene, blue foods like berries tend to be higher in anthocyanins, red foods like tomato are higher in lycopene, and yellow foods like corn have lots of lutein and zeaxanthin. Broccoli, greens, onions, oranges, garlic, and other fruits and vegetables have their own beneficial phytochemicals as well. Dr. Stu features free samples of the "Produce of the Week" in his office waiting room to encourage his patients (and their parents) to expand their fruit and vegetable palette. Posters

# What's a Serving?

Servings are so large at many restaurants now that people have lost track of what a normal serving looks like. Keep these amounts in mind whenever you are checking to see how well your kids are meeting their nutritional requirements.

For a preschooler, a serving is: ¾ cup low-fat or nonfat milk, ½ cup yogurt, ¼ cup cooked or ½ cup raw vegetable, ⅓ cup juice, ¼ of a fresh fruit, 1 slice of bread, ¼-½ cup of rice or pasta, 1 to 2 ounces of meat, or ¾ cup unsweetened ready-to-eat cereal.

For a school-aged child, a serving is: 1 cup low-fat or nonfat milk or yogurt, ¼ cup cooked vegetable, ½ cup salad greens, 1 small fruit, ½ cup grapes or berries, ½ cup juice, ¼ cup dried fruit, 1 slice of bread, ½ cup pasta or rice, 2 to 3 ounces meat or fish, ½ cup cooked beans, 2 tablespoons nut butter, 1 egg, or 1 cup ready-to-eat cereal.

*Information courtesy of the U.S. Department of Agriculture*

on the wall of the waiting room explain the health benefits of the week's fruit or vegetable.

*Protein.* Protein is essential for growth and development, and it's the basic building block for muscles and tissue. The amino acids that make up each protein molecule are also essential to a whole range of body processes.

Although children and pregnant women need more protein than average in order to build bodies, getting enough protein is not generally a problem in this burger-and-shake culture. Most Americans actually eat far more protein than they need. This puts a strain on their liver, kidneys, and digestive system, since protein is more difficult to digest and metabolize than, for instance, carbohydrates. About 4 ounces of protein a day should meet your child's needs. (As a guide, a 3-ounce piece of meat is about the size of a deck of cards.)

We would like to see folks move toward a more plant-based diet, so we do not call this protein category "meat" as so many other charts do. This spot on our pyramid therefore contains not just lean meats and fish but also dried beans, soy foods and nuts. Most of the saturated fats from red meat and chicken have been implicated in a host of unhealthy conditions including atherosclerosis (which may start in childhood) and cancer, which is why federal guidelines recommend no more than 10 percent of a day's calories come from saturated fats. In addition to the basic issue of unhealthy fats, we are also concerned about the additives found in most red meat, chicken, and even fish: antibiotics, growth hormones, and environmental toxins. Unless you are able to buy meats grown without antibiotics or hormones, we think that you should limit the amount of meat your young child eats.

Although it's fine to use small amounts of chicken or fish as flavoring agents, we think it's a far healthier strategy to make legumes, grains, and vegetables the focus of most meals. Try to use more low-fat or nonfat dairy products, soy hot dogs or hamburgers (which taste quite good these days), soymilk smoothies, bean burritos, and other yummy foods high in protein. Look for organic products when possible.

*Dairy.* Milk, cheese, yogurt, and other dairy products provide protein, too, but they are also important sources of the calcium and other minerals kids need to grow strong teeth and bones. Calcium needs vary by age, but range from 800 mg a day for ages one to five, 800 to 1,200 mg a day for ages eight to ten, and 1,200 to 1,500 mg a day for ages eleven to eighteen. (After age eleven, the National Institute of Health guidelines vary by gender.) These needs can generally be met with three servings a day of dairy foods or with enough servings from other sources (calcium-fortified orange juice or soy milk, tahini, cooked white beans, supplements) to meet recommendations.

You probably want to know where we stand on the tricky issue of whether or not to drink cow's milk. There are many who feel that it is "unnatural" to drink milk after the normal age of weaning. Some express concerns about the antibiotics, bovine-growth hormones (BgH), and other additives present in milk—additives which have not generally been tested for their long-term effects on children. Still others point out that many people in certain racial and ethnic groups are not able to digest milk properly because they lack an enzyme (lactase) that breaks down the lactose (milk sugar) in milk. And finally, there are suspicions that early exposure to cow's milk may trigger the development of juvenile diabetes, especially in children with a family history of diabetes.

We think all parents should educate themselves on this issue, talk with their pediatricians, and decide what choice is best for their own kids. We strongly recommend that you buy organic soy and pasteurized organic dairy products when possible. Soymilks are becoming more readily available, and many calcium-fortified varieties now contain nearly the same amount of calcium per glass as cow's milk does (although it may not be as well absorbed as the calcium in dairy products). Cow's milk is convenient, contains complete protein, and has a calcium-to-phosphorus ratio that maximizes absorption of calcium. Those concerned about lactose intolerance can buy lactose-free dairy products, or try yogurt and frozen yogurt. You may want to delay introduction of milk if there is a family history of allergies, or restrict the amount of milk your child drinks if he or she has had recurrent ear infections, asthma, skin disorders, constipation, or other signs of food intolerance or hypersensitivity. If your child is likely to have a familial susceptibility to diabetes, you may decide to avoid cow's milk altogether and get calcium from other sources.

What do we do in our families? Dr. Stu's kids drink nonfat, BgH-free cow's milk, and Dr. Russ's kids drink mostly water (and some organic nonfat milk on their cereal), which only proves our point that informed parents will differ in their choices for their kids.

*Fats and Sugars.* Fats and sugars are not up there at the tip of the food pyramid because they are evil and must be avoided at all costs. We don't believe in labeling food "good" or "bad," because doing so adds an extra level of tension and guilt to eating. We prefer to think of the items at the tip of the pyramid as foods to be eaten—and enjoyed—occasionally. Clearly, fat is an essential part of the diet, and sugar certainly feels like one. But you will get most of the fats you need and more than enough sugar from healthy foods listed elsewhere on the pyramid. This top portion is for the extras like salad dressing, jam, soda, and the full range of empty-calorie snacks.

Once again, the *types* of fats and sugars you eat make a big difference to your health. Let's start with fats, which your body needs to provide energy, absorb vitamins, and maintain body heat. The three basic divisions of fats are: saturated fats (animal fat, coconut and palm oil), monounsaturated fats (extra-virgin olive and organic expeller-pressed canola oils, nuts, avocados), and polyunsaturated fats (corn, soy, sunflower, safflower, and cottonseed oil). Most fats and oils are in fact a mixture of all three types of fats, categorized by their predominant form.

Monounsaturated fats are associated with a reduced risk of cardiovascular disease and some cancers, so you want most of your child's fat calories to come from foods high in monounsaturated fats. Saturated fats should clearly be minimized, as they tend to clog the arteries, raise levels of "bad" cholesterol, and increase the risk of certain cancers. Polyunsaturated oils were initially touted as being very healthy, but they are unstable oils that oxidize easily, promote inflammation, and, while they do lower "bad" cholesterol, they apparently lower levels of "good" cholesterol as well.

In addition to these three major fats, there are two important fatty acids, one to incorporate in your diet and one to avoid. Omega-3 fatty acids appear to reduce inflammatory processes and improve cardiovascular health. The modern American diet is low in omega-3 fatty acids, which are found in cold-water fish like salmon, and in walnuts, flaxseed, and flaxseed oil, so you should make a point to include these foods in your child's diet. Less healthy are the unnatural *trans*-fatty acids created when vegetable oils are solidified in a process called hydrogenation. Hydrogenated and partially hydrogenated fats—stick margarine and many fried or processed foods—appear to have the one-two punch of both raising "bad" cholesterol as much as saturated fats and lowering "good" cholesterol. Because these artificial fatty acids do not have to be listed as fats on nutrition labels, American children unknowingly eat a lot of *trans* fats "hidden" in products like baked goods. Look for the words "hydrogenated" or "partially hydrogenated" on package labels, and take special note of where the words appear on the ingredient list (earlier in the list means more of it).

# Ten Powerhouse Foods for Your Kids

Optimize your child's nutritional intake by serving foods like these that are packed with vitamins, minerals, fiber, and other healthy compounds:

1. *Oatmeal.* Like other whole-grain foods (bran flakes, whole-grain breads, brown rice), high in fiber, iron, vitamin K, magnesium, manganese, selenium, zinc, chromium, folic acid and other B vitamins

2. *Yogurt.* Rich in calcium, phosphorus, vitamin D, vitamin A, potassium, vitamin B-2, vitamin B-12, essential amino acids, zinc, plus probiotic bacteria

3. *Berries.* High in fiber, vitamin C, manganese, and antioxidant phytochemicals

4. *Broccoli.* Like other leafy green vegetables (dark green lettuce, cabbage, kale, chard, spinach) has fiber, vitamin A, vitamin C, vitamin E, vitamin K, calcium, potassium, magnesium, iron, folic acid, and disease-protective compounds like lutein and other carotenes

5. *Soy.* Like other dried beans (black, pinto, navy, red), has fiber, calcium, iron, magnesium, copper, zinc, potassium, vitamin K, folic acid and other B vitamins, plus heart-healthy plant compounds

6. *Salmon.* Contains vitamin E, vitamin D, calcium, magnesium, selenium, omega-3 fatty acids

7. *Calcium-fortified orange juice.* Has calcium, vitamin C, potassium, magnesium, folic acid, healthy phytochemicals

8. *Almonds and almond butter.* Good for fiber, vitamin E, calcium, magnesium, potassium, iron, copper, zinc, omega-3 fatty acids

9. *Tomato*. Has vitamin C, vitamin A, potassium, and carotenes
10. *Milk*. Rich in calcium, phosphorus, vitamin D, vitamin A, potassium, vitamin B-2, vitamin B-12, essential amino acids, zinc (See above for concerns about milk.)

Children under two have a greater need for fat than the rest of us, so we do not recommend that you try to restrict their fat intake (except for *trans* fats); their developing brains need fat to grow properly. After age two, the American Academy of Pediatrics recommends that fat intake gradually decrease so that by age five, total fat over the course of several days averages out to about 20 to 30 percent of calories. Saturated fat should be less than 10 percent of total calories, and cholesterol less than 300 mg a day. Once again, don't get too caught up in the numbers, but use them as common-sense guidelines.

As for sugar, let us count the ways we get it. Sugars are ubiquitous in processed foods; if you read the labels you'll find them not just in the expected baked goods and sweets, but also in "fruit" drinks, salad dressings, catsup, and even some spaghetti sauces. Sometimes it's hard to tell just how much sugar there is in a product because all the different forms of sugar are listed separately: sugar, brown sugar, corn sweeteners, corn syrup, honey, molasses, fructose, dextrose, maltose, sucrose, sorbitol, and mannitol. They all mean "sugar."

American children get too high a percentage of their daily calories from these nutritionally empty sweets. According to federal food surveys, added sugars (over and above the natural sugars in fruits, vegetables, grains, and milk) account for 16 percent of the calories eaten by kids aged two to five and 19 percent of the caloric intake of kids six to eleven—that's 15 to 23 *teaspoons* of unnecessary extra sugar every day from soda pop, juice drinks, candy, cakes, cookies, and heavily sweetened cereals. Unfortunately, children who load up on these calorie-rich but nutrient-poor foods don't have the appetite for the good stuff. Soda intake, for instance has a very direct effect on nutrition: Since the 1970s, soda intake by young children has risen 16 percent, while milk intake by young children has decreased by—you guessed it—16 percent. The children consuming the highest percentage of calories from sweets are also the most likely to be getting inadequate amounts of eleven vitamins and minerals, especially calcium. For all these reasons, we try not to even bring soda pop and other sugary foods into our own houses.

Let's face it, human beings like sweet things. But you don't want your children eating so many sweets that they miss out on healthier fare. That's why our first choice for dessert and sweet snacks is fruit, which delivers not just natural sugar but a whole range of vitamins, minerals, and fiber. Or try oven-roasted vegetables, especially squash, beets, sweet potatoes, and green beans, which have a natural sweetness missing in vegetables cooked other ways. Low-fat, low-sugar fruited and frozen yogurts also fill nutrient needs while satisfying a sweet tooth. Let these sorts of high-nutrient-value, flavorful foods be the mainstay of your kids' "sweets" intake, and you'll be able to cheerfully agree to the occasional soda or ice cream cone.

Even though we have just given you several pages of dietary guidelines, we also want to encourage you to be somewhat relaxed about diet. No child wants to live with the Nutrition Police. It's far more pleasant, and just as effective, to use more subtle tactics in your campaign to help your family eat better. The primary rule is: If you don't want them to eat it, don't bring it into the house. A lot of food arguments are avoided simply by only having foods in the house that you are willing to have your family eat. We recommend that you start by clearing your shelves of foods you want your family to eat less frequently. Then spend an hour at the grocery sometime when the kids aren't with you just reading the labels on all the foods, choosing the brands and varieties that seem healthiest and tastiest. Resolve to buy just those foods in the future—you can throw them in the cart without thinking about it since you've already done the research. Our secondary rule is: educate your children about foods so they have the information and incentive to eat well on their own. Then they become the police, not you.

*Try to incorporate lots of fruits and vegetables and whole-grain
foods in your family meals and snacks.*

*Rely on monounsaturated fats from olive, or canola oils rather
than saturated or* trans *fats.*

*Keep healthy options for snacking available and ready to eat.*

*Set a healthy example.*

*Remember, there are no "evil" foods—just foods that should only
be eaten occasionally.*

# Food Concerns

We have a number of scientific, cultural, and political concerns about
food that we'd like to touch on briefly. For instance, we think there are
good reasons to try to secure clean food and drinking water for your
family, but that's a big topic more deeply discussed in chapter 8. We
also think it is important to prepare and store foodstuffs safely to prevent food-borne illnesses like *Salmonella* and *E. coli* infections that are
becoming more prevalent (and more resistant to antibiotics). This subject is beyond the scope of our book, so we have listed sources of food-
safety information in the Resources section. Similarly, as we go to
press, the issues of genetically modified foods and irradiated foods are
looming large. We believe that these foods should be labeled clearly so
that parents have enough information to make their own decisions
about whether to buy them or not. We haven't room here for a discussion, so check the Resources section for more on genetically modified
and irradiated foods as well.

We think there are certain additives used in processed foods that
should be avoided. We suggest, for instance, that you avoid the excess
sugars and salt often used as cheap filler. In addition to overloading on
sugars, the average American child eats 2,948 mg of sodium a day, 23
percent above the recommended 2,400 mg maximum. We also share
concerns about some of the preservatives, colorings, and artificial flavorings used in processed foods. For instance, some children are very

sensitive to the flavor enhancer monosodium glutamate (MSG), the additive behind the facial tingling of so-called "Chinese-restaurant syndrome." MSG in food makes Dr. Russ's daughter so incredibly wired she almost bounces off the walls. The food dye tartrazine (FD & C Yellow Dye #5) may cause itching or hives in some children, and behavioral problems have been linked to it and other food colorings. We also suggest limiting the amount of cured meats, such as hot dogs, that your young children eat, as the nitrites used in curing have been associated in a few studies with the development of some childhood cancer and type-1 (juvenile onset) diabetes; soy dogs should be just as acceptable to your kids.

In addition to these scientific concerns, we are quite unhappy about the cultural messages our children get about food. First, there is the tremendous commercial pressure on our kids (and therefore on us) to eat unhealthy foods. Anyone who has ever watched TV with their children knows that kids' shows are filled with one ad after another for foods without nutritional value. We find this advertising extremely upsetting both as doctors and as fathers, as it seems to us to be harmful to the health of our children. Then the advertisers add insult to injury by subjecting parents to what we call "fast-food bribery" whenever McDonald's or Burger King or Wendy's offers a toy in their children's meal that is tied to a movie or TV show your child loves. In some areas of the country, fast-food franchises have even paid for the privilege of a spot in the school cafeteria and soft-drink giants have contracts for soda machines in school hallways.

The shows our children watch are interrupted every few minutes

---

*Be sure to store and prepare food safely.*

*Look for foods that are low in sodium and largely free of chemical additives.*

*Watch TV with your child so you can discuss the ads you see. Limiting TV time reduces your child's exposure to ads for unhealthy foods.*

for another snack-food ad, which encourages them to eat even when they are not hungry and to ask for "super-size" meals when they are. Portion size has also been increasing in this country, which raises expectations of what a serving is. In the 1950s a bottle of Coke held 6½ ounces of soda; now a "child size" take-out soda is twice that size. And can you remember when cinnamon rolls and muffins weren't as big as the balloons in the Macy's Thanksgiving parade?

# What Parents Can Do

Parents have the power to ensure that their children will have healthy attitudes about food. No matter what messages the surrounding culture sends, you are the people most able to influence your children by virtue of their love and respect for you. Don't waste this precious capital. If you can gradually integrate some of the following suggestions into your daily life, your whole family will win.

- Involve your children in all phases of food preparation. Grow some vegetables in pots on the balcony or plant a garden together. Go to a farmer's market or pick-it-yourself farm where you can choose your own fresh foods and learn something about them. Teach your kids how to cook simple foods and how to prepare the table for meals.
- Be adventurous. Try lots of new foods. Have your kids pick out a new fruit or vegetable to try each week.
- Become a nutrition educator. Read the labels on foods, and explain what they mean to your children. Explain the standards you apply while choosing food for your family ("I try to find a cereal that's low in salt and sugar, and ice cream that's low in fat because I love you and want you to be healthy"). Tell little children what's specifically healthy about a certain food ("spinach is really good for your eyes").
- Don't label foods as either "bad" or "good." Explain that some foods we need to eat often and some foods we need to eat only occasionally.

- Instill and model healthy attitudes toward food as a source of both pleasure and health. It's okay to go "yummmmm" when you eat!
- Clean out your pantry of foods you want to eat less often, and keep more desirable foods handy in ready-to-eat form.
- Be flexible and respect individual food preferences. Studies find that children have to encounter a new food eight or more times before they will willingly eat it—it takes time to get used to a new taste or texture. Put tiny samples of a new food on your child's plate along with the rest of the meal and require that he or she try a taste.
- Provide a variety of foods. Don't just focus on one macronutrient or a few stand-by menus. If your kids eat a wide range of healthy foods they'll probably get all the nutrients they need.
- Practice portion control. Provide your kids with servings appropriate for their size, age, and caloric needs.
- Don't skip breakfast and don't let your kids skip breakfast, either. The morning brain requires food—preferably carbohydrates—to get kick-started. Kids who don't eat breakfast don't do as well in school. For children, breakfast is also a major source of fiber, vitamins, and minerals; kids who skip the morning meal tend to have inadequate levels of these nutrients.
- Learn to cook or buy healthier substitutes for favorite foods that are too high in fats or sugar.
- Practice moderation. Don't jump to make major changes in your family's diet with every new nutrition book or TV news show. The media discovers a new nutritional hero or villain every week. Take the long view.
- Make meals pleasant occasions for the whole family. Establish meaningful rituals (saying grace, turning off the phone, sharing the high points of the day) that build family closeness. Studies find that children who eat dinner with their families eat more nutritiously all the time; teenagers who eat meals with their parents do better in school, and have fewer problems with drugs, alcohol, and unplanned pregnancy.

# Questions About Nutrition

*How do you get a kid to eat more vegetables and fruits?*

We admit this is often a difficult task, but we're glad to share strategies we've gleaned from our reading and from our experiences as parents. The first trick is to make fruits and vegetables more interesting. Involve your children in the entire culinary process, from planting the seed to growing and serving the food. Kids think it's a lot more fun to graze on snap peas in the garden or pluck a cherry tomato off the pot on the porch than to eat whatever green or yellow thing you stick on their plate.

Then be adventurous with foods. Enjoy trips to the nearest farmer's market or specialty food store, where there are often free samples to tempt kids into trying new tastes. Put samples of new fruits and vegetables on a toddler's plate until they look and taste more familiar; in fact, let your child help pick new kinds of produce to try (purple potatoes! yellow tomatoes! green cauliflower!).

And finally, make a variety of fruits and vegetable available at all times: Put little bags of dried fruits in an easy-to-reach cupboard and cut-up vegetables in the refrigerator, keep a filled fruit basket on the kitchen counter. Try the stealth strategy of adding fruits and vegetables to other foods (grated carrots in the spaghetti sauce, zucchini slices on the pizza, cucumbers and tomatoes in the sandwiches, blueberries in the pancakes).

*I've got a picky eater. How can I make sure she eats a balanced diet?*

Let's start with a new division of labor: It's your job to be a good role model for healthy eating and to serve a nutritious meal or snack. It's your child's role to eat what she wants from it. This avoids a whole lot of arguing over food. Offer a variety of healthy foods, including small amounts of new ones, and don't worry if she doesn't seem to eat much at certain stages of growth, or if she only seems to eat one thing. Food jags are common in young kids. Save what she doesn't finish for later, and keep healthy snacks such as produce, yogurt, and whole-wheat bagels on hand as well.

*Is fruit juice a healthy drink for my child?*

We don't recommend fruit juice in the first year of life as it may cause a child to develop a preference for sweet liquids that will reduce his intake of healthier beverages like water. We do not recommend apple juice for toddlers because it is high in a poorly absorbed sugar called sorbitol that often causes loose stools and abdominal pain. Children who drink too much juice (more than 12 ounces a day) in the first two years of life may lose their appetite for more nutrient-dense solid foods and grow poorly; those who drink too much calorie-dense fruit juice at later ages are more likely to be overweight. In our opinion, moderate amounts of diluted grape juice or orange juice are better fruit-juice options for older children, especially those with a tendency toward obesity.

*My four-year-old never clears his plate without a battle. What can I do?*

Take a deep breath and call upon all your patience. No one wants the dinner table to be a battle zone. Maybe you're over-estimating what he can eat; preschoolers aren't generally big eaters. Just offer small portions of a variety of foods, and ask him to take at least one bite of everything on his plate as "an adventure." Do not force an unwilling eater to clean his plate; you want your child to learn how to tell when he is hungry and when he is not, and eat accordingly.

Children will naturally eat as much as they need.

*What vitamins, minerals, or other supplements should I give my child?*

We'd much rather that your children got all their essential vitamins and minerals from food, but we are realistic enough to recognize that this isn't always possible. A good children's multivitamin is clearly no substitute for proper nutrition, but it is a way to hedge your bets. Look for a product that contains a range of vitamins and minerals and not too much added sugar. While there is no set rule regarding amounts of supplemental vitamins and minerals for children, a five-year-old should probably not be taking more than 50 percent of the adult Recommended Daily Intake of most vitamins and minerals.

More is not necessarily better when it comes to vitamins, especially the fat-soluble vitamins A, D, E, and K, which can be toxic in high doses. We have both seen children whose skin has turned orange from too much vitamin A. One boy was getting several times the recommended daily intake of A for children from the combination of his multivitamin and boxed juice drinks containing the adult RDA for the vitamin. Be sure to factor in all sources of supplementation. For safety's sake, keep all child and adult supplements where children absolutely cannot reach them; children commonly overdose on vitamins, especially those containing iron.

*How do I handle my child's sweet tooth?*

Use the power you have as the only people in the house with a checkbook and a driver's license to regulate what foods are available there. If you don't bring it into the house, it can't be eaten. Occasional sweets are fine as a treat, but we don't recommend you make a habit of stocking them.

*Are some sweeteners better than others?*

The debate continues about the potential adverse effects of artificial sweeteners, and even though there is no clear evidence of harm yet proven, we prefer to err on the side of caution. People with an inherited metabolic disorder known as PKU (phenylketonuria) clearly cannot use aspartame (Nutrasweet), and too much sorbitol, a sugar alcohol often used in sugarless gums and candies, can cause diarrhea in children. We are more concerned about long-term effects of chemical sweeteners, which is why we advise the use of natural sweeteners when needed—sugar, real maple syrup, honey, or a newly available herb called stevia that can be found in health-food stores (one or two drops should give you the sweetness you desire). Be aware, though, that raw honey should not be given to children under the age of two because of the risk of infant botulism, a very serious illness.

*What oils are best for my family?*

Look for oils that are liquid at room temperature; avoid anything partially hydrogenated. The oils with the best fat profiles are high in monounsaturated fats, and low in saturated fat. In order of monounsaturated content, the top oils are hazelnut, olive (our favorite), high-oleic-acid safflower (not regular safflower oil), avocado, almond, canola, mustard, flaxseed (very high in omega-3 essential fatty acids, but not suitable for cooking), and walnut. We advise our patients to stay away from products made from the fat-substitute Olestra, which can interfere with the absorption of fat-soluble vitamins A, D, E, and K and other fat-soluble nutrients.

*My daughter is a vegetarian. How can I make sure she gets the nutrients she needs?*

Children can thrive on vegetarian diets if they receive enough calories and care is taken to make up for essential nutrients such as vitamin B-12, iron, zinc, calcium, and possibly vitamin D that are normally derived from meat, eggs, and dairy products. Without these nutrients, vegetarian children are at risk for poor growth, anemia, and deficiency diseases. Vegan children (who do not eat any animal products) have to be even more careful about including alternative sources of micronutrients than do lacto-ovo-vegetarian children (who eat dairy and eggs but no meat). Parents of vegetarians should provide a wide variety of grains, legumes, and soy foods to make sure their children get all the essential amino acids. Concentrated sources of calories like nuts, seeds, soy foods, avocados, and dried fruits can help insure they get enough calories as well. Consider a daily multiple vitamin and mineral supplement as well as a safety net.

*What are some healthy snacks for kids?*

There's no end to the healthy snacks available for kids. For example, there's almond butter on a whole-wheat bagel, peeled baby carrots, air-popped popcorn (try it with brewers' yeast sprinkled on top), hummus on a warm pita bread, low-fat organic string cheese, frozen grapes, fruit-juice popsicles, yogurt, cut-up vegetables with a low-fat dip, fruit smoothies of soy or regular milk blended with organic strawberries and/or a banana, squares of soy cheese or a soy hot dog, a handful of almonds and dried blueberries—be creative.

# Chapter 6

# Don't Just Sit There:

## _Exercise and Physical Fitness_

**m**any American children are busy from dawn to dusk. They jump from bed to the school bus, spend five or six hours sitting in the classroom, come home for a few hours in front of the VCR or on the computer with their friends, lie on the floor doing homework, and finally, protesting their lack of sleepiness, stagger off to bed. Once a week religious instruction, music lessons, sports practice—or all three—might be squeezed into the schedule. Our kids' lives are so jam-packed that it's no wonder that we parents don't even notice that one essential factor for their good health is often missing.

This missing element—we'll call it Factor X—has amazing powers. It can sharpen the mind, reduce anxiety and depression, build energy, reduce weight, increase immune function, improve sleep, increase strength and flexibility, and lower the lifetime risk for diabetes, heart disease, osteoporosis, and certain cancers. If we told you a pill or nutritional supplement delivered all these benefits, you know you would jump at the chance to buy it for your family. And if we told you it was free? That remedy would be _flying_ off the shelves.

So how do you get Factor X? You move. The marvelous Factor X is simply exercise. People underrate the value of exercise, but remaining physically active throughout the day is an unbeatable strategy for good physical and mental health. And it's cheap. You really don't need much more than a pair of walking shoes, a jump rope, or a favorite dance tape to get all the exercise you and your kids need for next to nothing.

But, you ask, don't kids already get plenty of exercise? Aren't they busy all the time with all sorts of activities? Don't they get phys ed at school? We hate to be the ones to tell you, but despite all their busyness, our kids are just not moving their bodies around enough every day. Unlike children from earlier generations, they spend less time in vigorous outdoor play or physical chores. Many of them are "couch potatoes," immersed in many fascinating but sedentary activities. This inactivity is a prime factor in what experts at the Centers for Disease Control and Prevention (CDC) are calling "an epidemic of obesity" in American children. Sadly, obesity is now the number one childhood disease in America, and our children are on the way to becoming the fattest generation of adults in American history, with all the health problems that implies.

# Why Are Our Kids Overweight?

Before we continue with the topic of physical activity, we'd like to talk a little about this problem of obesity. This topic fits perfectly between our discussions of nutrition and exercise, because obesity is caused by taking in more energy in the form of food than is expended by physical activity. Although genetics plays a part in childhood obesity (we'll get to that in a minute), the reason American children are increasingly overweight boils down to two things: they eat too much of the wrong foods and they sit around too much.

Overweight is generally defined in one of two ways—as a measure of body composition called the body-mass index, or BMI (calculated by dividing weight in pounds by the square of height in inches, see page 93), or as a percentile that refers to the child's weight for height compared to other children of the same age. A child is generally con-

# Is *Your Child Overweight?*

In order to use the CDC growth charts below, you will first need to calculate your child's BMI. To do this, divide your child's weight in pounds by her height in inches, divide the result by her height in inches again, and multiply by 703. You might want to use a calculator.

For instance, if your child is seven years old, four feet tall, and weighs 50 pounds, her BMI would be 15, which you can see from the chart below is normal for a child her age.

*(50 divided by 48 = 1.04 divided by 48 = .02*
*multiplied by 703 = 15)*

If your child is seven years old, four feet tall, and weighs 70 pounds, however, her BMI is 22, which, as you can see from the chart below for girls, falls into the overweight zone.

*(70 divided by 48 = 1.46 divided by 48 = .03*
*multiplied by 703 = 22)*

Don't forget, this data is still generalized, and there are circumstances where the BMI arrived at will not be a true indication of a specific child's fat-to-lean mass. However, a BMI in the at-risk or actual overweight groups should at least trigger a discussion with your child's pediatrician.

sidered at risk for being overweight if he has a BMI-for-age above 25 or registers in the 85th percentile of weight for height on a growth chart. A BMI-for-age of over 30 or being in the 95th percentile of weight for height signals that the child is already overweight, a condition that is likely to persist into adulthood unless changes are made. Keep in mind however, that there are more variables to the BMI in children, whose actual percentages of fat-to-lean mass may vary by gender, race, stage of development, height, and sexual maturity. The BMI chart is a guideline only.

# BMI Values for Boys and Girls Ages 2–12 Years

*Calculating BMI Index:*
[Weight in pounds ÷ Height in inches ÷ Height in inches] x 703

| | | | |
|---|---|---|---|
| *85th–95th percentile* | | | |
| *>95th percentile* | | | |

| AGE (years) | BOYS | | GIRLS | |
|---|---|---|---|---|
| | *at risk* | *overweight* | *at risk* | *overweight* |
| 2 | 18.2–19.3 | >19.3 | 18–19.1 | >19.1 |
| 3 | 17.4–18.4 | >18.4 | 17.2–18.3 | >18.3 |
| 4 | 16.9–17.8 | >17.8 | 16.8–18 | >18 |
| 5 | 16.8–17.9 | >17.9 | 16.8–18.3 | >18.3 |
| 6 | 17–18.4 | >18.4 | 17.1–18.8 | >18.8 |
| 7 | 17.4–19.1 | >19.1 | 17.6–19.6 | >19.6 |
| 8 | 17.9–20 | >20 | 18.4–20.6 | >20.6 |
| 9 | 18.5–21 | >21 | 19–21.6 | >21.6 |
| 10 | 19.4–22 | >22 | 20–23 | >23 |
| 11 | 20.2–23.2 | >23.2 | 20.8–24 | >24 |
| 12 | 21–24.3 | >24.3 | 21.7–25.3 | >25.3 |

*Source: Derived from Centers for Disease Control and Prevention BMI Values for Children.*

How bad is the problem? According to national health surveys taken at regular intervals since the sixties, the number of overweight children in America has increased dramatically, especially in the past twenty years. Although interpretations of this data by various researchers differ, it appears that up to 25 percent of children and adolescents are overweight or at risk of being overweight. This parallels the doubling in the incidence of adult obesity over the same time period. Children of certain ethnic minority groups—Native Americans, African Americans, Hispanic Americans, and Asian Americans (especially Pacific Islanders)—are more likely to be obese.

However, as much as some would like to be able to blame the obesity epidemic on genes, it's just not possible. There is indeed a strong genetic influence on obesity. But human genes have not changed as much in the past twenty years as body weight has. The experts agree that this is just too swift a transformation in body composition to be genetic. Certain individuals and ethnic groups do appear to carry genes that make them more *susceptible* to obesity. Yet genetically susceptible children (and adults) who eat well and stay physically active can keep their weight within normal bounds. Activity seems to modify how the body regulates fat. Obesity that appears to run in families may reflect the passing down of poor health habits from parents to children.

There are five factors that are most often blamed by the experts for our national epidemic of childhood chubbiness:

1. *Less time spent playing, and more time spent in front of one kind of screen or another (TV/VCR, computer).* Toddlers in less-than-ideal day care situations may spend much of the day plunked in front of a TV show or video rather than doing the important developmental work of crawling, walking, tumbling, and otherwise honing gross motor skills. Older kids have become more passive and less able to entertain themselves in good old-fashioned play—running, jumping, climbing trees, or making up active games. There seems to be an actual dose-related response linking television viewing and obesity, with the greatest obesity seen in the children watching the boob tube most. Keep track of just how much time your children spend watching TV, videos, or the computer screen over the course of a week. We're betting you'll be surprised by the total.

2. *Too much exposure to advertising for low-quality food.* Except for the singing raisins, when was the last time you saw an ad for a fruit or a vegetable on kid's programming? There's a food ad every

five minutes during Saturday-morning cartoons. No wonder our kids are always grabbing us by the sleeve in the grocery store and begging for some sugar- and/or fat-filled food product.

3. *Less parental oversight on food choices.* Kids get an increasing number of their calories away from home, and when they *are* eating at home, there is often no adult with them to make sure they are eating well.

4. *More high-calorie drinks.* Kids, especially overweight ones, may get a lot of their daily calories from juice drinks and sodas. These beverages offer very little nutritional value for their calories, and they fill kids up too much to leave room for better foods.

5. *Fewer high-fiber foods.* Kids are eating fewer of the low-calorie, high-nutrient carbohydrates like fruits, vegetables, and whole grains, and more mixed-grain products made of white flour, sugar, and unhealthy fats. There is some evidence that fiber plays an important role in weight control.

Is chubbiness really so bad? At certain stages in their development—in infancy, or just before (boys) or during (girls) puberty—children naturally tend to be a little chubbier. But weight gain at other times should be a warning. For instance, children are meant to be lean from after the age of one until about age five or six, when they begin to put on weight again. This turning point around age five is called the point of adiposity rebound. New research suggests that kids whose adiposity rebound occurs too early, because they aren't encouraged to be active or because they overeat, are at double the risk to become obese adults.

Being overweight over the long term, especially when combined with a sedentary lifestyle, should also raise a red flag. Childhood obesity is linked to a scary array of health problems that appear in childhood: asthma and allergy, early onset of type-2 diabetes, high cholesterol, and high blood pressure. Of particular concern is the dramatic rise in type-2 (non-insulin-dependent) diabetes in children, especially minority children. Unlike the autoimmune, insulin-dependent form of diabetes that is known to occur specifically in children, type-2 diabetes was unheard of in kids until very recently. In fact, early reports of it appearing in juveniles were disbelieved by some medical experts, who considered this form of diabetes (then called adult-onset diabetes) solely the problem of overweight and sedentary older people. But they should not have been surprised. As adults have become more obese, adult levels of type-2 diabetes have skyrocketed, increasing six-fold in the past forty years alone. Our children are becoming less active and more obese as well. Why did we expect they would escape the consequences? The appearance of type-2 diabetes in children is particularly alarming, because it puts them at higher risk for all the complications of diabetes— atherosclerosis, hypertension, kidney failure, blindness, and impaired circulation—at an earlier age. Overweight children who become over- weight adults are at greater risk for other health problems including gall bladder disease, breast cancer, and colon cancer. It's clear to us that the best way to protect your children's health is to keep them fit.

## How Parents Can Help an Overweight Child

We don't want you to obsess unnecessarily about your child's weight; there's enough obsession with weight and body image in our society already. But we do want you to take your pediatrician or family practi- tioner seriously if he tells you that your child is heavier than average for his or her height. If other culprits, such as endocrine disorders, have been ruled out, use this warning flag as a signal to do an evaluation of your family's nutritional intake and energy expenditure. It could be you've let some good habits slip and merely have to re-institute them. Or you might need to begin to make a few changes to move your fam- ily toward a healthier lifestyle. The most effective programs for child obesity do not single out the overweight child, but are intended to instill healthier behaviors in the entire family, starting with the *parents*.

Since childhood obesity is easier to prevent than it is to cure, we recommend you follow these tips for all children, even those of "nor- mal" weight, to ensure they stay that way:

- *Take a good look at yourselves.* Eighty percent of overweight children have overweight parents, and genetics is not the only reason. Consider whether you encourage your children to be sedentary or to eat poorly, either directly or indirectly. According to one study, only 28 percent of moms and 36 percent of dads exercise regularly. Parental influences—for good or ill—are decisive, because the dietary patterns set in childhood tend to be permanent. Be prepared to make changes in your own behaviors to become a good role model. You might even want to turn the tables and ask your kids to give *you* stars or stickers for exercising more, or making better food choices!

- *Breast-feed your child.* Even just a few months of breast-feeding lowers a child's risk of obesity. In a large German study, school-age children who had been breast-fed for at least six months were 40 percent less likely to become obese than those raised on formula.

- *Teach your child how to tell when she is hungry.* Learning to recognize the sensations of hunger and satiety may help a child avoid the kind of mindless eating that causes excess weight. That's why we often advise parents to respect natural hunger instincts and not insist that young children finish everything on their plates. Remember, it's your job to put healthy food on the plate, it's their job to decide what and how much to eat.

- *Get more active, in big and little ways.* Studies have found that even fidgeting helps maintain normal weight, so clearly any amount of exercise can have a beneficial effect. Start small—take the stairs rather than the escalator, park a block away from your destination, get off the bus one or two blocks early—and work up to a total of 45 minutes of exercise done all at once or scattered through the day. Once again, don't underestimate the power of your own example on your children; if you take a positive approach toward movement, they will too. Even the mundane household physical chores—sweeping, washing the car, vacuuming—can seem like fun.

- *Cut back on TV, video, and computer time.* Here's a scary fact: American kids spend more time watching one screen or another than they do at any other activity except sleeping. Several studies have linked this viewing with obesity, with one finding that kids who logged more than five hours a day at the TV/VCR/computer were almost five times more likely to be obese than kids who spent two hours or less there. Unless you're willing to hook a stationary bike up to the TV and computer and make your kids work for their screen time, you'll have to limit viewing to open up time for exercise.

We believe no child should have a TV in his or her bedroom. In fact, we'd really prefer it if the TV was in the family room or *your* bedroom, where it is generally out of sight and you can monitor its use. We recommend you limit your children's free-time use of the TV, video, and computer to just one hour a day during the week; you can loosen up a little on weekends. This not only frees up time for physical activity, but also reduces the number of ads for junk food and junk behavior that your children see.

- *Stress high-value over low-value foods*. Overweight children might not eat a greater volume of food than normal-weight children, but their choices may be higher in empty calories from added fat and sugar. You can educate your child as to which foods are for every day, and which are for occasional consumption, through the casual conversations you have while buying, preparing, or eating food together.
- *Make sure there are always "everyday" foods available in the house and in the car*—low-calorie, high-impact foods like carrot sticks, nonfat yogurt, and apples. You might even put a fresh fruit plate out during the hours when snacking is most likely to occur.
- *Eat meals together*. Do you make a point of eating meals together or do family members just wander through the kitchen grabbing their own food choices? We hope you sit down together at the table, as you not only gain more control over what your children eat, you also improve everyone's chances for a nutritionally complete meal. Family dinner is most important, but don't forget some oversight at breakfast, too. Kids not only need a morning meal to be able to function well in school, but

breakfast is often their main source of fiber, vitamins, and minerals. Once again, parents can be role models by eating a good first meal, too (only half of all parents eat breakfast now).

- *Don't fall for big-eyed pleas for nutritionally poor breakfast cereals, snacks, and packaged meals.* Too many parents do not have the backbone to insist that a child eat a healthy breakfast or lunch, giving in to the heartfelt appeals for the latest high-sugar cereal with a TV character on the box, high-fat Lunchables™, nearly juiceless "juice drinks," and the darling little individual bags of candies and snacks that "everybody else has." An occasional treat is fine, but your message about better choices in food should be a consistent one.

- *Think about serving size.* In this world of "super-size it," people have lost sight of what constitutes a single serving. Toddlers, for instance, really need only small amounts of a variety of foods, not big heaping servings.

- *Don't buy soda except for special occasions.* Overweight children especially get too many calories from sodas and fruit drinks. Water tastes great, is good for the body, and contains no calories. As alternatives, you can add a little fruit juice to sparkling water for a refreshing drink or blend nonfat milk or soymilk with fruit and yogurt for a great-tasting healthy milkshake.

- *Don't make kids diet.* Growing children—even overweight ones—need enough energy and nutrients for development, so any reduction in calories to lose weight should be small. Instead of talking about weight *loss*, we talk to kids about weight *maintenance*, encouraging overweight kids to stay at the same weight as they grow taller until they reach a healthier weight-to-height ratio. We put the focus on making better food choices rather than restricting intake, and on increasing the number of calories burned in physical activity. Fitness is really the goal here, not thinness. This is an important distinction, because our culture tends to equate thinness with acceptability—a terrible lesson for a child. Our children are already exposed to unachievable body images (Barbie's 18-inch waist, G.I Joe's 55-inch chest) that make them feel inadequate. The weight maintenance approach allows children to monitor their own height and weight and feel good about themselves and their bodies. It also decreases the chances of tipping a child—especially a girl—into an eating disorder or depression.

- *Treat obesity as a family issue.* Research suggests that obesity in children is difficult to control unless the whole family is involved. Don't single out the overweight child for special treatment—everyone in the family should be eating well and exercising. In fact, a recent study found that obese kids lost more weight when the program focused on the parents as agents of change than when it focused on the overweight child. Remember: Children don't change, families do.

- *Take an active role in improving nutrition at your child's school.* Possible areas for improvement: school meals, snack machines, and school-based advertising for unhealthy foods. We're thrilled that pockets of parents around the country have begun speaking up with some success for school meals with less fat, less sugar, more fruits and vegetables, and more whole-grain foods. Improving cafeteria food is especially important for the many children who depend on school breakfast and lunch for much of their daily caloric intake. Parents in some towns have also insisted that coin-operated machines in the schools dispense not soda and salty or sugary snack foods, but bottled water or fresh fruit. Maybe you can do something about the prevalence of advertising in the classroom or on school grounds for foods we try to teach kids to avoid in health class.

# The Exercise Prescription

It may sound flip, but exercise, in one form or another, really is good for whatever ails you or your kids—and it's fun too. It can improve conditions as varied as obesity, high cholesterol, depression, stress, back pain, and even fatigue. It can give a kid a real boost of energy when she feels like her tail is dragging. In fact, Dr. Stu has been known to require his teenaged patients with mononucleosis to walk to his office for their visits because he knows how much more quickly they will recover with a little exercise. Exercise can also help prevent such chronic conditions as diabetes, osteoporosis, hypertension, and atherosclerosis—all of which can have their roots in childhood.

We believe strongly in encouraging children to be physically active, for both the immediate benefits of exercise and the long-term health protection it provides. Parents are really key players in this effort, because 95 percent of kids who are physically active have parents who are, too. You're not an athlete? No problem. You only need to be *active*; you don't need to be *good*. It's the effort that counts more than the results. Besides, we're convinced that there's a sport or activity for every taste and talent. Your preference could be walking or dancing, lifting weights or swinging a tennis racket, riding a bike or pushing a lawnmower at top speed. Pick whatever's fun. Those who require variety might even do a little of everything.

When we use the word "exercise," we don't mean boot-camp calisthenics or 26-mile marathons. We just mean physical activity. Walking around the neighborhood, shooting a few hoops, working in the garden, rolling around on the lawn with the dog, washing the car, jumping rope, dancing to your favorite CD, playing hide and seek or Sardines, tossing a Frisbee or a baseball. None of these activities require planning or expense—just get up and go.

And yet, we don't do it. And, as a consequence, our kids don't either. In fact, less than 25 percent of our kids get 20 minutes of vigorous exercise every day. Fewer than 25 percent get 30 minutes of *any* type of exercise every day. *That means that three out of four kids are not getting enough regular activity to protect their current and long-term health*. Our children get less active with age, especially girls, who by the time they are ten are getting only half the exercise they did when they were six.

Why are our kids so sedentary? The reasons range from the cultural to the personal, but the end result is that they are at increasing risk for a wide range of *largely preventable* health problems. Pediatricians, fitness experts, and government agencies are calling this lack of activity a public-health emergency, and we want parents to understand

# Ten Reasons Why Our Kids Are Couch Potatoes

1.  Our kids have poor role models: Half of American adults get *no* regular exercise.
2.  We have many new ways of distracting ourselves while sitting down. Video games, cable television, and the Internet allow us to stare at the tube 24/7.
3.  Labor-saving devices such as automobiles, TV remotes, garage-door openers, trash mashers, etc. have reduced the opportunity to burn off small amounts of energy in everyday living.
4.  You can now get the same adrenaline rush that used to be available only through physical activity by punching the remote or moving a joystick.
5.  We are becoming a high-tech culture of spectators.
6.  We train our kids to be sedentary by using electronic baby-sitters such as TVs, VCRs, and computers to sedate or amuse them; in fact, kids between two and five spend more than 25 hours a week in front of the TV.
7.  Schools are cutting physical education classes.
8.  Streets and playgrounds are often unsafe for unsupervised children.
9.  Fewer parents are home after school to watch their kids and shoo them outside.
10. Children may not have room in their heavily scheduled lives for free play.

just how vital it is that this unhealthy trend be reversed. Our children's future health depends on it. Exercise is especially important for girls—the children most likely to slack off as they get into their teen years. Girls who are active are able to build the strong bones they will need to protect them through life, and they may be reducing their risk of breast cancer in adulthood as well.

American kids are spending less time playing. There is an oft-cited University of Michigan survey showing that American kids age twelve and under have nearly doubled the time they spend at sports since 1981, from an average of 2½ hours a week to 4½ hours a week. That would be good news except for the fact that the study actually found a net loss in activity, because kids are "playing" less. The number of hours spent in unstructured play and outdoor activities (as opposed to organized sports) declined from 16 to 12 hours a week, wiping out the gain in sports-related activity.

But how important is play anyway? Pretty darned important, as it turns out. Play is children's work—more fun than our own perhaps, but just as vital. Play is the way young children educate their bodies and minds and exercise their creativity. Free play—unorganized and uncontrolled by adults—gives them a chance to develop and refine their motor skills, learn about the world, become aware of how their bodies move through space, learn to get along with others, learn to amuse themselves, and use their imaginations. When you plunk a young child in front of a TV or video, you stop this process and encourage passivity. It's a harsh reality, but parents who use TV as a babysitter are also setting their children up for poor health later.

Young children love to move around, so your principal role in the early years is not to discourage them. Allow them to be free of restraint as much as is safely possible, out of their strollers and playpens and into the world. Sure, it's more trouble for you, but it's very good for them. As they get older, you can help them find activities that are fun for them and encourage them to try all sorts of exercise, from tumbling to team sports to dance and movement. They may only be able to handle short sessions of ten minutes or so at first, but kids age five to twelve should be getting at least 30 minutes a day of physical activity of various types. There is some evidence that forcing children to exercise backfires, producing adults who refuse to move a muscle, so rather than shoving a recalcitrant child onto the playing field, you may be better off focusing on more indirect strategies: finding activities that interest your child, rewarding increased activity, providing more active family experiences, and being a positive role model yourself.

What kind of exercise is best for children? You want cardiovascular exercise as well as activities to build strength and flexibility. Children need weight-bearing, high-impact activity, too—such as tumbling, dance, or jumping rope—to build bone mass during this crucial period. We feel strongly that for safety's sake, all children should also learn to swim. We advise you to include some form of all three of the major forms of exercise in your family activities. For instance:

1. *Aerobic exercise.* Aerobic exercise, sometimes called cardiovascular exercise, works the heart and lungs as well as the muscles. The goal is to raise heart rate, increase oxygen intake, and improve stamina. Running, swimming, soccer, basketball, bicycling, aerobic dance, and brisk walking are all forms of vigorous aerobic exercise. Even playing run-and-chase with your little ones counts. We both squeeze lots of aerobic activity into our children's lives in little daily bits and in longer weekend outings.

2. *Resistance exercise.* Resistance exercise, or strength training, increases muscle strength and endurance by working a muscle against resistance in the form of weights, elastic tubing, or a person's own body weight. Generally a certain number of repetitions ("reps") of an exercise are done at a certain weight, gradually moving on to heavier weights or more repetitions as the exercise becomes easier. Methods include Nautilus-style machines, exercises with stretch bands, push-ups and pull-ups, and weightlifting with dumbbells. Young children can get resistance exercise most easily by doing exercises like modified push-ups that use their own bodies as the weight; older children who are large enough to use free weights or machines should be well-supervised and stick to light weights and more reps. Machines and free weights should only be used with supervision.

3. *Flexibility exercise.* Stretching exercises, yoga, and tai chi stretch

muscles, tendons, and ligaments to improve flexibility and balance. Dr. Russ' kids love to do yoga with their dad.

be sure to teach your children to warm up with gentle exercises, jogging in place, or stretches before any extended period of vigorous exercise and to cool down in the same manner after the session.

In addition to different forms of exercise, there are different intensities as well. For instance, the activities of daily life—strolling to the car, climbing stairs, taking out the garbage—are generally considered to be light exercise. Walking and other activities that expend calories without working up too much of a lather are considered moderate activities. In contrast, running or circuit training—exercise that makes you sweat and boosts your heart and breathing rates—is considered vigorous. All three intensities of activity are beneficial. More intense workouts provide more benefit, but the fact remains that any exercise is better than none. Once you and your family make the big decision to become more active, you can start small, and gradually work up to more active time as everyone starts to experience how good it feels to move around more.

We think that children should stick with free play until age five or six. After that age, you can start them in more structured community sports programs whenever their motor skills and cognitive skills are ready for the activity and the teamwork. This is very individual, so just because the neighbor's child is ready, don't assume yours is. As a parent, make sure the focus during the elementary school years is on learning basic skills (how to kick or hit a ball) and on fun, not competition. The fun part is important: 20 million kids start organized sports, but 6 million drop out by age thirteen. Those who drop out are often sports-loving kids with limited to moderate skills, who end up spending too much time on the bench or feel too much pressure from coaches and parents if the emphasis shifts from having fun to winning at any cost. Encourage kids who display an interest to continue to play school or league sports as they get older. Aside from keeping them fit for at least a season, these sports programs teach fair play and provide an opportunity for social interaction, the experience of teamwork, a chance for mentoring by a caring adult, a sense of belonging, and an identity ("I'm a runner"). If you're lucky, the kids will be too busy with sports to get into trouble, and the habit of exercise may carry over into adulthood.

We're strong supporters of team sports when started at the right age and with the right attitude, because sports were very important to both of us growing up. Dr. Russ played just about every sport (some more successfully than others) in pickup games, youth leagues, and school teams, and still plays in adult basketball and baseball leagues when he can. A shared love of baseball deepened his relationship with his family. In fact, don't get him started on the meaning of baseball to his family, or you're in for nine innings of stories about men and boys tossing a ball back and forth over the course of three generations (and a mom who can hammer a ball a country mile!). Dr. Stu was hockey-mad as a kid; he played street hockey, roller hockey, ice hockey, even improvised games of indoor hockey in his dad's store using a roll of tape as a puck. Give him a ball and a stick and he's still a happy man. Both of us (and our wives) participate in and support our kids in all their physical activities, knowing how much sports have meant to us.

# The Importance of Physical Education

Walk into any of the schools that feature the new PE, and you'll regret every minute you ever spent waiting in line to toss the ball in the basket during your own school years. These kids are all active, engaged, and having fun. The first-graders are in a huge circle stretched along the perimeter of a huge rainbow-colored parachute. They raise it together and in waves, lower it, dance under it and back out again, run clockwise and counterclockwise, laughing and gazing in delight at the billowing cloth. Later, older kids jump rope, Double Dutch, in a display of fancy footwork you can only dream of emulating, before moving on to juggling—an equally impressive show of hand-to-eye coordination. In other classes kids enjoy everything from folk dancing to traditional sports like basketball and soccer, but with a difference—everybody plays.

This is the kind of physical education we want for our kids. The tide is turning against programs that keep kids on the bench or waiting in line for half the period, that focus only on competitive team sports, that drill for outmoded physical fitness tests, that separate kids into the "cans" and "cannots," that seem more like boot camps than fun. The new PE encourages full-time movement in a variety of forms to meet current developmental needs and promote life-long physical activity. This change for the better is coming not a minute too soon. Despite Department of Health and Human Services Healthy People 2000 goals to increase the number of students getting PE daily and increase the amount of time they are actually active in those PE classes, only one state in the entire country—Illinois—requires daily PE. Very few states meet CDC and National Association for Sport and Physical Education recommendations for 150 minutes a week of PE for elementary students (30 minutes a day) and 225 minutes a week for middle-school students (45 minutes a day). As a result, only 50 percent of kids in first through fourth grades, and even fewer kids in fifth and sixth grade, get PE as often as three times a week. Just over a quarter of high-school students have PE every day, so even those kids who do develop the PE habit in grade school are left in the lurch as they get older.

PE is being squeezed out of the core curriculum by a number of factors: the belief that physical exercise is a "frill," a lack of financial resources in strapped school districts, and a lack of time as more and more required topics are added to the academic program. But parents need to speak up to school administrators and school boards about the value of PE. Clearly good PE classes encourage healthy behaviors that benefit our children now and save society health dollars in the future. PE helps protect our children from cardiovascular and other chronic disease, controls weight, teaches teamwork, improves sleep, builds self-esteem and feelings of competence, relieves stress, and passes on the idea of fair play. Physical education classes provide a safe place to exercise, an important issue in some areas where the parks and playgrounds may be unsafe for kids, and provide access to equipment and venues that families may otherwise not be able to afford. Daily PE even appears to help with academic learning.

We list some resources for parents in the back of the book, but parents should know how to evaluate their children's PE program. We are big fans of new PE, which puts the emphasis on personal fitness rather than competitive sports, with the goal of acquiring life-long skills and habits of exercise, so that will be our bias. In our opinion, there are ten things that a good PE program should do. It should:

1. occur daily for 30 minutes for grades 1 to 4 and 45 minutes for grades 5 and 6.

2. offer a variety of developmentally appropriate and enjoyable activities that spur the learning of fundamental motor and social skills.

3. focus on cardiovascular fitness, flexibility, agility, and muscle strength rather than on specific sports.

4. keep students moving for most of the class period. Provide a warm-up before class and cool-down at the end.

5. focus on cooperative rather than competitive games (no losers).

6. teach skills and activities that foster life-long fitness.

7. include different types of activities over a period of time so kids with different abilities and interests all get a chance to shine.

8. partner with parents. Teachers may send home a quarterly newsletter or periodic individual reports that highlight a student's weak areas and suggest family activities to address them. Some PE teachers hold parent fitness nights at the school as well.

9. promote healthy nutritional and exercise behaviors outside of class. The teacher should make sure that the students are adequately hydrated during class, too.

10. be fun. Are the kids and teacher smiling?

In addition to organized physical education classes, elementary school kids need breaks for movement during the school day. The precious 15 to 20 minutes of running-around time morning and afternoon that we call recess is the only thing that makes sitting in class all day bearable for many kids. Yet, responding to a push for stronger academics, schools across the country are eliminating recess. Atlanta, Georgia, abolished recess in all its classrooms a decade ago, and in fact new schools built there do not even have playgrounds. We can't understand why parents aren't up in arms about it. Adult workers get coffee breaks—even the Marines get hourly breaks in their training—so why should we expect our children to do without a refreshing break?

We think eliminating recess is a disturbing trend that undercuts public-health campaigns promoting activity and flies in the face of all the developmental research on the importance of play to learning. As integrative doctors, we look at education integratively as well. We think it is important to educate not just the mind with academics, but also the body with PE and recess and the soul with the arts. Exercising the body and the soul may enhance the work of the mind, as well. There is some evidence that recess helps kids burn off excess energy, increases alertness, stimulates brain development, exercises their imaginations, and improves their socialization skills. In fact, we also see a possible connection between the loss of opportunities for activity in the school day and the increasing use of medications for problems of inattention.

If your children's elementary schools are cutting back on recess, we urge you to work with teachers and school administrators to bring it back. Maybe parents can volunteer to help oversee playgrounds during these breaks. We include some recess-preservation resources at the back of the book.

# What Parents Can Do to Keep Their Kids Active

- *Add more activity to your own day.* Children admire and want to emulate their parents. What lessons do you want to teach them?

- *Make some family time active time.* Why not take a regular walk together after dinner, play a game of catch after work, or bike together on the weekend? You'll help your kids, and yourself too—15 minutes of active play 7 days a week can help mommy or daddy lose 7 pounds in a year.

- *Limit TV/ VCR/ computer time.* The American Academy of Pediatrics suggests none for kids under two, and no more than 1 or 2 hours a day for older children. We would go further, and advise just 30 to 60 minutes of free-time screen time on a weekday. If your kids are before the screen for longer than that, insist that they get up every half hour (set a timer) and move around for 5 minutes or so.

- *Toss away the remote controls.* Make them walk over to change the channels.

- *Discover what kinds of physical activities your kids enjoy.* Kids who are forced into sports or activities they don't like may be turned off exercise for life.

- *Encourage children to walk more.* If safety is an issue, walk with them. You'll get both a little exercise and a little extra time together.

- *Ask your kids what they do in PE class.* If it doesn't sound like enough, observe a class. Do they look like they're having fun? Are they all in motion at least half the time? If necessary, lobby with teachers, principals, and your school board for a better program.

- *Make sure your kids stay hydrated when they exercise.* Thanks to sports bottles, drinking water throughout the day can become as automatic a habit for your children as clicking on their seat belts.

- *Teach kids some of the simple outdoor games you used to play.* Red Rover, Capture the Flag, Duck Duck Goose, Simon Says, Running Bases, and Sardines are fun for all ages.

- *Assign your children chores that keep them moving.* Dusting, vacuuming, weeding, and taking out the compost or the garbage all count as exercise.

- *Share an interest in your children's sports activities.* Attend games as often as you can, practice with them, offer positive feedback, and make sure that the experience remains fun and not a source of stress for your child.

- *Avoid labeling your children as "athletic" or "unathletic"* at too early an age. Many kids considered "unathletic" at age eight or nine do quite well in sports later. Concentrate on making sure they are fit and happy, because a foundation of fitness will allow late-bloomers to reach their peak potential.

- *Get involved in community efforts* to increase the number of parks, playgrounds, recreation centers, and playing fields available for the children in your town or neighborhood.

- *Think of the long term.* Commit yourself to keeping your children fit to protect them from adult problems like osteoporosis, diabetes, and atherosclerosis that have their roots in childhood.

# Chapter 7

# Just Sit There:

## *The Importance of Rest and Relaxation*

ah, the bliss of a stolen afternoon at the ball game, an evening laughing with friends, a walk along the beach, or even twenty minutes of peace and quiet in the shower, enjoying the hot water on tight end-of-the-day muscles. These moments of relaxation are essential for our physical and emotional well-being, no matter how fulfilling our lives. Taking time to play or rest nourishes the soul and helps us cope with the stresses and strains of daily living.

Right about now you're probably thinking, "Relax? *Relax?* I'm too busy to relax." You're juggling jobs, chores, and parenting duties while trying to maintain all the personal relationships that are important to you. If you're a single parent, you are *beyond* busy. There aren't enough hours in the day to do all that has to get done, and we're asking you to take time off to do . . . nothing?

Yes, that's exactly what we're doing, and we're doing it in the full knowledge that we do not always practice what we preach. We do try hard to make room for the things that sustain us—prayer, meditation, family fun, keeping a journal, spending time amidst the beauties of nature—despite the fact that we are doctors and card-carrying members of a society that values busyness. When we don't make room for this kind of nourishment, our kids do it for us. If they think he needs to rest, Dr. Russ's young son and daughter pull him over to a chair and cover him with their precious blankies. Dr. Stu's kids lure him outdoors for a fast game of hoops when he's been working too hard. Our co-author Lynn's son notes her posture when he passes her desk and stops to massage her shoulders if they look tight. Sometimes we are not even aware of the tension we're carrying until our kids reflect it back to us.

Even though this is a book about your children's health, we are going to take a moment to focus on their parents first, because we cannot tell you how to protect your children from the physical effects of stress without addressing the role of stress in your own lives. Like obesity, anxiety is often a family affair. Our kids absorb a lot of anxiety from us. Although we like to think that we are protecting them from our adult worries, they do sense tension in us and can respond with anxiety of their own. Once you recognize the two-way flow of anxiety, anger, and other stress-related emotions between parents and kids, you can start to modify your responses and make the whole family healthier. For instance, learning how to control your anger (a big risk factor for heart attack in adults) not only improves your own health, but offers a healthier model for your children as well.

Although we believe that raising healthy children is the most fulfilling role of our lives, many of us hide a guilty secret: There are days we fantasize about a child-free vacation in a South Pacific paradise where there are no last-minute class projects, no picky eaters, and no carpooling minivans. We should not be afraid to admit that parenting can be very stressful. Parents have heavy obligations, no time for themselves, and not enough hours in the day to satisfy everyone. They are sleep-deprived and always on call. As the enforcer of unpopular decisions, they may get no respect. They postpone their own needs and desires to insure that they are present for their kids, and they often feel inadequate as they juggle their responsibilities and try to do everything as well as they did before they had kids.

Every parent feels stressed at some time or another, especially stay-at-home moms and dads. We encourage parents to talk freely about the pressures and follies of raising children, and feel strongly that they should be able to do so without fear of being labeled a bad parent. When it seems appropriate, we may suggest parent support groups, parenting classes, or family therapy to deal with deeper or more ongoing issues. The message here is: Don't be afraid to talk about stress and ask for help when you need it.

We are more than willing to admit that our own lives are filled with stresses, and there are times when we feel overwhelmed. Yet we choose to be caring fathers and mothers anyway, knowing (or hoping!) that the tremendous rewards of raising children will balance out the daily irritations and occasional nasty shocks. We know that we will face not only "good" stresses brought about by change and accomplishment, but also "bad" stresses like pain, grief, anxiety, and frustration. Since we cannot eliminate all sources of distress from our lives, we must develop coping skills that allow us to change the way we react to stress so that we can be patient and supportive parents and partners.

If you are always tired, snappish, and overwhelmed by your responsibilities, eventually your body will pay the price. As integrative doctors, we know that mind and spirit have incredible effects on the body—for good or ill. Just as physical problems can affect your mental state, your thoughts and emotions can affect the workings of your body. (See chapter 10 for a fuller discussion of mind/body medicine.) In our experience, stress is too often ignored as a contributing factor to illness. This is partly because of the negative connotations of the term "stress-related illness." Most people hear the phrase and think, "The doctor is telling me it's not a real illness, that it's all in my head. Everyone will think I'm weak or faking it if I don't have a physical reason for all this pain." People are so unwilling to accept the fact that stressful situations may be affecting their children's health (or their own) that they will push for more tests and more advanced medications rather than look more closely at their own lives. They would rather start down the slippery slope of invasive procedures and pharmaceutical side effects than admit that stress may be at least partially to blame for ill health. We have had parents stalk angrily out of the office at the suggestion that something in a child's home or school environment may be creating or worsening a physical problem. This is a shame, because it is far more effective to treat the root cause of a chronic illness than its symptoms, far kinder to try the gentler approaches before the more invasive ones, and far less expensive to try to deal with possible factors like stress before diving into a sea of diagnostic testing. Parental insistence on "medicalizing" what may be a stress-related response reinforces the child's role as a sick person, and makes it that much harder to uncover and deal with the emotional issues triggering the problem.

Here's an example. Dr. Russ helped care for a young boy with juvenile rheumatoid arthritis whose mother was excessively concerned about every detail of her son's health. Her anxiety and constant attention to his illness created a corresponding anxiety in her son that expressed itself in flare-ups of joint pain. At first she did not appreciate hearing that her own emotional state was affecting the course of her son's illness, but eventually she came to agree that her boy had less pain and moved more easily when she relaxed and gave him space to just be a kid.

Let's face facts: Everyone has stress; it's how you deal with it that matters. Admitting to stress is not a sign of weakness or personal failure. Denying stress does not make it go away. We have to learn how to recognize stress in ourselves and how to defuse it before it does damage. When stress is chronic, or when it is not well managed, we suffer from side effects, such as neck and back pain, digestive problems, and headaches. One theory is that our subconscious mind resorts to provoking physical discomfort to get our attention when we repress unwelcome emotions. These pains are a signal that we need to take the time to deal with an issue we are trying to ignore. Our culture doesn't allow us time off, though, unless we are "sick," so a pain in the back or the neck provides a legitimate excuse to slow down. We like this theory because we have seen for ourselves how often muscular or stomach pains disappear once their real causes are understood and addressed.

Although stress is generally emotional, it has well-understood physical effects on the body. When you are stressed or overstimulated your heart beats faster, your muscles tighten, you become more alert, maybe your palms get sweaty. These are all responses that for millennia kept us alive by preparing us to either go on the attack or run for cover when our safety was threatened. These instinctive reactions, commonly called the "fight-or-flight" response, are triggered by the release of chemicals from the adrenal gland—adrenaline (epinephrine) and cortisol together dilate the blood vessels to increase pumping capacity, move blood from the intestines and toward the muscles to prepare for action, and pour glucose and fats into the bloodstream for fuel. The fight-or-flight response is meant to last just long enough to deal with the situation at hand. After that the body is supposed to return to its normal state.

Unfortunately, the fight-or-flight response is called upon so much more often in our fast-paced modern world that some people are in a near-constant state of overstimulation and physiological stress. Over time, this chronic stress takes its toll, and the physical strategies meant to be protective become destructive instead. The elevated blood pressure caused by adrenaline ultimately damages the blood vessels. Sustained exposure of the blood vessels to excess sugar and of the brain to high levels of cortisol predispose toward cardiovascular disease, diabetes, and some dementias.

Study after study has documented the effects of stress. Caregivers, exam-taking students, and other people in stressful situations have been found to have a reduced immune response that makes them slower to heal and more vulnerable to colds and flu. They are more likely to suffer digestive disorders, as the bowel is exquisitely sensitive to psychological stressors. In adults, stress contributes to cardiovascular disease, hypertension, obesity, eating disorders, infertility, erectile dysfunction, and a host of other disorders. We see many adolescents whose immunity is lowered by the pressure of academic demands; they show up with recurrent infections of all varieties, especially during the dark months of winter. In children, stress is associated with a wide range of problems, including frequent colds, diarrhea, bed-wetting, abdominal pain, cough, headaches, motor tics, and asthma attacks. Children are especially vulnerable to the effects of long-term exposure to stress hormones, which can slow down growth, brain development, and sexual maturation.

It's not just the acute crises in life—illness, death of a loved one, divorce, moving—that cause trouble. The cumulative effect of the little stresses of daily life—the reactivity to all of life's petty frustrations from losing a toy to a misunderstanding with a friend—can create physical distress too.

# The Relaxation Response

In the 1960s a Harvard researcher named Dr. Herbert Benson started talking about something called the "relaxation response," the cascade of physiological activity that returns the body to a normal state after the need for hyperalertness has passed. The relaxation response counters the fight-or-flight response point for point—decreasing heart rate, blood pressure, and muscular tension and producing a feeling of deep relaxation. In his research on the effects of meditation, Benson discovered that people could indeed be taught how to reduce their own response to stress. In the years since, Benson and other scientists have shown that many physical

---

## Mini-*Relaxation Exercises*

Practice these exercises with your children and encourage them to do them on their own when needed. Brainstorm times when a "mini" may come in handy.

1. *Atten-SHUN!* Close your eyes and focus your attention on your breathing. Is it fast? Slow? Ragged? Strained? Try to make it as slow and regular and relaxed and easy as you can.
2. *Backwards Count.* Close your eyes and exhale. As you inhale, say the number 2 to yourself; as you exhale, say the number 1. Continue slowly and evenly, focusing your attention on the flow of air through your nose or mouth and your counting.
3. *Hamster Twitch.* Take three quick breaths through your nose. (You'll look like a cute twitchy-nosed hamster when you do.) Then exhale through your open mouth with a *whoosh*.

symptoms can be minimized or resolved by regular practice of the relaxation response. Benson's Mind/Body Medical Institute at Harvard even offers training in stress reduction to educators so that both teachers and students can use these techniques in (and outside of) the classroom. Their studies show that such training facilitates learning, improves grades, reduces tardiness and absenteeism, increases self-esteem, and reduces aggressive behavior.

There are many ways to evoke the relaxation response, among them meditation or prayer, breath work, biofeedback, hypnosis, guided imagery, and progressive muscle relaxation. We'll discuss the specifics of these relaxation techniques in the chapter on mind/body medicine, but the box on page 188 lists a few quickies that can be used anytime and any place.

## Children and Stress

You may not believe that children can suffer from stress, but it's true. In addition to the stress in their own lives—standing at the free-throw line in a close game, taking an exam, having to give an oral report, losing a favorite doll, trying to win friends, dealing with divorce—our kids also absorb anxiety from us. We like to think they are unaware of the big issues we are dealing with—problems in our marriage, financial tension, job insecurity, substance abuse—but they sense it all, and are sometimes more stressed because they do not have the experience or the full information to quiet their fears. If you've ever doubted that parents transfer their stress to their children, just work in a doctor's office for a week. An irritable infant, for example, often has parents who are either very stressed out or have unresolved fears of doctors or doctors' offices. We've learned from experience that nothing will soothe an anxious child until the parents' worries are addressed and the big folks relax. We have actually seen children with inflammatory bowel disease suffer less pain and fewer bouts of diarrhea after their *parents* have been taught breathing exercises and other stress-reduction techniques.

In some ways our children are more stressed than recent generations. They are exposed to more violence and sexuality, spend less time with their parents, are overloaded with more information, live in a faster-paced world with less free time, are measured against standards of beauty that are difficult to achieve, have earlier sexual experiences, and are growing up in a more money-oriented society. Many fear for their personal safety. True, they don't have job, financial, parenting, or marriage worries, but they do have to deal with the same anxieties about living up to expectations that we all have. And many parents have set the bar high, pressuring their children to succeed in all things. Family therapists now see elementary school children with chronic stress-related headaches, stomachaches and free-floating anxiety from parental pressure to excel at school or sport.

A state of stress has become as normal to many children as it is to adults. The sources of stress and the way it is expressed may differ, but both adults and children should always be open to the possibility that stress is involved in medical and behavioral problems. Many primary-care providers believe that up to 70 percent of adults have stress-related disorders. We estimate that 30 to 40 percent of the sick children we see are there for conditions caused or worsened by stress.

How do you recognize the signs of stress in your child? Often you'll see the same signs you may recognize in yourself: nervousness, muscle tension, irritability, depression, fear, insomnia, headaches, and neck, back or abdominal pain. Children also have symptoms of their own. If your child is whiny, clingy, fearful, withdrawn, staggered by even minor change, or hyperactive, he may be stressed. If he is suddenly stuttering, wetting the bed, sucking his thumb, acting out, or changing his eating habits, he may be stressed. If he suffers from recurrent colds or sinus infections—signs of a depressed immune system—he may be stressed. Children tend to internalize stress to protect their parents. We often say that the pediatrician's office is where parents trying to hide stress from their kids meet kids trying to hide stress from their parents. If doctor and parent are willing to consider the possibility that stress is a factor, a child's physical problem may become the spark that sets off parent-child discussion of issues previously unnoticed or repressed.

If no organic cause is found for a child's symptoms, do not assume that the symptoms themselves are not real. The pain your child feels from, say, a stress-related abdominal problem, is as real as that of

## Explaining Stress to Your Child

Once a child understands that his or her symptoms are an attempt to cope with stressful thoughts or events, she can begin to alleviate them. We start by explaining what stress is and how it differs from fear or excitement, which share some of the same physical signs. We ask, do you remember how you felt when you stepped up to the plate with the bases loaded or rode on a scary roller coaster, or sat down to a test in a subject you didn't quite get? Remember how your heart beat faster, your palms got all sweaty, your muscles got tight, or butterflies jumped around in your stomach? Remember how those feelings went away as soon as the ride or the test was over? Well, stress causes the same kinds of body symptoms when you're worried about something you can't talk about, or under a lot of pressure. It's like a message from your brain to your body, telling you that you need to slow down, relax, and get a handle on whatever is upsetting you. Once you figure out what the problem is, and start to deal with it, you can tell your body that you got the message, and it doesn't have to act sick anymore. Then it usually fixes itself.

In his practice Dr. Stu sees lots of thirteen-year-old boys with what he calls "pre–Bar Mitzvah syndrome." In the weeks and days before this important and stressful religious ceremony, many of them come to see him with headaches, abdominal pain, and acute infections. Many of these symptoms disappear once he explains the role of stress; all of them disappear after the ceremony.

appendicitis. The child is not faking the pain. Stress may be causing the pain or may be worsening the pain of an underlying physical condition, but the pain is still real, and the parents should treat it as such. If your child's doctor raises the possibility that stress may be a factor, be open to the suggestion. Some parents are unable to accept the idea that their child would sense and respond to stress in so physical a manner; others resist the mind/body approach because they think it implies their child has a mental problem. In fact these stress responses are quite normal and show an awareness of one's circumstances and environment. Simple acknowledgement by parents of the role of stress (theirs or his) in their child's health problem will go a long way toward expediting healing. Once the parents accept this diagnosis, parents and physician can help the child understand the symptoms are actually coping mechanisms and everyone can work together to discover the root of the problem.

The top three stress-related conditions we see are abdominal pain, headache, and cough. Many parents are quite familiar with "school-day tummy," but few realize that chronic cough can have an emotional component as well. Take, for example, Marina, whose parents were unwilling to accept Dr. Stu's diagnosis that her intractable cough was stress-related. They took Marina to a specialist who put her in the hospital for a week of tests—a series of chest X rays, an invasive throat probe, blood tests, sputum cultures for various organisms, a bronchoscopy, an allergy consult, and an ear, nose, and throat evaluation. All tests were negative, but Marina was still wracked by coughing spasms. Now her parents were willing to entertain the idea that some other factor might be at work. They brought her home (against the pulmonologist's orders) and began to talk as a family about issues that might be concerning Marina. Within a week Marina's cough was gone and she was back at school.

If you suspect your child is stressed, there are several things you can do. First, examine the stresses in your own life and consider how they might be affecting your child; take steps to bring your own stress under control. Then, talk to your child in an open-ended way about things that might be bothering her. Explain what stress is (see box on page 121), and help her identify any stress reactions she may be having. Brainstorm ways to relieve his stress. Teach him coping skills or relaxation techniques to use in stressful situations (see chapter 10). If physical symptoms persist, make an appointment with his pediatrician or family practitioner to discuss them. Be wary if your child's doctor suggests psychotropic drugs. In fact, unless your child has a developmental disability, *don't do it*. In the interest of convenience, many doctors and parents appear more willing to use drugs than get to the emotional root of the problem. Both hyperactivity and depression can be symptoms of stress in children. We are frankly appalled that, according to a recent study in the *Journal of the American Medical Association*, prescriptions for hyperactivity medications such as Ritalin increased threefold in children under five between 1993 and 1997, and the use of antidepressants in these preschoolers doubled. Apparently 3,000 prescriptions for Prozac were written for children under the age of *one* in 1994 alone. Keep in mind that we do not even know yet if these drugs are safe and effective in children, nor do we have any idea of the long-term effects of regulating chemicals in the developing brain. We strongly urge you to not to jump into medicalizing what may well be a stress-related problem.

# What Parents Can Do to Manage Family Stress

We understand that it is not easy to find time or space to relax. In fact, we appreciate how hard it might be even to find the time to read this book. So once again, our advice is just to try to do what you can. Knowing that there are steps you can take to relieve stress, and knowing when to take them, is a good first step. Trying to make one stress-reducing change in your life is a good second one. We're betting that once you've learned the power of a mini-meditation, or a moment of prayer, or a vanilla-scented foot massage to modulate your reaction to stress, you'll be motivated to try a few more of these ideas. We hope

# The Restful Home

We all have busy lives, and the everyday world is not going to magically become less stressful. However, we think it is important that your home provide a sort of sanctuary from all the rush and pressure of the outside world in order to allow your family a chance to rest. Consider ways to make your family's time at home more relaxing. You might use colors in the house that make you feel happy or soothed; instead of all white walls, consider peach, soft blue, sage green, golden yellow.

Experiment with scents that you find relaxing. Lavender, sandalwood, lemon, rose, vanilla, and apple are usually considered sedative. Reduce the clutter in your house and you'll reduce both the frustration when you cannot find something and the wearing sense of continual disorder. Try silence or some soft music at certain times. Bring in more flowers, plants, or other signs of the natural world. If you live in a noisy place, think about buying a white-noise machine or a pleasantly gurgling indoor fountain. Set up one area—even if it's small—where family members can go for peace and quiet. Make it comfortable for reading or noodling around with arts or crafts. Remind your family of all the people who love them by displaying photos of grandparents, aunts, uncles, cousins, and special friends.

eventually you will come to realize that stress management is as important to health as exercise and good nutrition.

- *Learn a relaxation technique yourself and use it regularly* (see chapter 10). Teach one to your children as well, and explore with them the times it might be helpful for them.
- *Try to cut back on the demands on your time.* Practice saying "no" to more than you can handle. Put a family calendar of activities in

a prominent place, and make sure no one is overscheduled. You might consider limiting the number of activities each child does in the course of the school year, and have them choose their favorites.

- *Leave lots of space for free time.* We all need time to dream, to reflect on our day or our week, to improvise with a crayon or play a musical instrument.

- *Spend at least some small amount of time one-on-one with each child every day.* You can catch little worries before they become big stressors.

- *Sit down for family meals together as often as possible.* The entrée can be pizza, but take the time to light some candles and express your gratitude to set the tone. There is some research evidence that older children who eat frequently with their families are more motivated in school and less likely to be involved in risky behaviors as teens.

- *Unplug the phone during dinner* and other times you do not want to be interrupted. (Admittedly, this is harder to do if you don't have an answering machine.)

- *Limit the amount of time you and your children spend in front of a screen.* We suggest TV/video/computer time be limited to an hour a day. These forms of entertainment/ education are generally fast-paced and high-adrenaline, so avoid them close to bedtime. Be tough about the media that your children are allowed to see.

- *Establish relaxing rituals that are meaningful to you.* In some homes, prayer at certain times of the day reinforces the importance of other values and senses of time. In others, a stroll after dinner may do the trick. Relaxing bedtime rituals like reading aloud or reviewing the gifts of the day can help kids (and their parents!) unwind.

- *Take time for yourself.* It may be the 15 minutes you always spend decompressing in the shower as soon as you get home from work, or 30 minutes of do-not-disturb time you carve for yourself from another part of the day. This is not a luxury, but a necessity, for keeping your own stress levels under control and preventing your kids from picking up your anxiety or speediness.

- *Avoid caffeine.* Frankly we cannot understand why parents would even consider offering their children caffeine-laced soft drinks such as Pepsi, Coke, and Mountain Dew, but they do. Caffeine is an addictive drug that raises anxiety levels.
- *Teach everyone in the family how to massage* heads, hands, backs, shoulders, and feet. (See chapter 11 for more details.)
- *Plan ahead so you don't have to rush.* Try to slow the pace if everyone in the family seems to be speeding around unnecessarily.
- *Relax your standards.* Make human values your priority. Which is really more important: to scrub the windows or spend time listening to your kids, to find the perfect curtains or visit with a lonely neighbor?
- *Make sure everyone gets enough sleep*—yourself included.
- *Be mindful of your world.* There's beauty all around us, if we only look for it. Try doing just one thing at a time so you can give it your full, unstressed attention.
- *Teach your kids the body cues to monitor their own stress levels*, and simple tools to manage stress, such as breath work. (Turn to chapter 10 for more information.)
- *Give your children the emotional vocabulary to explain and understand their feelings.* Get the older ones journals where they can vent and explore these feelings.
- *Laugh more.* When the tension level in your family is mounting, do something to help blow off steam—a funny walk contest, a pillow fight, or a totally goofy movie. Your kids will have a good time and the child in you will get a chance to be silly for a while. We never outgrow our need for play.
- *Take a day off for pure relaxation.* Even if faith does not require you to set aside Sabbath time, you can experience the same refreshing time-out from the world by establishing the "one-in-seven rule" and dedicating one day a week to fun family activities.

# Chapter 8

# It's Not Only What They Breathe:

## Protecting Your Children from Environmental Hazards

When you hear the words "environmental hazard," do you think only of things like water pollution and pesticide exposure? If so, you are seeing only part of the picture. When we talk about environmental hazards, we don't just mean problems with the capital-E "Environment," but also risks to your children's safety in their immediate physical environment—the places where they live, play, and study. Your children's health may be affected not only by chemicals on the lawn or pesticides on the food, but also by the failure to use a seat belt or a bicycle helmet. Although we most often think about air or water pollution when we talk about environmental threats, failing to buckle up in the car may actually be an even greater threat to your child's life.

As integrative physicians, we are well aware of the positive and negative health effects of the various facets of a child's physical or social environment (more on the latter in the next chapter). We've seen children born with fetal-alcohol syndrome (FAS) and extremely-low-birth-weight babies born to heavy smokers. We've treated children with abdominal pains, seizures, learning disabilities, and mental retardation from exposure to lead. Children gassed by carbon monoxide from an inadequately vented heater. Children whose asthma gets worse every time the air pollution index is up. Children poisoned by household cleaning products and those struggling to breathe after chlorine has been spilled at the neighborhood pool. We've cared for a boy who was severely asthmatic in his native Russia, where he lived in a town with a huge rubber-processing plant, and who is perfectly healthy here; and a girl whose worsening asthma was painstakingly traced to the mold growing in a damp wall in her classroom.

We hope in this chapter to explain to you what we think are the greatest environmental threats to your children, and what you can do about them. We don't want to frighten you so you freeze like a bunny in your tracks, or overwhelm you so you throw up your hands in despair. We just want to give you the information and the tools to protect your kids—and yourselves—from the problems that hit closest to home for your own family. Our major areas of concern are the personal safety of children and the safety of the food they eat, the water they drink, and the air they breathe. We leave it to you to determine your own priorities among these issues and how best to act on them. Because we do not have the room to go into great depth on any of these topics, we are including a list of helpful organizations, books, and Web sites in the Resource section at the back of the book.

# Environmental Pollutants

You may be tempted to skip this section. After all, you want to know how to keep your kids healthy, not how to stop global warming. But unfortunately, the health of the environment has a lot to do with the health of the people who live in it. You can make sure your kids eat right and exercise, but if the water they drink is tainted with chemicals, or if the air they breathe is too high in ozone or full of toxic particles, your best efforts will be undermined. Your children are indeed what they eat—and what they breathe and drink, as well.

A great deal of environmental progress has been made since the first Earth Day teach-ins in 1970. So are we done yet? Unfortunately, no. Although many of our past environmental messes have been cleaned up, others linger, even fifty or sixty years later. DDT and other toxic chemicals banned years ago are still so pervasive that they can be found in the tissues of nearly every human on Earth. In addition to these old environmental insults, we are drowning in a sea of chemicals, combined in an endless number of ways in new products, which are allowed to be marketed even though the manufacturers have not done studies of their long-term effects, alone or in combination. These toxic substances so far have been linked to miscarriages, infertility, neurological disorders, developmental problems, cancers, birth defects, intellectual deficits, behavior disorders, and respiratory illness. So, yes, there's still work to do.

Our children are exposed to toxins and carcinogens daily, yet our society still places more value on economics—the right to sell chemical products of uncertain safety or the cost of cleaning up brain-damaging lead from old housing stock—than on our children's health. Consider the fact that fewer than 20 percent of the 70,000 synthetic chemicals registered with the Environmental Protection Agency (EPA) have been assessed for their potential to harm children—who are uniquely vulnerable to their effects—yet they can be marketed and used. Consider that we know that exposure to lead in old house paint severely impacts young children, yet we don't make lead-abatement a budget priority.

Why aren't we putting children first? If you think about it, it *is* surprising that our safety standards for nearly all environmental toxins are set for adults. After all, pound for pound, children take in more air, more food, and more water—and whatever contaminants they contain—than do adults. They have different (and sometimes weaker) mechanisms for getting rid of toxins, and absorb toxic elements (such as lead) at proportionately higher rates than do adults. Not only are they exposed to more toxins, but they are at greater risk of an adverse response to them, as well. Their little bodies are in a constant state of development in which major growth and maturation may be triggered by the very slightest hormonal or nutritional nudge. It is well known that toxic exposure has more long-lasting effects the earlier in life it is sustained, and that exposures during key periods of development are more likely to be irreversible.

Exposure to the environment begins even before a child meets the world first-hand. There is a growing body of evidence that toxic damage can occur before birth, and even before conception. That's why we recommend that all adults of childbearing age follow on-the-job safety procedures, and limit their exposure to toxic metals and chemicals as much as possible. Pregnant women should be especially careful of the new life developing within them. The fetus is exquisitely sensitive to chemical and toxic influences because its cells are dividing, differentiating, and growing so rapidly.

Alcohol and tobacco smoke—two common substances we do not normally think of as environmental pollutants—readily cross into the placenta to cause developmental and physical damage such as physical abnormalities, mental retardation, and learning and behavioral problems. Low levels of lead, mercury, or certain chemicals transmitted by the mother can also affect the future child's intellect and development. The brain is especially vulnerable in these early stages of development because the blood/brain barrier—the protective mechanism that restricts toxins in the blood from gaining access to the central nervous system—is not fully functional until six months after birth. There are also concerns, based on studies of wildlife, that hormonally active agents such as pesticides, dioxin, and polychlorinated biphenyls (PCBs) may cause reproductive, nervous, or immune system problems in developing children exposed to them. Several studies have found these chemicals, also known as HAAs, in the amniotic fluid of pregnant women. HAAs act as hormones, and so may interfere with the development of organ systems, which are normally triggered by very subtle variations in natural hormones at very specific times.

It is not clear how many of these pollutants are passed to an infant through mother's milk. The average woman's breast milk does usually contain the pesticides, dioxin, and PCBs that are so ubiquitous in the environment that they are considered "background" contamination. **Experts agree, however, that it is far better to breast-feed than not to breast-feed.** Human milk contains so many valuable compounds that breast-feeding still provides a net benefit (except in cases where the mother is on certain medications toxic to the infant or has a transmissible viral illness such as HIV).

Throughout their childhood, kids have greater exposure to environmental pollutants than adults in a number of ways. In addition to eating more food and drinking more water per pound of body weight than adults, they also eat *fewer* foods, increasing their exposure to the specific pesticides and other chemicals used on those crops. For instance, the average toddler eats 21 times the grape juice, 16 times the raisins, and 6 times the green beans of an adult (adjusted for body weight). They eat comparatively more dairy foods, which potentially exposes them to more recombinant bovine growth hormone (rBgH) as well. The average infant who drinks formula reconstituted in water takes in several times more water each day per body weight than a grown man, getting that much more exposure to possible contaminants such as lead, chlorine, nitrates, or pesticides that may be in the drinking water.

Children live closer to the ground, where they breathe in or absorb through their skin solvents and pesticides in carpets, lawn chemicals, and the many pollutants found in common household dust. They suck their thumbs, bite their nails, and put everything in their mouths, including old paint chips and other soil contaminants. They play outside more, where they can breathe particulates and ozone into developing lungs that take in more air (and more pollutants) per pound of body weight than adults' lungs.

A number of childhood diseases have increased dramatically over the past 20 years, and there are those who point the finger at environmental pollutants. Childhood asthma has risen 40 percent, learning and behavioral problems appear to be skyrocketing, and two of the most common childhood cancers (acute lymphoblastic leukemia and a form of brain cancer called glioma) are up 10 to 30 percent. According to data from the National Cancer Institute's Surveillance, Epidemiology and End Results (SEER) program, cancer rates in children from birth to age fourteen rose 1 percent a year from 1974 to 1991.

We believe that our children are at special risk from environmental pollutants, and we are not alone in this belief. Scientists doing research in this area invariably tell us of the scope of the problem and their frustration with their inability to rouse any public interest in it. Dr. Phillip Landrigan, head of the Center for Children's Health and the Environment at Mt. Sinai Hospital in New York City, expressed this same concern when he wrote in a recent article, "By default we are conducting a massive toxicological experiment in the United States, and our children are the experimental animals."

# Three Major Pollutants

We've arbitrarily divided the environmental pollutants that most concern us into three categories: heavy metals, solvents, and pesticides. We would like to explain a little about the dangers of each, how your child is exposed to them, and what you can do to reduce their exposure. We haven't room to touch upon any of these issues in great depth, so remember to check the Resources section at the back of the book for other sources of information.

The toxic heavy metal that concerns us most is **lead**. Although lead poisoning has decreased dramatically since the metal was eliminated from gasoline in the 1970s, it is still the number-one environmental hazard for children, affecting 1.7 million kids, or about 1 in every 25. How are our kids exposed? Mostly through dust, dirt, and water. In older neighborhoods and near heavily trafficked roads, lead from car exhaust and fine particles of pre-1978 lead-based house paint has been deposited in the soil over the years. Children are at greater risk of this form of exposure because they play close to the floor where lead tracked in from outside is more likely to accumulate, they chew on anything (even painted wood) at certain ages, and they are always putting their hands in their mouths. They may also ingest lead through drinking water that travels through old lead water pipes and faucets, and even from the fumes from candles with lead wicks. In the past, anti-lead campaigns have been aimed at protecting poor children in the dilapidated housing of inner cities, but middle-class parents remodeling older homes are now discovering to their shock that their children may be at risk as well. It was estimated in 1990 that more then 4 million children lived in lead-contaminated buildings.

The neurological consequences of lead poisoning can be great: lowered IQ, learning disabilities, hyperactivity, and aggressiveness. A two-to-three-point loss of IQ has been associated with every 10 micrograms per deciliter (mcg/dL) increase in blood lead level. We know that developing embryos are more likely to have poor developmental outcomes if their mothers have elevated levels of lead in their blood (often from lead stored in their bones since their own childhood and released into the blood during pregnancy). We also know that children—especially preschoolers—are at far greater risk of lead toxicity than adults because lead can interfere with the growth and development of their brains and nervous systems at a time when they are most vulnerable.

The optimal level for lead in the blood is zero. Although federal safe levels were originally established at 60 mcg/dL of blood, more recent research has caused the EPA to lower that level to 10 mcg/dL. It is not clear if damage occurs at even lower levels. There is also compelling evidence from Dr. Herbert Needleman of the University of Pittsburgh and other researchers that childhood lead exposure may be a major factor in the increase of attention disorders, antisocial behavior, and even juvenile violence. Needleman's prison studies have consistently shown significantly higher lead levels in juvenile and adult violent offenders than in noncriminals; a recent study found that lead levels in adult offenders were 1,300 percent higher than in nonincarcerated controls.

Reducing our children's exposure to lead will be an expensive undertaking that may require government subsidy, but it must be done or we risk losing too many fine minds. As a society we were willing to ban lead from gasoline; we must also be willing to clean up our toxic mess from the past to finish the job. In the meantime, we list a few steps parents can take to protect their own children below, and additional resources at the back of the book.

Protection from **mercury** exposure is also important. While we're not convinced that mercury-amalgam dental fillings raise a health risk, we are concerned about mercury pollution from other sources. Mercury compounds released into the air from coal-fired power plants and waste incinerators drift down to pollute soil and the water. Aside

# Protection Against Heavy Metals

• *If you live in an older home, check for the presence of lead in the paint or the soil around the house (see the resource section in the back of the book).* If lead levels are elevated, research and implement lead-abatement measures (sheet-rocking over painted surfaces, hauling away tainted soil) to seal or get rid of the lead. Move out during any remodeling, and have the house carefully cleaned after the work is done. Wipe down walls and other surfaces regularly with a damp cloth to remove lead-laced dust. Take off shoes before entering the house to reduce the amount of dust tracked in. Wash toys frequently, especially those that end up in your child's mouth.

• *Consider having your child's blood-lead levels checked.* Your child's doctor should perform a lead assessment once a year from ages one to six. We recommend having your child's blood tested for lead at about the age of ten months. If you suspect your house or soil might contain lead, follow up with another test later. If both tests are normal, you and your doctor can decide whether to continue with annual tests. Americans adopting children from abroad should realize that lead problems are much more widespread in other countries. We recommend that you test the blood-lead levels of adopted children, especially those from China, so that detoxification therapies (chelation) can begin as soon as possible if they are necessary.

• *Make sure your children eat foods rich in calcium and iron, as low levels of these minerals appear to speed the uptake of lead.* Pregnant women should be sure to get adequate levels of calcium (1,500 mg a day) so lead is not drawn from their bones into the blood supply they share with their fetuses.

• *Take precautions if your house has lead plumbing pipes.* Test your water for lead. There are inexpensive and easily available screening kits for this. If the pipes appear to be the problem, and they are accessible, replace them. Otherwise, get a water filter, or run the cold-water tap for a minute before using water for drinking or cooking. (Use the first minute's water on your plants.)

• *Dispose of thermometers, batteries, and all other sources of heavy metals properly as hazardous waste.*

• *Evaluate the need for a lead-abatement program in your area.* Work with neighbors and local officials to safeguard children.

• *Reduce intake of some forms of fish when you are pregnant.* Children and pregnant women who eat too much big ocean-going carnivorous fish—such as swordfish, tuna, or shark—or too many fish from local lakes and rivers may be exposed to high levels of mercury or other toxic metals. Check the state-by-state fish warnings listed at **www.epa.gov.** Consider varying the menu if your child demands tuna sandwiches frequently; the advocacy group Physicians for Social Responsibility estimates that one 7-ounce can of tuna a week provides nearly double the EPA "safe" dose of mercury (0.1 microgram per kilogram of body weight per day) for a 50-pound child.

• *Avoid thimerosol.* Tell your doctor or health department that you want your children to be immunized with vaccines free of the preservative thimerosol, which contains mercury.

• *Do not give your children patent remedies from China, India, or the Caribbean.* Some contain heavy doses of lead, mercury, and other toxic metals.

• *Be cautious with candles.* Some candle wicks use lead as a stiffener. When they burn, they may put enough lead into the air to exceed your child's safe daily lead intake. Look for candles that are guaranteed lead-free and don't overdo their use in tightly closed rooms.

from the immediate risk to neighbors of these plants, the greatest exposure may come through eating large predatory fish at the top of the food chain whose fat contains concentrations of the toxic metal from smaller fish they have eaten. Other potential sources of exposure: vaccines that contain the preservative thimerosol (currently being phased out), broken mercury thermometers, illegal dumps, and certain folk medicines and charms, especially from the Caribbean. Exposure to mercury compounds can lead to neurological deficits.

**Organic solvents** are the volatile compounds found in gasoline, dry-cleaned clothes, home-cleaning products, chlorinated water, plastics, carpets, plywood, and many other everyday products. Solvents are especially dangerous because they evaporate at room temperature and so are easily absorbed by inhalation, skin contact, or ingestion. Organic solvents (also called volatile organic compounds or VOCs) are often to blame for what is called "sick-building syndrome." Our children are exposed to VOCs at the gas station, at the dry-cleaners, and at home and school, especially when there is remodeling, redecorating, or new construction taking place. VOCs also show up in drinking water, especially in industrial areas.

Exposure by either parents or children to organic solvents has been linked to a number of health problems: infertility, miscarriage, birth defects, low birth-weight, and childhood cancers. For instance, studies show a connection between a father's occupational exposure to industrial solvents and brain tumors in his children. Women of childbearing age should protect themselves from exposure to similar occupational solvents. Exposure to perchlorethylene (PCE) and other solvents used in dry cleaning, for example, cannot only cause miscarriage in pregnant women, but they are also rapidly expressed in the breast milk of nursing mothers. Despite the dangers of these volatile compounds, the most worrisome organic solvent is still ethanol; drinking alcohol during pregnancy can cause serious lifetime defects in the resulting child.

Solvents like chlorine combine with organic materials in the environment to create a large family of hazardous chlorine by-products. Among them are dioxin (best known as a product of the paper-bleaching process) and other organochlorines, which are all hormonally active agents (HAAs). This means they have the ability to mimic or interfere with the normal actions of human hormones that determine how a body develops and functions. In wildlife, and in laboratory testing, hormonally active agents (sometimes called endocrine disruptors or environmental estrogens) have been associated with long-term effects on the nervous, endocrine, and reproductive systems. Among the effects: motor delays, behavioral problems, learning disabilities, cancer, breathing problems, decreased reproduction, gender abnormalities, and precocious puberty. It seems likely that HAAs such as dioxins, PCBs, and pesticides have their greatest effects on the developing fetus or the very young child, stages when the body is very sensitive to hormonal cues in developing the major body systems.

High levels of the chlorine compounds created in the process of disinfecting drinking water have been linked to a number of other health risks, including cancer. We are certainly not in favor of eliminating chlorination of water—it's essential to protect us from waterborne diseases such as cholera—but we do think you would be wise to filter out these compounds before using the water or let your drinking water sit overnight in the refrigerator to give the volatile compounds a chance to dissipate. Put a filter on the showerhead, too—a 10-minute shower provides more exposure (via skin and lungs) to chlorine by-products than you get from drinking *two quarts* of the same water. Pregnant women should be especially careful, as excessive exposure to chlorine by-products has been linked to a higher rate of stillbirths.

We use the term **"pesticides"** to mean all synthetic chemicals that kill insects, weeds, fungi, nematodes, and rodents. Pesticides concern us not just because trace residues permeate our foods but also because they contaminate the water we drink and the very soil we walk on. We already have a certain level of constant exposure to the most persistent of these chemicals, but we would like to protect our children from any additional exposure as much as possible. We are going to suggest a few simple actions you can take to do so. But first we'd like to explain the issues.

There is clear evidence that pesticides lower immune function, increase the risk of some cancers, and cause neurological and developmental problems in those with the most direct exposure to them. In agricultural areas, where exposure to pesticides begins before birth and

# Protection from Volatile Organic Compounds

● *Do not allow your children to pump gas for you.* We suggest using the automatic-fill lever and keeping everyone inside the car while the gas is pumping into your tank.

● *Let all dry-cleaned items hang outside or in the garage until they lose their chemical smell.* Excuse pregnant women from dry-cleaning pickup chores. Look for a cleaner who uses the new nonsolvent techniques.

● *Give new carpets and other remodeling materials that contain solvents time to "outgas" before moving your family back into the home.* Leave the windows open and turn on fans to speed the process.

● *Look for and learn how to use nontoxic citrus or vinegar-based cleaners in the home.* Limit your use of chemical cleaning products, disinfectants, and deodorizers.

● *Consider installing a filter on your faucets and showerheads to reduce exposure to chlorine by-products.*

● *Avoid painting while children are around.* Paints, especially spray paints, contain solvents to help them dry faster. Be cautious with other arts and crafts supplies used by your children, too, especially markers and airplane and instant glues, which should be used under supervision and in well-ventilated areas

● *Don't microwave foods in plastic wrap or plastic containers.* Hormonally active chemicals called phthalates (*tha-lates*) can migrate into your food.

● *Be careful about rubber duckies.* Buy children's bath toys, squeeze toys, and teethers that are labeled free of the phthalates DEHP and DINP, hormone-disrupting chemicals commonly used in the soft rubbery toys that kids love to chew.

● *Don't drink alcohol while pregnant.* As far as we're concerned, this is non-negotiable.

> • *Don't smoke tobacco in the house.* In addition to carbon monoxide, nicotine, and carcinogenic tars, cigarette smoke contains solvents like formaldehyde. Children who live with adults who smoke indoors have higher rates of respiratory illness, decreases in lung function, and heightened risk for smoking themselves.
> • *Don't buy produce from roadside stands alongside busy streets.* Fumes and toxic dust can contaminate the food.

continues through childhood, pesticides cause such neurodevelopmental problems as memory deficits, decreased stamina and motor ability, and slowed intellectual development. Drawings by children heavily exposed to pesticides are dramatically different from those made by children with less exposure; they look, in fact, much like the drawings of people with Parkinson's disease. (The latest research links garden-chemical exposure to Parkinson's in adults.) Although there is less research on the long-term effects of the lower doses of pesticides to which most of us are exposed, it's not a huge stretch of the imagination to think that agricultural chemicals designed to poison, destroy reproductive capacity, damage nervous systems, and disrupt endocrine systems of pests might affect humans adversely.

We are very concerned that allowable pesticide residue standards do not yet include enough protection for pregnant women and for children. In 1988 Congress charged the National Academy of Sciences with looking into the risks of pesticides to children. Their 1993 report concluded that we just didn't have the information we needed to assess the long-term effect of pesticide exposure on the developing reproductive, nervous, and immune systems of children, who were clearly more vulnerable for a number of reasons. They suggested various avenues for research and action, and, as a result, government agencies are now required to consider the special vulnerability of children while setting safe pesticide levels, consider all possible routes of exposure (and not just food), and take into account the possible synergistic behavior of exposure to multiple chemicals (as generally happens in the real world). This process is moving very, very slowly, although the EPA has recently banned two of the six most commonly used organophosphate pesticides (methyl parathion and chlorpyrifos) and phased out or restricted the use of two others (azinphos-methyl and diazinon) because of concerns about children's exposures.

**We don't want to scare you so much about pesticides that you cut back on the fruits, vegetables, and whole grains that your children need.** Produce contains a wide range of known and as-yet-unidentified compounds that are necessary for good health. Some of these compounds can even help balance out any potentially harmful effects from pesticide exposure. But we do urge you to consider making a few changes in your shopping and eating patterns to reduce your child's exposure. For instance, you can wash your produce, or buy certified organic produce when possible. According to food-industry statistics, 73 percent of supermarkets now offer organic foods. If yours doesn't, try educating your produce manager about the increased popularity (meaning sales) of these foods. If you can't afford to buy organic produce all the time (and most of us can't), decide whether you can grow some yourself, buy organic just for younger children who are still developing, or buy organic versions just of the foods your children eat most. Remember, children eat a lot more of some foods than adults do, and so have increased exposures to any contaminants on or in them. That's why we are more concerned about the high number of pesticides used (and left) on apples, for instance. The typical one- or two-year-old child drinks 30 times more apple juice, eats 13 times more applesauce, and eats 5 times more apples (relative to body weight) than the typical adult. Apples typically carry residues from seven to nine pesticides in or on them. If your children consume a lot of apples in one form or another, you might consider looking for organic apple products even if you cannot afford or find any other organic produce.

Just knowing which fruits and vegetables are the most likely to carry a heavy burden of pesticides is a good start. According to USDA and FDA measurements (taken after the produce is washed and prepared for consumption), pesticide residues are highest on apples, spinach, peaches, pears, strawberries, Chilean grapes, potatoes, red raspberries, celery, Mexican cantaloupe, and green beans. Some of these crops carry residues from six or seven different neurotoxic or carcinogenic agricultural chemicals. We don't even know what the effects of multiple exposures are, as federal agencies and manufacturers are not testing for this. On the bright side, other fruits and vegetables that have very low levels of pesticide residues can be substituted. The Environmental Working Group regularly publicizes a list of the "dirty dozen" and their "cleaner"alternatives (see Resources section for their Web site). The EWG says that such substitutions can halve your exposure to pesticides. A recent list of low-residue crops included corn, cauliflower, green peas, asparagus, broccoli, pineapple, domestic cantaloupe, kiwi, onions, bananas, watermelon, and Chilean cherries.

Our children are also exposed to pesticides through chemicals used at home, in school, and in parks. These are areas where parental involvement can make a huge difference. Recently Senator Joseph Leiberman (D-Conn) called for the EPA to start gathering information on pesticide use in schools. After all, he said, we have limits to pesticide exposures for adults at work, why are we not similarly concerned about the places where our children spend their days? Pesticides and herbicides are routinely used in many school districts to control insect and animal pests, maintain athletic fields, or beautify the landscape. In some cities and states, school officials are already required to use less toxic alternatives when available or to notify parents before use.

Then there's the home. The United States produces 5 to 6 billion pounds of pesticides per year. Three-quarters of it is exported, and much of the rest of it is used, as expected, by commercial agriculture. According to the EPA, about 71 million pounds of these insecticides, herbicides, and fungicides are used by families in their homes and yards. That means that parents can drastically reduce their children's exposure to pesticides (and the solvents that are also included as "inert" ingredients in many of these products) merely by cutting out home use. There have been a few studies linking the use of home pesticides to cancer and neurological disorders in children. Among the resources at the back of the book are several that will help you find

# Protection Against Pesticides

• *Have your drinking water tested for pesticides, solvents, and other chemicals, and filter it if necessary.* This is especially relevant if you live in an area that is currently or formerly agricultural. People in new subdivisions built in former fruit orchards, for example, have found high levels of agricultural chemicals in their soil and water. The EPA can tell you how to get your own well tested and how to get access to testing results for your local water company. Install a home water-filtration system if necessary. Be sure to filter the showerhead as well as the taps. Let water run for 30 to 60 seconds before using, and never use water from the hot-water tap for drinking or cooking.

• *Peel and/or wash your produce.* You cannot do much to avoid systemic pesticides that are taken up throughout the cells of a plant, but you can wash surface residues off your produce. Just put a drop or two of Palmolive or other liquid dish detergent in a big bowl or pot and swish fruit around, then rinse with fresh clean water.

• *Buy organic when you can.* Organic produce can be more expensive or hard to find. If you can only buy some items that are organic, focus on fruits and vegetables like apples and imported grapes that are generally high in trace residues, or on the kinds of produce your kids eat the most. Substitute "cleaner" crops for "dirtier" ones—for example, kale for spinach, domestic grapes for imported ones, or blueberries for strawberries.

• *Make sure your family eats a wide variety of produce.* This reduces their exposure to pesticides specific to certain foods.

• *Reduce your intake of saturated animal fat in meat or dairy products.* Animal fat is a storage place for dioxin, pesticides, and other pollutants. Consider buying pasteurized organic nonfat or low-fat milk to avoid exposure to pesticides, bovine growth hormone (rBgH), or antibiotics fed to the animals.

● *Dispose of all home and garden chemical pesticides and herbicides at your local hazardous-waste site.* Substitute nontoxic alternatives for bug and weed control. Consider lowering your standards—does every dandelion have to die? Seek out safer alternatives to chemical flea collars, flea bombs, and pet-care products as well. Look into the use of pesticides and other chemicals at day-care centers, schools, parks, playgrounds, and other places where your children spend time.

● *Avoid the use of pesticide-based shampoos for treatment of head lice.* We offer alternatives in chapter 23.

● *Leave your shoes at the door.* The dirt and dust on our shoes tracks in lead, pesticides, herbicides, and other toxins found in the soil.

safer substitutes for bug sprays, lawn chemicals, flea collars, head-lice shampoos, etc.

## Is Your Water Safe to Drink?

Since drinking water can contain any or all of the three classes of contaminants we've been discussing, we're making a special place to talk about it. The quality of drinking water varies dramatically from one community and region to another and from source to source. A typical contaminant in one place might be rare in another, and vice versa. For instance, an agricultural town dependent on groundwater from wells might have problems with nitrates from fertilizers, whereas a more industrial area might find solvents seeping into their drinking water source. Communities that rely on rivers or lakes might be more vulnerable to industrial pollution or biological contaminants like bacteria or viruses. Water that is alkaline, or "soft," might be more likely to leach heavy metals from older plumbing within the house.

Many public systems provide excellent drinking water. You can find out if your provider is one of them by checking the Consumer Confidence Report (CCR) it is required to file with the EPA on a regular basis (see Resources). If you have concerns about the possible presence of compounds not being tested for, you can check the water yourself through one of the laboratories recommended by the EPA. If you live in an older home, you might also want to check the water that comes out of your own taps to reassure yourself that it is not contaminated with lead. If you have doubts about the quality of the water, investigate and install a home water-filtration system.

Be aware that bottled water is not necessarily better than what comes out of your own faucet. Some of the four billion gallons a year sold in bottles is, in fact, just tap water that has been "polished" for better flavor. A 1999 study by the Natural Resources Defense Council of more than a thousand bottles of 103 brands of bottled water found that while most of it was of good quality, nearly a third violated some chemical or bacterial guideline in at least one sample.

# Think Globally, Act Locally

If you're feeling depressed about the enormity of our environmental problems, remind yourself how far we have come in environmental consciousness, education, and action in the past thirty years. Impassioned individuals and environmental groups like the Sierra Club, Environmental Defense, Mothers and Others for a Livable Planet, and The Nature Conservancy have helped make everyone more aware of the connection between environmental health and human health, and brought many important issues into the mainstream. At the time of the first Earth Day, recycling was considered an eccentric activity of long-haired hippies and frugal New Englanders. Thirty years later, some municipalities will fine you for *not* recycling, and school children are routinely taught the ecological facts of life. Thanks to federal legislation passed in the 1970s, DDT has been banned, lead has been removed from gasoline, the air over many of our cities is cleaner, and rivers that once were clogged with industrial waste run more clearly.

There is still a lot to do. Even if you have cleaned up your home or your neighborhood, there are still larger issues to be addressed. Foremost among them is the exposure of our poorest children to the greatest number of toxins; levels of lead, pesticides, solvents, mercury, particulates and other forms of air pollution are all worst in low-income neighborhoods. For instance, 27 percent of children in inner cities have elevated blood-lead levels, and only 2 percent of surburban children, a clear example of environmental injustice. We need to keep our eyes on the big picture and act both nationally and internationally. Pollution respects no boundaries, so by helping others, we help ourselves as well.

We consider environmental awareness to be a component of both integrative pediatrics and good parenting. Working for a cleaner environment affects not just our children's health today, but their health as adults, and the health of their children and grandchildren. We hope that all parents would try to protect their own children, and other children around the world as well, through whatever personal or political actions seem most suitable to their interests, time, and talents. Even the smallest steps help. For instance, the batteries you toss in the hazardous waste rather than the household trash now may prevent your grandchild's illness in the future. (Better yet, buy solar-rechargeable batteries.) The integrated pest-management program you help set up at your children's school to help reduce or eliminate the use of pesticides and herbicides may protect hundreds of kids now. The local campaign for lead abatement you devote some weekends to may allow generations of kids to reach their full intellectual potential.

# Physical Hazards in Your Child's Environment

The environmental threats to your children's safety don't all come with polysyllabic chemical names. Some of them can be understood simply by imagining yourself an inexperienced, physically weak, low-to-the-ground being who is intensely curious about the world. Taking on that attitude as you stroll (or better yet, crawl) through the house will help you spot the unsafe things that can be opened, yanked on, pulled over, climbed up, fallen on, and otherwise interacted with by a youngster. If you maintain that attitude as you move around the yard or through the neighborhood, you'll see the greater risks they face because of their innocence, curiosity, or smaller size and strength.

We've both seen the tragedies that come from ignorance or denial of simple safeguards. Here are twelve tips to raise your awareness about the greatest hazards in your children's physical environment.

1. *Assess your child's exposure to violence.* Work with parents and teachers at your children's school to include the teaching of conflict-resolution and anger-management skills. Work with the neighbors and the police to create a safer neighborhood environment. Be vigilant about who spends time with your child; abuse by family, friends, and caretakers is a major cause of physical and emotional trauma for children. The presence of firearms is an environmental hazard that might be peculiar to the American home; twelve times more American kids under fifteen years of age die from firearms than do kids in twenty-five other industrialized countries. More than 8 million children live in homes with at least one unlocked gun, which creates a risk not only of accidental shooting but also of suicide (60 percent of adolescents who commit suicide do so with a gun). Any firearms in a home with children should have trigger guards and be locked away unloaded, with the ammunition in a separate locked location.

2. *Make sure your child is buckled up in the car.* Even a moderate-speed crash can turn untethered children into projectiles. If you insist on proper protection in the car, buckling up will become an unconscious habit. Infants and children up to four years of age should always be in approved car seats in the back seat. Children up to 4'9" and 80 pounds need to use approved booster seats with their seat belts. Young children

using adult seat belts alone are four times more likely to suffer head, brain, and abdominal injuries in a crash than those using car seats or booster seats designed for them. Make sure you put them in the back seat away from airbags, and install seats properly. Drive carefully, and do not drive while impaired.

3. *Buy your children bicycle helmets and insist that they wear them.* The new helmets are so cool looking, your kids may not even complain. Helmets should be buckled securely and worn so they protect the forehead. We've seen kids die in bike accidents, so as far as we're concerned, you're a neglectful parent if you allow your child to ride without a helmet. You should wear your own, as well, and don't forget to teach your kids the basics of bike safety.

4. *Avoid accidental poisonings.* Keep all toxic or caustic chemicals locked up, and that includes beauty aids like hair relaxers. Switch to nontoxic products when possible. Keep supplements (even kiddy vitamins) and medications where children cannot ever reach them. Avoid poisonous houseplants until the kids have stopped putting things in their mouths. Always keep the 800 number for poison control by the phone.

5. *Drown-proof your kids as soon as possible.* Teach them how to stay afloat and then how to swim. If you have a pool, restrict access to it with a gate that locks. Put floatation devices on everyone on a boat. Always supervise young children in the bath; a child can drown in just a few inches of water. Carry a cordless phone with you to the pool or the bathtub, so you won't be tempted to leave a child alone in the water if the phone rings.

6. *Make sleep safe, too.* Lay your child on her back ("back to sleep") on a firm crib mattress—no soft mattresses, sofa beds, or water beds. (Let her be on her belly when awake to help strengthen neck muscles and keep her head shaped properly.) Use only breathable blankets, rather than pillows or heavy quilts and blankets that can suffocate.

7. *Protect your child from fires.* Lock up matches. Keep fresh batteries in all smoke detectors, and install a carbon monoxide detector as well if you have a gas heater or appliances. Label

your child's bedroom window with a special window decal that alerts firefighters to a child's potential presence. Practice fire drills as a family so everyone knows how to exit the house safely.

8. *Kid-proof garage doors.* Either reduce pressure levels on old-style automatic doors so a child cannot be injured seriously if trapped beneath them, or install doors with electric eyes that halt the descent of the door when anyone breaks the beam of light.

9. *Do a safety survey of your home, looking at it from kid level.* Are there electrical or venetian-blind cords hanging, heavy potted plants or ornaments that can be tipped onto little heads, drawers or cupboards that do not lock? Are pot handles hanging out over the stove where kids can reach them? Have you locked up prescription and over-the-counter medications (including vitamins) or stored them beyond the reach of even the most daring kids? Is the hot-water heater set below 120 degrees to prevent burns?

10. *Don't buy a child a toy that is not safe for her or his age.* Watch out for foreign toys that may not meet U.S. safety standards.

11. *Use sunscreen on any child over six months of age* to protect them from burns now or skin cancers late in life. (Keep younger ones out of the sun except for short periods.) Apply about a shot glass of SPF 15 to 24 sunscreen containing zinc oxide or Parsol 1789 to a child 15 to 30 minutes before exposure, and every two hours thereafter. Remember that sunscreen does not provide unlimited protection. Even with sunscreen on, children should wear hats, sunglasses, and other physical protection, especially between the hours of brightest sunshine from 10 A.M. to 2 P.M. Remember that 80 percent of lifetime sun damage occurs before the age of eighteen—you don't want your kids to blame you for every wrinkle when they're middle-aged!

12. *Check out playgrounds and playing fields for safety.* More than 200,000 preschool and elementary students have to go to the

ER every year for accidents sustained at playgrounds, and 36 percent of their injuries are serious ones. Avoid concrete, and look for more forgiving surfaces like sand, bark, or the new rubberized asphalts. Make sure your children know how to use all the equipment safely, and that they are supervised at all times.

# Aliens Are Brainwashing My Kids!:

## Protecting Your Child from Unhealthy Aspects of the Culture

b *efore you start this chapter, we'd like you to turn to the authors'*
*photos on the book jacket. As you can see, we're fairly young guys.*
*Hold this picture in your mind as you read this chapter so you*
*don't dismiss us as a couple of cranky old fogies unable to accept change. We are*
*just fathers and doctors deeply committed to protecting the minds, bodies, and*
*spirits of vulnerable children from harm.*

We move through a sea of cultural attitudes and directives throughout our day: "You deserve a break today," "Look out for Number One," "Never trust a man (or a woman)," "Coke is it." We are rarely even conscious of them, yet these cultural messages form our character, influence our physical and mental health, motivate our actions, and contribute to our hopes and dreams. They have an even greater effect on our kids, who are more vulnerable to psychological manipulation. To adults much of this is just background noise—a sort of social static—but children have fewer defenses.

We are very concerned about the messages that American popular culture gives our children. As integrative practitioners, we believe some of these cultural influences threaten the health of our youth, and we feel that it is important for doctors who care for children to speak out on this public-health issue. For instance, the glorification of violence even in media aimed specifically at children has the end result of desensitizing many young people to the effects of violent behavior. (The preschool Dr. Russ's children attend had to finally ban Pokémon games because too many children were being injured in imitative play.) The restaurant industry's suggestions that we "super-size" our meals contributes to both the obesity and the malnutrition of our children. Dolls with unattainable dimensions (think Barbie) and ubiquitous advertising that features waifish models make girls more susceptible to eating disorders. Similarly, unnaturally pumped-up action figures and buff male models put pressure on older boys to use steroids to achieve an idealized "manliness." And most of all, there is the stress of noise and overstimulation, of the pace of life and the pressure to be perfect.

Cultural messages—either blatant or subtle—strongly affect the physical, mental, and spiritual health of our children and our society. Parents, doctors, and other advocates for children need to act together to protect our children from the cultural pressure to think or act in unhealthy ways. We counter this "mental pollution" in our patients and our own children by trying to instill healthier messages about themselves, their families, their communities, and their world. It takes firmness and commitment, but we believe there are lots of ways that parents can ensure that *they* are the ones who have the major impact on their children's values and attitudes, not the mass media or the ubiquitous "everyone" (as in "Everyone says . . . ," "Everyone else has . . . ," and "Everyone else gets to . . .").

Mass media is a fairly new phenomenon. Our grandparents got most of their news and information from print sources such as books, newspapers, and magazines, and eventually from the radio. Many of these sources were local or regional, so the messages, products, and perspectives offered in them differed depending on whether you lived in, say, Massachusetts or Mississippi. It is only with the advent of television and corporate news empires that a more national popular culture has taken shape. Now we all read the same news, see the same shows, hear the same advertising, and shop in the same stores. Nearly every aspect of our lives has been commercialized and milked for profit. This commercialization has led to a skewing of values, so that in many cases the messages that bombard our children contradict the important values we are trying to pass on to them.

There's no doubt that our kids are barraged with media images. The average child sees an estimated 360,000 television advertisements before graduating from high school—and that doesn't even count all the ads from the radio, the Internet, magazines, billboards, materials used in school, and even the logos plastered all over professional athletes. Children watch hours of television every day, much of it of poor quality or not intended for them. As they get older they are influenced as well by the Internet, by radio shows and by popular music. How much does the trash-talking that comprises much of our public discourse today influence the way they think and act? How do kids make sense of all this information and manipulation? We think it's the role of parents to protect very young children from exposure to unhealthy messages and to teach older children how to analyze and understand the images beamed at them. (We list several good resources for teaching media literacy at the back of the book.)

The first fact of life we have to accept is that the messages sent by the mass media are generally motivated by profit rather than a concern for what's best for our children. That's not evil—it's just the way it is. Our kids are a very desirable market, because all their income is disposable. Few parents realize the strength of this buying power. American children twelve and under spent nearly $28 billion dollars of their own allowances and earnings in 1999, and they influenced nearly $249 billion of their parent's purchases as well. So we have a dangerous combination here—kids with spending money who may not yet have developed the ability to discern fact from fiction. Many kids under the age of eight are developmentally unable to tell the ads from the TV shows, and cannot grasp the concept that what they see in an advertisement may not be literally true. They don't have the tools to screen out the hyperbole and exaggeration that adults pretty much expect and ignore. Advertisers count on this developmental weakness and create materials to take advantage of it. In addition, kids see plenty of media messages supposedly aimed at adults; for instance, it's been estimated that 90 percent of the time children are watching TV they are looking at shows not intended for children.

The second fact of life is that images transmitted in the media have changed since we were children. There is certainly far more violence, sexuality, drug use, and bad language and attitudes in even PG-rated movies than there used to be, and TV shows and computer/video games have also ratcheted up the adult content in programs aimed at children and families. For instance, air time for war cartoons increased almost thirty-fold from 1982 to 1986, and the number of violent acts per hour just in children's shows jumped almost 40 percent in the 1980s. That's why it's so important to be familiar with the TV shows, songs, magazines, video games, and Internet sites to which your child is exposed. If you had assumed that the material on these media is what it was twenty or thirty years ago, when you were a kid, you'll be surprised by what you find. Dr. Stu, for instance, was flabbergasted to see a singer who spends a lot of time in the courts on charges of violent behavior featured on a children's holiday concert on TV. Yet Nickelodeon apparently thought the singer was a good role model for kids. Even professional sports has changed, becoming more aggressive and more commercial and, in the case of professional wrestling, adding a sexual subtext where none existed before.

# Countering Unhealthy Messages

As parents and community members we must make it a priority to model and instill in our children healthy values and behaviors. If we do not, they will assimilate the values and behaviors conveyed by the media and popular culture. They will grow up thinking that rich people are better, senior citizens are doddering fools, women are helpless, all family conflicts can be resolved in the ten minutes before the next commercial, and buying Nike shoes or drinking Gatorade will enable them to shoot and score like Michael Jordan.

We thought we would briefly tackle the cultural messages that we find most unhealthy and suggest ways parents can intercept or counter them. You may not agree with our choices—every family has its own values—but this short list is at least a way to start the conversation. It may also inspire a bit of soul-searching of your own. All of us are affected by these toxic cultural influences, too, and odds are our kids have picked up on them.

THE PROGRAMMING: *Money is everything.*

What's the number one value in America today? We'd have to say "money," because that is so often the ultimate standard by which political, governmental, social, and commercial decisions are made. The bottom line determines whether we protect children from lead or not, whether we use fillers like sugar and salt in food or not, whether we add violence or sex to the movie or not, whether we pay day-care workers and teachers well or not, whether we outlaw automatic weapons or not.

It is inevitable that children growing up in a society that worships the almighty dollar will receive this message in a thousand ways. As a result our kids seem to want to accumulate lots of the newest and most exciting "stuff." They scorn those who are not financially successful as "losers." They want to grow up to be rich and famous, preferably before the age of thirty and with the least possible expenditure of effort. But we don't want them to know the price of everything and the value of nothing, do we?

We are a nation that considers the word "consumer" synonymous with "person," where shopping is a major leisure-time activity. Popular culture tells us that we are what we buy, so many kids become overly concerned about having the "right" jeans and shoes, and going to the "right" school. In a culture dedicated to consumption like ours, children are the ultimate marketing targets, because brand loyalty established in youth will continue for decades. It's no wonder that the most popular cigarettes among underage smokers used to use advertising images like Joe Camel that are attractive to the young.

This cultural emphasis on the things that money can buy is especially harmful to those with limited financial resources. Struggling parents may find it painful or embarrassing that they cannot buy everything they would like to for the children they love, and that their children are teased or ignored by their peers for not having the right "stuff." We think it's very important that parents who are financially comfortable teach their own children to offer kindness rather than derision to kids who cannot afford the latest fad.

Money doesn't automatically bring happiness, and it may not bring good health either. The latest research indicates that those who place great value on money and personal possessions are more anxious and depressed, have more physical complaints, and smoke and drink more than those who put more importance on their relationships with family, friends, and community.

DEPROGRAMMING: Help your children separate their "wants" from their "needs." Tell them you'll take care of their needs as you are able, but they may need to purchase things they want by saving their own allowances or earnings (or waiting till their birthdays). Find free activities to do as a family, like going to a park or a street fair. Encourage making rather than buying gifts. Share the beauty of simple things—a fresh blueberry, a sunset, the smell of new-mown grass, an interesting detail on a building down the block. Strengthen their moral and spiritual values in whatever ways you can. A child with a strong spiritual center is less likely to worship money and material things.

Simplify your life. Gather together things you just don't use (including toys) and donate them to a charitable organization. Involve your children in the service work you do and explain to them why you do it. Better yet, pick a special service activity for the entire family. Tell them stories about people who have performed admirable acts of charity. Don't audibly judge people by their possessions, or lack thereof. In a society that is increasingly breaking into "haves" and "have-nots," where one in six children live in relative poverty, it's important to teach your children compassion and understanding for those less fortunate than themselves. In our own homes, our children get excited about putting money into a jar for charity each week and deciding where to give the money when the jar's full.

Watch TV with your kids and comment now and then about what a product portrayed in an ad realistically can and cannot do to improve their lives. Teach your children how to be savvy shoppers so they don't confuse price for value, and show them that the most expensive item is not necessarily the best.

THE PROGRAMMING: *Speed is of the essence.*

Thanks to computers, e-mail, fax machines, and cell phones we are now living in an age when it is impossible to be out of touch, and there is no longer any time to mull over an issue or an idea. We have become impatient with delay or with the slow pace of normal human interaction, and often choose to do things quickly rather than with thought. We've watched fifth and sixth graders carry on three or four Internet "instant message" conversations at a time, a feat we thought extraordinary until we noticed that they were moving so fast that they were not really "listening" to their correspondents or thinking about what to say in return. Like many adults, they focused on the destination and forgot to enjoy the journey. Maybe that's why we're all so impatient with delay, why we push in lines and complain whenever we have to wait for anything.

As we discussed in chapter 7, fast-paced living can be very stressful, especially if we do not make time to rest and rejuvenate. This applies not just to our day-to-day living, but to our longer-term goals as well. Lots of parents are pushing their children to achieve more and faster in school, on the playing fields, in the arts—in nearly every area of their lives. They fill their children's lives with lessons and coaching and practice and tutoring. We say: give kids some time to be kids. They don't have to learn every possible skill and have every possible experience before they're eighteen. They need room to dabble, to try out new talents and experiences, to discover their own individual strengths and passions without the pressure to be the best or the most skilled. A tight focus too soon can actually stunt their creativity and resourcefulness.

A corollary to "speed is of the essence" is "you shouldn't have to wait for what you want." Granted, immediate gratification has its attractions, but a steady diet of getting whatever they want whenever they want it is a sure way to spoil kids. We're not talking about love and attention here, but about material things.

DEPROGRAMMING:   See if you need to slow down the pace of life at your house. Let your children experience the emotional power of real, unhurried human interaction. Take the time to write them little notes or letters occasionally to express your delight or pride in something they've done. Restrict time spent with highly stimulating TV and video games. Read aloud, do puzzles, and play games together instead. Audiotapes, which require imagination and visualization to bring the story to life, might make a better, slower-paced babysitter than videos. Let your kids' interests and passions dictate how far or how fast they move in their endeavors.

Try not to indulge all of your child's material desires, as their wishes often change from day to day. Talk to your kids about your own long-term planning, about things you have struggled or worked for. Introduce school-age kids to the concepts of budgeting and saving. Even preschoolers can get the point; Dr. Russ's kids know that any request for a new toy will be met by suggestions of work that can be done around the house to "earn" it. Require your children to put part of their earnings and allowance into short- or long-term savings and encourage them to save for a higher-priced item they really want.

THE PROGRAMMING: *The good life revolves around junk foods.*

The makers of unhealthy foods have a lot of power over our kids, who generally know very little about good nutrition. The advertising slots on children's programs are jammed with junk-food ads, creating a toxic health environment for our kids that encourages them not only to eat unwisely but to eat too often as well. The restaurants themselves are everywhere (you know you live in a rural area if the nearest McDonald's or Wendy's is more than 15 minutes away). If that's not enough, there are playgrounds, special meals, and cheap toys to pull in the kiddies as well. Our kids are exhorted through the ads and reminded by the ubiquitous brightly colored buildings that food that is high in sugar, salt, fat, and calories and low in nutritional value is fun, tasty, and available all the time. As parents, we have to balance our children's longings for a quick trip to the drive-thru with our knowledge that fast foods are linked to cardiovascular disease, diabetes, obesity, and cancer. Are we the only ones that find it ironic that McDonald's sponsors a foundation dedicated to children with serious health problems?

DEPROGRAMMING: Educate your children about nutrition in the ways we suggested in chapter 5. Help them learn how to deconstruct advertising appeals by the makers of junk foods. Find tasty, healthy snack foods that appeal to your children so they do not feel deprived by not having whatever new junk food is currently being heavily advertised. Work to get pop machines out of the schools.

THE PROGRAMMING: *It's cool to be negative and disrespectful of others.*

The mass media is full of negative words and images, and depicts a world where the really cool kids are flip and uncaring and there's no percentage in being nice to anyone who can't do something for you. If you believe popular culture, only babies and other hopeless innocents have a positive attitude. As a result, kids may think it's far more "adult" to be cynical and dismissive of traits like sincerity, kindness, courtesy, and joy, and to look for a negative motivation behind every action. In fact, the primary method of communication for many older kids appears to be the put-down.

Aside from the unpleasantness of dealing with a child who is always looking for the worst in a person or situation, negativity has real health effects. A cynical and disrespectful attitude fosters an unsupportive relationship with peers, family, and community that undermines physical and emotional health. On the other hand, a positive attitude toward life is consistently associated with longer life, better health, and a more effective immune system,

DEPROGRAMMING:   If you take an optimistic approach to life yourself, your children are likely to imitate it. We're not suggesting you deny life's difficulties, but merely that you pass on more of an "if life hands you lemons, make lemonade" attitude. That sort of thinking results in a more resilient person, one who is better able to survive and thrive despite the ups and downs of life. Encourage your children to treat people of all ages, backgrounds, and genders with respect, and insist that others treat your kids with respect, too. Praise acts of kindness. Don't make excuses for bad behavior, whether it's that of your own child or others.

THE PROGRAMMING: *Looks are everything.*

This is not a new message, at least for females, who have for generations been under pressure to conform to certain (ever-changing) standards of beauty. However, this message is no longer aimed solely at adults, but at adolescents of both sexes and younger kids as well. Now they, too, measure their worth by their appearance rather than attributes such as character or kindness. By giving them big-breasted, tiny-waisted Barbie dolls and G.I. Joe action figures with giant pecs and biceps we set unattainable standards for body shape and set the stage for eating disorders and illegal steroid use during the teen years. The conflicting messages to stay slim *and* eat in unhealthy ways may well explain why so many American girls diet, and why the percentage of girls who feel "happy with the way I am" drops from 60 percent in elementary school to 29 percent in high school.

DEPROGRAMMING:   Expand definitions of beauty. Point out to your kids not only the physical kinds like a man's attractive eyes, a woman's strong arms, or an elderly person's well-earned wrinkles, but also the less obvious beauties of a sharp mind, a sweet voice, or a courageous spirit. Be more concerned with your child's fitness and health than with whether he or she conforms to current standards of beauty. Make it clear you value strength of character over physical beauty.

THE PROGRAMMING: *Violent behavior is acceptable.*

Violent behavior is the norm in some places in America, and children suffer from it. Our inability to regulate guns puts too many children at risk at school and in the streets. Our inability to get a handle on child abuse means some are not even safe in their own homes. But even if they live in more peaceful surroundings, our children are still strongly influenced by the pervasive violence in the books, magazines, television, music, and movies that surround us. Too many kids adopt the music, haircuts, clothing, gang signs, and attitudes of musicians (both white and black) who send a clear message that guns are cool, "attitudes" are cool, and violence not only is cool, but is the only way to maintain respect and keep your woman in line.

A heavy exposure to violent images can affect a child psychologically in three ways: it may make a child overly fearful of the world, it may make a child more aggressive, or it may desensitize a child to the pain and suffering of others. Children tend to copy violent or aggressive behaviors in their play and in their attempts to resolve conflict. These violent images aren't just coming from certain kinds of music, but from almost all forms of "entertainment." In our experience, teaching your children (especially boys) not to love violence is a very difficult thing, because that culture is so seductive. Through toys and video/computer games, powerless little kids get to blow up planets and yank the spinal columns out of "enemies." No one really gets hurt in this "play," but unfortunately the attitudes and actions practiced during these games can carry over into real life. Violent video and computer games are worse than violent TV and movies because they require the player to identify with and assume the role of the aggressor, conditioning kids to seek violent solutions to conflict.

Nurturing aggressive behavior has physical as well as psychological effects. Far from being a healthy outlet for aggression, violent video games raise levels of the same neurochemicals released by anger and hostility, emotions associated with lowered immunity and a wide range of cardiovascular problems. A recent study even found that hostile and aggressive young adults are more likely to already have changes in their arteries symptomatic of early atherosclerosis.

DEPROGRAMMING: Choose with your children the TV shows, videos, and computer/video games that they will watch. Turn down the sound during commercials and talk about what you've seen. Pay attention to the lyrics of the songs your child listens to and discuss those that concern you. Let your children's friends' parents know not to show your child, for instance, a PG-13 or R-rated video without your permission.

If your child displays aggressive behavior, track down and deal with its inspiration. Teach your kids skills for resolving or avoiding conflicts. Let them know that anger is a natural emotion that can and should be controlled or channeled. Teach them to express it appropriately and to defuse it by counting to ten, going for a run, or writing in a journal. Show them lots of love and affection. Know where they are and who they're with—all the time.

Support programs (such as Tribes or Peace Keepers) in your children's schools that teach children how to care for one another and give them the skills and the motivation to resolve conflicts without violence.

THE PROGRAMMING: *Cigarettes, alcohol, and certain drugs are glamorous.*

This has been an issue for decades, but we now have irrefutable medical evidence of the harm done by substance use and abuse. Yet somehow the message hasn't gotten through; only half of eighth graders surveyed understood that there was a health risk to smoking or chewing tobacco. It hasn't gotten through to popular culture either, or we'd see fewer sports figures with drug and alcohol problems, fewer celebrities smoking cigarettes, and two thirds of children's animated films would not include the use of alcohol or tobacco.

You may think that the use of tobacco, drugs, and alcohol is not an issue for your child, but school counselors can tell you that these problems are occurring at younger and younger ages and across all social strata. It is not uncommon for middle-school students—even the ones from so-called "good" families—to enter treatment for problems with alcohol or other drugs. Every day 5,000 kids under seventeen smoke their first cigarette; some of them are still in elementary school. In a study done at the University of Washington, 25 percent of sixth graders in that state had smoked cigarettes, 40 percent had tried alcohol, and 7 percent had experimented with marijuana. A similar federal study of eighth graders done in 1997 found that 47 percent had smoked cigarettes, 54 percent had tried alcohol, 23 percent had tried marijuana, and 21 percent had tried inhalants ("huffing," or sniffing spray paints and other aerosols). These are frightening statistics, not only because inhalants and alcohol can be lethal, but also because exposing the developing brain to these addictive substances may create a long-term need for the drug. The earlier you get hooked on tobacco or alcohol, for instance, the harder it is to quit. Don't think the tobacco companies don't know this.

DEPROGRAMMING: Evaluate your own use of alcohol, tobacco, and other drugs, and commit to being a good role model. Because kids may not understand the short- and long-term effects of substance use, educate them about the dangers. They may not realize the permanence of some of these impulsive decisions. For instance, of the 5,000 kids who start smoking each day, 3,000 will become regular smokers and 1,000 will eventually die of a tobacco-related disease. Counter advertising that links smoking and drinking with popularity and desirability with the real effects of these drugs on their bodies—everything from bad breath, vomiting, and stupid behavior, to diseased organs and death.

At a good time, ask your kids about their use, and their friends' use, of controlled substances. Protect your children from peer pressure to try or use alcohol or tobacco by making sure their parties are always under parental supervision, and letting them know that it's okay to blame you for their not partaking. ("My dad would be *furious* if I did. And you know my dad—he'd find out.") Know your children's friends. Form alliances with other parents to provide safe drug- and alcohol-free places for kids to hang out, and let them know that you want to be told if they suspect your child has been smoking or drinking.

You cannot relax about substance abuse just because it was not an issue when you were a child. Alcohol, tobacco, and other drugs are now far more pervasive in the culture, are stronger, are less frowned upon, and are readily available—even in the schools.

THE PROGRAMMING: *Winning is everything.*

We love competitive sports, but as dads and coaches, we are often appalled by the messages parents and other adults send children about sports and sportsmanship. We have seen fathers (unfortunately, it is usually the men) shout belittling comments to their kids on the field, throw tantrums over how many minutes of game time or what position their kid will play, suggest ways to evade the rules, and even threaten violence against players on the opposing team. In Florida the problem of bad adult behavior became so great at youth games that one youth sports league now requires all parents of potential players to take a one-hour class in appropriate conduct before their kid can even set foot on the playing field. Adults need to back off and allow the children to enjoy themselves. Sports give them the chance to experience the satisfaction of teamwork, the joy of camaraderie, and the thrill of achieving personal goals. The playing field is where they learn how to function in a group, to look out and care for each other. The sense of sportsmanship and the enjoyment of physical activity they develop will stand them in good stead throughout their lives. It's a shame to spoil it all with a misguided desire to win at any cost.

DEPROGRAMMING: Remember sports are play, and play is supposed to be fun. Make sure all kids get a chance to play, and that players rotate positions so they all get a chance at the key ones. Watch your own behavior on the sidelines, and feel free to criticize that of parents displaying the wrong attitudes. Praise good sportsmanship. Emphasize the specifics of play—a nice pass, a well-placed kick, good teamwork, the perfect double play—over the final score. Heap praise on children, on your team or the opposing team, who throw themselves fully into the game, regardless of whether they scored three times or not at all.

THE PROGRAMMING: *Americans are better than everyone else.*

Americans are like little children—we tend to think that we are the center of the universe. We act as if we are bigger, stronger, smarter, richer, and more beautiful than everyone else. This attitude, understandably, often irritates people in other countries. As America becomes more diverse culturally, more of us have to drastically change our image of how an American looks and sounds. All Americans are not—and never were—white people from Europe.

DEPROGRAMMING:  Encourage your children to be tolerant of differences in race, culture, religion, gender, or abilities; we have a lot to learn from each other. Read about how people live in other countries in magazines like *National Geographic World* or *Faces*. Visit ethnic fairs and celebrations; try out new dances or foods. Discuss who is and isn't included in TV shows, movies, and other offerings from the mass media. Is everyone in America thin, white, gorgeous, and in their twenties?

In this chapter we have tried to raise your awareness of what messages your children are picking up from the popular culture. If this leads to action as well, so much the better. Consider spending a little time looking at the world through your children's eyes to understand what unhealthy messages they may be receiving. You may decide to monitor their media input more than you did before, or change some of your own responses. Maybe as a result of reading this chapter you'll find the strength to not just throw up your hands in resignation and give in when your child keeps pressing for that 42-ounce Coke, the $50 name-brand jeans, or that R-rated teen-scream video. You may not always be the most popular parent in the house (or on the block), but parenting is not a popularity contest. Keep repeating the values you hold dear; and maybe, eventually, they will sink in.

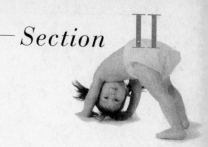

# Complementary Therapies for Children

I n these next six chapters, we introduce forms of healing that may be new to you. Some of them may turn out to be familiar concepts under new names, some are imports from other cultures, and a few push the boundaries of medical understanding. We believe that all of them, however, may have a place in integrative pediatric medicine.

The healing modalities we will be talking about run the gamut, and include relaxation techniques, osteopathic manipulation, clinical hypnosis, acupuncture, homeopathy, massage, guided imagery, healing touch, chiropractic adjustment, herbal remedies, and prayer. We offer them to you as complements to your child's conventional medical care. None is a substitute for a trained physician who specializes in the health of children and families. However, we think you should become familiar with these useful tools and techniques, because your child's doctor may suggest them or because you may want to explore their use.

What's the evidence for the effectiveness of these forms of healing? In some cases, it's as good as that for conventional medicine. In other cases, while the therapy might be new (and unstudied) in this country, it has been used successfully to treat many people in other countries for generations. A number of the therapies we'll discuss have become nearly conventional for such things as managing pain with children; more than 70 percent of university-affiliated pediatric pain-management programs use at least one form of complementary medicine, most commonly biofeedback, relaxation, massage, art or music therapy, or Therapeutic Touch.

In most cases, the therapies we recommend have at least some supportive research evidence and always have anecdotal evidence of efficacy. If a potentially effective therapy is safe and relatively inexpensive, we don't feel a need to wait for further research to explain how it works—it's enough for us to know that *it works*. Because most of the therapies described in this chapter are gentle and noninvasive, with minimal side effects, we feel that their benefits outweigh the risks. There are some cautions with each of these therapies, of course, but when used correctly, most of them fall into the "could help, can't hurt" category. We recommend them generally for mild illnesses and for chronic conditions for which conventional medicine offers limited benefits (and additional risks).

In the pages that follow we will try to tell enough about each therapy so that you will be able to understand how and why it might be used to improve your child's health. We will try to explain the thinking behind each form of healing, and what to expect from a practitioner. We'll tell you how we've made use of the therapy with our patients and our families. Most of these therapies are safe and gentle, but we will tell you of any concerns or cautions we have. Although we consider ourselves experts in the integration of these complementary therapies into conventional care, we are not ourselves expert in all of these specific forms of healing. Be sure to check the Resources section at the back of the book for more information and sources. And don't forget the cardinal rule: Always tell your child's pediatrician about any other therapies, remedies, or supplements that your child is taking so he or she can coordinate care, caution about interactions, and be on the lookout for side effects.

# Chapter 10

# Little Bodies, Big Minds:

## *Mind/Body Medicine for Children*

**m**any parents may be put off by the term "mind/body medicine." It does sound a bit "fringe," a little too "woo-woo." So let's demystify it: "Mind/body medicine" simply refers to a group of therapies designed to activate the power of mind and spirit to help heal the body. A mainstay of integrative medicine, mind/body techniques are also used by open-minded conventional doctors who have learned that they can maximize the good effects and minimize the side effects of a conventional treatment—and even *treat* many conditions—by teaching their patients how to enlist their emotions, attitudes, and thoughts for the service of healing. Pediatricians have been especially open to mind/body therapies, many of which were first used to alleviate the pain or side effects of cancer therapy or chronic disease in children.

A certain amount of mind/body medicine is a part of every healing encounter—conventional or integrative. When your child's doctor tells her that a medication will make her feel better fast or sings a silly song to distract her from an incoming injection, that is mind/body medicine, whether the doctor is aware of it or not. When you watch a funny video to help you forget about what ails you, or when you take a few deep breaths before a stressful experience, you are practicing mind/body medicine yourself. If you delivered your child using Lamaze or similar natural-childbirth methods, you have practiced mind/body medicine. Likewise when you kiss your little boy's "owie" to make it better, or hand your little girl her special "sleepy-time" teddy bear to help her fall asleep.

Doctors are now using mind/body techniques such as biofeedback and self-hypnosis to help children change unhealthy habits, ease pain, relieve anxiety, and reduce the symptoms associated with such problems as head- and stomachache, chemotherapy-induced nausea, asthma, irritable bowel syndrome, warts, and insomnia. Mind/body medicine is a hot area of research where knowledge changes every day, so we'll just give you a broad, very general look at the field and an idea of how it might be used by an integrative pediatrician.

Western medicine—unlike Chinese, Indian, and many folk medicines—treats the mind and body as two completely separate entities, like this [M] [B]. Integrative medicine sees mind and body as connected, like this **M—B**, with the causes of many medical problems falling on some point on the continuum between mind and body. Some health conditions may have a greater physical component, and some may have a greater emotional and psychological component, but most have some of each. How can they not, when our brains, organs, and immune systems are in constant communication with each other? The idea that what happens to the mind affects the body and vice versa is not so revolutionary. After all, many parents have seen stomachaches disappear as soon as the magic words "you can stay home from school today" were spoken—a fine example of physical pain caused by a stressful state of mind being cured when the source of anxiety or tension is resolved. On the other hand, a physical problem can affect mental state. For example, an active child with an injury that precludes sports or play may become anxious or depressed when she cannot do all the things she is accustomed to doing.

Clearly, what we think or feel can have a physical effect. Want proof? *Imagine holding a fresh, juicy lemon that you have just picked from the tree. Smell the lemon, drinking in its strong lemony aroma. Imagine that you are slowly cutting the lemon in half, and that the juice is flowing down the sides of the fruit and onto your hand. Picture the bright yellow lemon half with drops of juice dripping from it. Now imagine biting into the sour, juicy flesh of the lemon.* Your mouth is watering now, right? Just visualizing the lemon evoked a salivary response from your body. In the same way, your heart beats faster and your senses become hyperalert when you read a Stephen King thriller late at night, even though there is no real danger threatening you. And haven't there been times in your life when repeating the familiar affirmation from *The Little Engine That Could* ("I think I can, I think I can . . .") helped you do something you didn't think you had the strength or stamina to do?

The concept that *all* healing has a mind/body component can be a tough one to get across to both patients and conventional doctors. Our entire medical system is based on the image of the body as a machine that can be fixed with the proper tool or intervention whenever it breaks down. There's no room in this picture for the effects of attitude or emotion. Although some scoff at the idea that their thoughts or emotions have anything to do with their physical health, disease does not exist alone; it affects and is affected by a person's attitudes, lifestyle, and thinking. You (and your doctor) may not choose to recognize it, but you cannot deal successfully with the body without impacting the mind, and vice versa. Good doctors know this and frame their health advice carefully. Effective healers of all sorts know the power that belief—or lack of it—has in treatment.

Doctors know that their patients respond better if they believe that their physician is skilled and caring. This is an example of the "placebo effect," the well-proven phenomenon that some people will improve even when given a fake or inactive treatment if they believe it will work. A placebo (Latin for "I will please") is a therapeutically inactive treatment, like a sugar pill, given in the old days to placate patients. Surprisingly, the placebo often caused an improvement or cure. The simplest example of a placebo response is how much better children often feel once they head for the doctor's office. We don't know how often parents have said to us, "You wouldn't know it to look at her, doc, but this child was sick as a dog just twenty minutes ago at home." Maybe it's the fresh air on the trip over, or the toys in the waiting room, but we prefer to think that the child's immune response has been activated by the sense that she is on the road to healing.

Because of the power of the placebo effect, the best clinical trials to determine the effectiveness of new drugs or treatments are "placebo-controlled," that is, some people in the trial will get an inactive but similar pill, injection, or therapy while others get the real deal. In order to be considered useful, the medical intervention being tested has to work significantly better than the placebo. However, a certain percentage of people (15 to 70 percent, with the greatest effect coming from pretend pain medications or sham surgical procedures) will feel better from nearly any medication or therapy, regardless of its actual effect on the body. In fact, the total effect of any given medication comes from the combined effects of the active ingredient and the placebo response.

Studies on the placebo effect have been fascinating. Placebos have worked as well or better than the tested medications in trials of sedatives, antidepressants, and blood pressure drugs. In one placebo trial, people with asthma were told that one bottle of harmless salt-water spray contained an allergen and another bottle of salt water contained a powerful allergy medicine. Thirty percent of the subjects went into full-blown asthma attacks and another 18 percent suffered airway restriction when they were exposed to the "allergen." Even more amazingly, in most cases their symptoms went away after they used the "drug."

The placebo effect offers the purest example of a person's own innate healing capability, one that doctors usually take for granted. If you're wondering how a placebo can affect physical health when it is both harmless and inactive, you're not the only one. We think it's ironic that Western medical science dismisses the placebo effect as a nuisance that gets in the way of studying a drug that is likely to have side effects instead of studying how to maximize the effectiveness of the placebo that has no negative side effects. If we could harness or strengthen the placebo response, we would likely need to use fewer pharmaceutical drugs—or at least lower doses of them—and risk fewer side effects.

# What Mind/Body Therapies
# Can and Cannot Do

Research into the mind/body continuum is really just coming of age in America, but we are slowly amassing good data on the beneficial effects of such therapies as meditation/relaxation, biofeedback, hypnosis, guided imagery, and yoga. In addition to these clinical studies, researchers in a new field called psychoneuroimmunology are looking more closely at the biochemical connections between the nervous, immune, and endocrine systems—body systems formerly thought to work independently of one another. It turns out that these three systems are actually in constant communication via hormones, brain chemicals, peptides, and other biochemical messengers. These signals go both from body parts to the mind and from the mind to the body, causing every physiological change in the body to be accompanied by a change in the mental and emotional state as well, and vice versa.

Using mind/body techniques, people can influence processes controlled by the autonomic (involuntary) nervous system that were once thought to be outside our control. For example, we can indeed alter such "unconscious" actions as blood pressure, breathing, heart rate, and circulation by learning to shift activity from the stimulating sympathetic arm of the autonomic nervous system to the more relaxed parasympathetic arm. We can influence other parts of the nervous system as well, changing our brain wave patterns or reducing or increasing our perception of pain. We can change the hormonal output from our endocrine systems and change the balance between various immune cells.

Mind/body medicine can sometimes be used to cure, especially those problems related to stress. It can also be used as a complement to conventional medicine to reduce pain, ease symptoms or drug side effects, and improve compliance with treatment plans. But it has its limitations, and some people go too far with the idea. While we strongly believe that the mind can influence the workings of the body and can certainly affect the immune system, we do not believe that the mind can *cause* disease—for instance, that we cause our own cancers solely by having pessimistic thoughts. Certain mind states such as stress may make a child more susceptible to disease, but his attitudes, beliefs, and emotions are not solely to blame when he gets sick; there are many other factors in ill health, including genetic susceptibility, viral or bacterial threats, environmental toxins, nutritional deficiencies, and lack of exercise. By the same token, if a child does not get better after using mind/body techniques, it does not mean that he has failed, or not tried hard enough. Every one of us is different, and what works for one may not work for another. Norman Cousins and Norman Vincent Peale to the contrary, the power of positive thinking cannot heal everything (though it may improve your quality of life).

Mind/body medicine is often referred to in pediatrics as "self-regulation." We like this term, as it suggests the power that a child holds in his own hands. The focus on mind/body medicine is on magnifying and directing the effects of *his own* thoughts and attitudes to improve his own health, on enlisting all his powers to the service of healing. It can be tremendously empowering for a child to realize that he is not helpless but might be able to change the way he experiences an illness or might gain mastery over body processes he had thought to be beyond his control. In fact, just realizing that fact is enough to make some people begin to feel or function better.

Mind/body medicine should be a key component in any pediatrician's bag of tricks because every childhood illness has an emotional/psychological component that must be addressed. We often see children with physical symptoms that upon examination have no medically explained physical cause, symptoms that we recognize as signals of psychological distress. For instance, stomach pain is a common complaint in children, who carry stress in their bellies, rather than in the head, neck, or back as adults do. Our patients are not faking or intentionally causing their tummy aches, but through mind/body techniques they can be taught how to consciously prevent or ameliorate them. Children are especially receptive to the idea that they have the power to help themselves, and are generally better at the therapies than adults because they are more imaginative and more open-minded. Their inexperience leaves them with no preconceived notions—there's no reason, to a child, why a special soothing pink seashell under the pillow won't bring sleep.

We think it is helpful to introduce children to the concept of mind/body medicine when they are healthy so they have the proper mind-set in place and tools in hand when these techniques are needed medically. Any child can benefit from knowing mind/body approaches to reduce stress and anxiety when they arise. If you need to use mind/body techniques for treatment, however, keep a few cautions in mind. Organic causes of illness must be ruled out before you go treating, say, a child for "school-day tummy" when she may really have appendicitis or inflammatory bowel disease. Mind/body techniques should be considered a complement to—and not a replacement for— drug or other medical therapies required by children with serious chronic diseases like asthma or juvenile rheumatoid arthritis. The choice to participate in any mind/body treatment must come from the children themselves, without parental pressure, because empowerment is an important aspect of healing. Children who have post-traumatic stress disorder, a history of abuse, or psychosis should use the mind/body techniques of hypnosis and imagery only with the guidance of a specially trained therapist who knows how to handle any unsettling emotions or images that may come up.

Be aware that a certain percentage of children tend to experience psychological distress as physical symptoms. Children who frequently experience headache, fatigue, dizziness, stomachaches, or chest pain for which no organic cause is found may be "somatizers" who are actually suffering from anxiety, depression, or antisocial disorders. The source of their distress needs to be uncovered through counseling, after which the child can be taught mind/body strategies to help her cope.

# Mind/Body Techniques

Use of mind/body therapies has become more commonplace in pediatrics in the past twenty years. Some experts estimate that 10 to 25 percent of the problems presenting at a pediatrician's office are psychophysiologic, and therefore amenable to mind/body therapy. We use mind/body medicine in some form or another in every encounter with a patient, even if it is only in the way we phrase questions or advice to elicit the greatest healing response. We harness the powers of the placebo by the attention we pay, the efforts we take to increase our patients' control over their conditions, and our confidence in the efficacy of the treatment we have advised. It's important to ask our small patients what they think the cause of their problem is—and what they think might help—in order to discover and utilize their hopes and fears in our therapy. These insights can, for example, help a patient with chronic problems alter the experience of the illness, and thereby alleviate some of its symptoms. In addition, we use specific techniques, such as breath work, hypnosis, or distraction, to lower anxiety or perceived pain during medical procedures like blood draws or shots. We also use or refer patients to other practitioners for various mind/body therapies to treat specific conditions, as we will discuss in Section III.

We believe that techniques such as breath work, relaxation, meditation, hypnosis, guided imagery, yoga, and the creative arts all have a place in relieving the pain and trauma of medical procedures and in giving children enough mastery over their bodies to ease or sometimes even cure their health conditions. We have already talked about the power of the placebo, and in the following pages we'll explain several of the more common mind/body modalities. We want to be clear that we are not ourselves expert in all the techniques we'll be discussing. We do practice some of them, and are well enough versed in the others to be able to devise an integrated treatment plan and refer our patients to skilled practitioners. We'll tell you what each technique is and how it is used. Where we can, we'll give you a sample activity so you can get a taste of the therapy. Some of these techniques require training, some require the presence of a therapist or technician (see Resources), but most can be done by you and/or your child whenever and wherever suits you. Using these tools will let your child—the one who always says, "I want to do it for myself"—be the boss of his own body.

We do want to repeat that mind/body therapies are not fringe medicine or New Age religious practices, but techniques backed with a great deal of research and clinical evidence. However, your religious or worldviews may preclude your being comfortable with some forms of mind/body medicine. Some folks believe that turning inward for healing calls out the Devil, while others are unable to separate the use of meditation for stress reduction from its place in Buddhist and Hindu practice. We offer these modalities solely as ways of evoking a healing response.

The most important factor in successfully using a mind/body therapy with children is the whole-hearted support of both children and parents. We try to be sensitive to signs of parental apprehension or disbelief, so we can discuss these concerns openly with the parents and answer all questions. We want to make sure that the parents understand the cause of their child's health problem and are supportive of our proposed treatment. In the same manner, parents and children need to feel confidence and trust in the person conducting the mind/body sessions. If there is not good rapport between child and practitioner, the child may not be able to relax deeply enough to focus on the training.

# The Mind/Body Toolbox

For ease of discussion, we have divided mind/body therapies into three categories of tools. First in the Mind/Body Toolbox are the pocket tools that are always with your child and can be used any time. Then there are the tools that are kept in the drawer because they require some parental supervision or assistance, at least in getting started. And finally there are the power tools, techniques that should be learned under the direction of a trained practitioner. In our experience, many parents need all these tools as much as their children do, so consider practicing some of these mind/body techniques as a family.

## Pocket Tools

In this category we include methods of stress reduction that children can access and use on their own at any time, such as breath work, intentional muscular relaxation, social and family connection, journaling, and exercise. In addition to these specific therapies, it is helpful if parents and other mentors can teach children attitudes and skills that increase their ability to solve problems and give them a sense of mastery. A feeling of mastery is important in developing the optimistic attitude associated with longer life and better physical and mental health. Caring adults can also teach children how to be their own coaches, engaging in positive self-talk ("I can do it!") that encourages an upbeat, healthy attitude.

**Breath work.** Even though we talk about "the breath of life," many of us do not pay any attention to our breathing. We breathe shallowly and high in our chest, which does not provide much oxygen for our body's cells and tissues or keep breathing muscles like the diaphragm toned. Some of us forget to breathe at all, especially when we are concentrating. For example, think about the last time you tried to thread a needle. We bet you were holding your breath without even realizing it.

Yet it turns out that the simple act of breathing in and out can have powerful effects on the body. For this revelation, we should thank the yogis of India, who pioneered the study and practice of breath work, learning to control body functions such as hunger, thirst, blood pressure, heart rate, and temperature as part of their spiritual practice. In India the word for "breath," *prana*, is also the word for "spirit." Breath has been associated with the spirit as well as the body in other cultures as well; in fact, the English words "spirit" and "respiration" share the same Latin root.

The breath, being a part of both the voluntary and involuntary nervous systems, is able to affect both the body and the emotions. Proper breathing can calm the nervous system, slow the heart rate, stimulate the immune system, and even switch your mind over to another form of brain wave. As the esteemed yoga teacher B.K.S.

Iyengar once said, "Regulate the breathing and control the mind." Imagine—you can control how you feel physically, emotionally, and mentally *with your breath!* That's a lot of power. Breathing in certain ways can make you feel more positive, more alert, and more energetic, or it can make you feel calmer and more relaxed. The trick is to pay attention, to be aware of your breath, of how you breathe and how fast. When you breathe in and out slowly and deeply, you relax and let loose of anger and muscular tension. When your breath is quick and powerful, you feel more stimulated.

Breath work can be used to relieve stress, pain, panic, or anxiety and can make you become more aware of what's going on in your own body. When we give a shot or draw blood, we have children pay attention to their breath or blow bubbles to distract them from fear and pain. We teach slow deep breathing to kids with asthma to help them deter or reduce the severity of asthmatic attacks. We use what is called diaphragmatic breathing, or belly breathing, to help children slow

## Belly Breathing

Have your child put her hand gently over her belly button. Ask her to imagine that she has a balloon underneath her belly button that will blow up when she inhales. Ask her to breathe in through her nose slowly to the count of three or four, pulling the air deep into her lungs and feeling her belly expand like a balloon blowing up. Make sure her shoulders are loose and relaxed. Now ask her to breathe out through her mouth slowly to a count of six or eight, feeling her belly deflate like a balloon. Tell her to take her time. Young children can do this for a minute or two, gradually working up to 10 to 20 minutes as they get older.

*Adapted from Rebecca Kajander,* Diaphragmatic Breathing *(1997)*

their heart rate, reduce pain perception, and calm their nervous system. It's simple and easy to learn (see the box on page 179), as long as you remember to let your stomach relax and pooch out a little rather than holding it in. We also described several breathing exercises in the box on mini-relaxation exercises in chapter 7.

**Intentional muscular relaxation.** Many children—and their parents—unconsciously spend their days with their muscles clenched. This muscle tension inhibits circulation and allows toxic waste products to build up in the tissues, causing pain and slowing healing. Intentional muscular relaxation techniques help you discover where tension is being held in your body and allow you to release it. The techniques themselves simply call for tightening and then relaxing the muscles in the body. Many people find that these exercises offer them a chance to finally feel what it's like to be totally relaxed.

**Exercise.** We devoted an entire chapter (chapter 6) to the healthy effects of exercise, but we would like to remind you again that moving the body can affect the mind and the emotions. Exercise is a proven stress reducer and mood elevator that builds a child's self-image and sense of mastery at the same time that it optimizes physical health. When your child is stressed, depressed, or angry, suggest a quick walk to blow off steam, dancing to favorite music, or ten minutes of charging up and down the stairs.

**Journaling.** Keeping a diary or a journal can help reduce stress and ease physical and emotional pain by allowing a child to disclose or explore worrisome thoughts. Your child might want to have his own journal (don't peek), or you might keep a private family or parent/child journal that allows family members to express themselves emotionally when it is hard to do so face-to-face. (There are wonderful examples of interactive journals such as these in Henriette Anne Klauser's excellent book, *Put Your Heart on Paper.*) Younger children may enjoy journaling in the form of a poster that keeps track of progress (dry nights, servings of fruits and vegetables eaten) toward certain goals with stars or other fun stickers or stamps. This form of positive reinforcement can be very helpful in changing behavior.

**Connection with others.** Study after study has found that people who are loved by their families, supported by their friends, and

## Letting Go of Tension

*Floppy Raggedy Ann or Andy.* This is a good exercise to help a child become aware of just how a relaxed body feels. Ask your child to imagine herself a floppy rag doll. Everything should feel loose and comfortable. Tell her to let herself be all floppy like Raggedy Ann. Pick up an arm and praise her for the way it flops down when you pick it up. Now check the other arm, and praise its floppiness. Encourage her to be loose and floppy like Raggedy Ann all over.

*Progressive muscular relaxation.* We recommend playing this as a kind of "Simon Says" game with your child. First, ask the child to lie down in a comfortable position. Ask him how the muscles in his body feel: Are they loose? Tight? Tell him he will be clenching each part of his body for five to seven seconds and then releasing, taking a nice big breath before he moves on to the next. Start with the toes, then gradually do the feet, ankles, calves, stomach, fanny, chest, fingers, hands, arms, shoulders, throat, and all parts of the face. Then have him tighten everything at once for seven seconds and release. Ask him how his muscles feel now.

*Raggedy Ann exercise is adapted from Karen Olness and Daniel Kohen*, Hypnosis and Hypnotherapy with Children *(1996).*

involved in their communities live longer and healthier lives. Positive social interactions with others bring not only value and meaning to our lives, but they relieve stress, build support systems, and prevent isolation. Some people with chronic health problems even find that they feel less pain while having fun with friends or doing volunteer work. There are a million ways to build healthy connections within your family through religious rituals, family meetings, meals and trips taken together. Children can also build their own social and emotional support systems through team sports, extracurricular activities, volunteer activities, and correspondence with "mouse pals" (the e-mail successor to pen pals) or distant friends and family.

## Tools in the Drawer

Tools in the drawer require a little guidance or training. You and/or your children might need to take a class to get started, or turn to the Resources section at the end of the book for lists of organizations, books, tapes, or Web sites that may be helpful to beginners. We heartily recommend both yoga and meditation as activities that are even better when done as a family.

**Yoga.** Here in the West, most of us do not use the full range of yoga practices but focus instead on the use of meditative awareness, breathing exercises, and physical exercises (called postures, or *asanas*) to help reduce stress and improve fitness, flexibility, and mood. In its native India, however, yoga is a lifestyle that includes these exercises as well as spiritual practice, vegetarian diet, and a mandate to do good in the world.

Although the health benefits of yoga have been long studied in Asia, we are just beginning to do research on the subject here. So far in the West, yoga has been shown to be of benefit in the treatment of asthma, carpal-tunnel syndrome (a common problem for those who spend a lot of time at computers), and some cases of chronic pain. There has even been a published study on the use of yoga to improve the IQ scores of mentally retarded children.

Yoga can be fun with kids of any age. Kids love the dramatic possibilities of the postures named after animals and the fun of imitating mom or dad. You might find, to your chagrin, that your own little lions and cobras are far more flexible than you are. Very young children can do yoga for short periods; as they grow older they can hold the poses longer and with greater precision.

**Meditation.** You don't need to find a guru or go to a monastery to meditate. In fact, although forms of meditation are an important part of several religious traditions, when doctors and researchers talk about meditation, they usually have something less religious in mind. They are referring to the self-directed process of focusing on a sound, an image, or a thought to still the mind and relax the body. Dr. Herbert Benson of Harvard University's Mind/Body Institute called his meditative technique "the relaxation response" specifically to divest this stress-reduction tool of any religious implications. You can choose to meditate in a way that delivers a spiritual benefit as well (Benson himself thinks that deepens its effect), but that's up to you.

Studies of meditation in adults have found that regular meditation can lower blood pressure, improve heart health, relieve pain, and reduce anxiety. As integrative doctors, we have recommended medita-

## Abby and Jonathan's Favorite Yoga Poses

*The Tree.* Six-year-old Abby loves this one best—she calls it the "talking on the telephone" pose. Stand up tall and straight on a firm surface. Feel yourself growing right out of the floor. Put your weight on your left leg, and slowly pick up your right leg, bent at the knee, and place the sole of your right foot against the inside of your left thigh. Place your palms together in front of your face, and then raise them over your head if you can. Hold this pose as long as you can, then gently put your right leg down and do the pose with your left leg raised.

*The Cross-eyed Lion.* Four-year-old Jonathan loves to roar. Sit on your folded legs with your butt resting on the back of your heels. Rest your hands on your knees. Take a deep breath and, keeping your head straight, open your mouth wide and stick your tongue out as far as you can. Look at the tip of your nose. Give a mighty ROAR! Take another deep breath and roar, repeating four times.

# Basic Meditation

Sit in a quiet place in a comfortable position. Close your eyes, and relax your muscles. Breathe slowly and repeat your focus word or phrase silently in your mind. If your attention wanders, draw it back to your focus word. Don't be worried or irritated, just gently return to saying your word in your mind. Do this for five minutes at first, then extend the time as you are able. When the time is up, open your eyes. Sit for a minute or two to enjoy the feeling of relaxation before going on about your day.

tion for reduction of both pain and stress, as well as for complementary therapy for autoimmune and breathing disorders. There is little clinical evidence on the effects of meditation on children, but in our experience (and that of other practitioners) children can also benefit from regular meditative practice, which then becomes a tool they can take into their adult lives.

There are many ways to meditate, and no one way is the "right" way. You have to discover what's right for you and your child. Many people meditate in a comfortable seated position, but some meditate while walking. Some meditators focus on a meaningful word or phrase ("peace," or "love," for instance); others on an image, like a starry sky or a loved one's face. Those practicing what is called Mindfulness Meditation don't focus at all, allowing thoughts to drift across the mind without getting involved in them. Meditation can be done alone or in groups, at a regular time of day or whenever it's needed, seated or walking, in long stints or short bursts, with music or in silence.

Dr. Russ first introduced his kids to meditation by popping a favorite (instrumental) tape he uses when teaching yoga into the tape player in the car and asking them to close their eyes and breathe in and out gently. He then asked them to picture the sky, a river, or a favorite animal while the tape played. After three to five minutes he asked them to open their eyes again. This imaginative time-out is a nice way to introduce the idea of a focused quiet time to young children.

A child's ability to meditate increases with age. A preschooler may only be able to handle a few minutes at a time, whereas a middle school child could meditate for 10 to 15 minutes once or twice a day. Very active kids might enjoy the Chinese exercises known as tai chi, which are often considered a form of moving meditation. Consistency of practice is important; the more you meditate, the better you get at it.

## Power Tools

Power tools call for the help of a trained practitioner. Once a child is trained, however, he or she will be able to use the skills at will. Although there are other useful techniques—such as art, dance, and music therapy—that also fall into this category, they are not often used in primary care and so we are less familiar with them. We will be focusing instead on biofeedback and the various forms of self-hypnosis and visualization—power tools that we use extensively in caring for our patients.

**Biofeedback.** This is a heavily used therapy in pediatrics, and there's a lot of clinical evidence of its effectiveness. The power of biofeedback comes not just from teaching kids how to make actual physiological changes in their bodies but also from the graphic proof it provides children that they can have mastery over their physical conditions—that they are not the powerless victims of their bodies.

Biofeedback uses sensitive machines to monitor body processes and display the information via sounds or pictures. Biofeedback machines can be set up to respond to increases or decreases in heart rate, muscle tension, peripheral body temperature, sweat-gland response, or brain-wave activity. The machine makes visible what is normally invisible, so that a child can see what is happening in her body and learn how to control it. The various systems of our body communicate with each other all the time; biofeedback allows us to open these messages and, with an increased awareness of body sensations, change what they say. Once a child learns how these self-regulatory skills feel, and has practiced them both with and without the machine, the machine is no longer necessary except for an occasional brushup of skills.

In a first biofeedback session a health professional trained in biofeedback will talk with your child about the goals of treatment—for instance, to reduce the severity of asthma attacks. He will explain what body function the child will be trying to affect, and will apply sensors hooked to the computer to various parts of the body depending on what physiological factor will be measured (muscle tension, respiration, etc.). The computer may communicate this information through a readout, a sound, or—increasingly for children—through a video game. The child then attempts to change the body function in the desired way, using the computer feedback.

Children learn especially quickly with biofeedback, which is often described as "a video game for your body." In fact, the computerized games used in many biofeedback programs for children make sessions both fun and more involving. For instance, kids can learn how to tense and relax specific muscle groups to determine the path of a computer spaceship trying to avoid asteroids. Children may become competent in self-regulation after a month of once-a-week, 40 to 60-minute biofeedback sessions (younger children will have shorter sessions), and maintain their skills through home practice and the occasional follow-up.

Biofeedback is recommended for a variety of pediatric conditions, often in combination with self-hypnosis or relaxation. The self-regulation skills learned by children through biofeedback have been found to help reduce the number, severity, and duration of migraine and tension headaches; improve circulation in their hands and feet to counter the effects of Raynaud's syndrome; ease problems of muscular tension; relieve the pain of cancer, burns, or arthritis; and manage anxiety. We'll discuss some of these uses in Section III.

**Hypnosis, Visualization, and Imagery.** We discuss these three therapies together because there is so much overlap in their use and effect. They all evoke a trance state of higher alertness that focuses concentration and allows access to the unconscious mind. While training and credentials vary in this field, all three therapies take advantage of the fact that images created in the mind can seem as real to the body as those actually experienced. By allowing mind and body to "talk" to each other through words and images, these therapies offer children a child-controlled, child-centered way of managing habits, regulating some aspects of body function, and activating their own healing powers. Hypnosis may rely more on the words of the therapist for its effects, and visualization/imagery may depend more on the patient's own images and perceptions, but in truth there are more similarities than differences in these techniques. In fact, a practitioner of clinical hypnosis may use imagery both to invoke a trance state and to offer suggestions during it. We do advise parents to look for a physician, psychologist, or other health professional trained in clinical hypnosis or guided imagery (see Resources), but we realize that realistically your choices may be limited by what's available in your area. Look for people with the most training and most experience working with children; children with post-traumatic stress and children undergoing chemotherapy will require more advanced levels of training.

A few words about the trance state—a trance is not as exotic as it sounds. Kids move in and out of trance states all day, using their vivid imaginations to conjure up fantasy play, daydreaming, becoming so involved in what they're doing that they lose all track of time. When your kids sit open-mouthed in front of the TV or computer screen, they're in a trance state. When they are so engaged in a book or a piece of music that they don't hear you call them for dinner, they're in a trance state. Hypnosis and imagery merely take advantage of this state of relaxed body/alert mind by using your child's imagination and concentrated attention to intentionally heal or to change behavior.

A practitioner trained in clinical hypnosis will not make your child stand up and bark like a seal or implant a post-hypnotic suggestion that will make her do something stupid or embarrassing later. That's show biz, not medicine. The kind of therapeutic hypnosis we're talking about uses your child's own imagination, values, and desires to program his or her brain. Hypnosis and imagery are just tools that allow communication with emotions and thoughts buried in the unconscious that may be affecting your child's health or behavior. Children can come out of or change the content of imagery or hypnotherapy sessions whenever they want, just as they can change their daydreams. Practitioners should always give children the chance to go wherever they want to go. One patient described the process to Dr. Karen Olness (a leader in the field of pediatric self-hypnosis) as being ". . . like watching a movie, only you're in it and you're the director."

In pediatrics, we say that all hypnosis is self-hypnosis. Our goal is to teach a child how to access the trance state and to discover which of a child's own thoughts and images can then be used *by the child* while in that state to regulate his or her own body functions or behavior. Children have so few filters and such active imaginations that they can usually get into a receptive state very easily. In fact, there's already a component of hypnosis in your child's encounters with the doctor. We're not talking about Jedi mind tricks here, but the fact that chil-

---

# Finding Your Safe Place

A visualization session may start with a relaxing exercise like this one:

Allow yourself to imagine a comfortable place, a peaceful place. It might be a place you've been before or somewhere that's just coming into your imagination now. Just pick the first place that comes to mind.

Allow yourself to imagine that you are in that place right now. Describe what you notice. What do you see? How do you feel? What is the temperature? What time of day is it? What do you hear or smell? How does the ground feel under your feet?

Find a spot in that place where you feel most comfortable. Spend a few minutes enjoying the sensations you experience there. . . . (session continues from this point).

dren are usually very focused on the doctor from the minute they walk into our examining room. Whether it's from fear, curiosity, or respect, that intense focus makes them very susceptible to our suggestions. As young doctors we used to be puzzled by parents' reports that our off-hand advice to their children about simple problems like wetting the bed or sleeping in their own beds invariably led to improvement. With experience and professional growth, we have come to see that we were overlooking a powerful tool.

Many doctors and other medical/dental professionals have learned to use simple imagery exercises to relax children or relieve the pain of a procedure. In addition, they may refer patients in need of more time to people trained in clinical hypnosis or guided imagery. Professionals skilled in hypnosis or imagery can give a child the tools to relieve pain, reduce anxiety, heal faster after surgery, reduce the side-effects of chemotherapy, stop bed-wetting and other bad habits, sleep better, ease asthmatic breathing, and make warts and other skin problems disappear. Dr. Stu's son Yoni uses self-hypnosis to relieve growing pains. By imagining himself on a roller coaster, he has been able to reduce both the severity and the frequency of these episodes so that pains that used to occur three or four times a week are now rare.

Rather than taking control away from a child, the purpose of hypnosis or visualization is to help strengthen self-control. The specialist is merely the coach who teaches the child how to regulate her behavior and body processes. During a session, this "coach" will first spend a little time developing rapport with your child and discussing the problem to be addressed. Then your child will be relaxed into a trance state in order to access those emotions and thoughts that cannot be reached through the conscious. This state may be accessed through simple diaphragmatic breathing and/or an imagery exercise that mentally takes the child to a favorite place or activity. In hypnosis, questions will be asked, and suggestions to help the child achieve goals of self-regulation may be offered. These will be suggestions, not directives; your child remains in control. Someone who specializes in visualization or guided imagery will rely on sensory information—images, taste, smell, sound, and touch—rather than words, in the belief that the brain communicates more easily through images. The images will be explored for their meaning. Using words or images, the child can learn how to be more aware of what's happening in her body and then be coached into visualizing step-by-step the successful achievement of a behavioral goal (staying dry all night) or the physical changes she wants to occur (bronchial tubes as wide-open superhighways, wounds healed up without a scar). She can also be taught how to imagine herself in a safe favorite place whenever she needs to separate herself from pain. After training, your child can do her visualization exercises or self-hypnosis alone, with your help, or with an audiotape. In studies, even children as young as three have been able to learn these techniques, although skill increases with age.

# How to Give Your Child a Magic Feather

In the classic Disney cartoon, Dumbo the big-eared baby elephant cannot fly until he is given a "magic" feather. He always has the ability to fly, but he has been grounded by his lack of belief in himself. There may be times when your child needs a "magic feather." He may have school-morning tummy, or sleeping problems, or difficulties sticking with a prescribed regimen for asthma. She may be nervous about the big game or a move to a new home. A little mind/body medicine may help. Here are a few tips for helping your child activate mind/body responses:

- Make it clear that you have faith in your child and his ability to prevail over adversity. Your support is the most powerful "magic feather" a child can have.
- Have audible faith in the healing program your pediatrician has proposed. Encouraging your child's belief that she will be cured optimizes the healing response by calling upon the power of the placebo.
- Encourage a sense of health. Congratulate your child on having a strong and healthy body. Point out how quickly his cuts heal.

- Ask about feelings and emotions when children are ill or anxious. Help them understand that sometimes our emotions are expressed through our bodies. What's going on at home or school? Talking to a teacher or school counselor may be helpful.

- Establish healing rituals. Use prayers, symbols, mantras, or imagery sessions to support your child's wellness.

- Take a positive approach to healing, using affirmative statements rather than negative ones. The unconscious mind does not recognize negative words like "no" and "not" and so is likely to hear, "I *will not* pee in my bed in the middle of the night," as "I *will pee* in my bed in the middle of the night." Far better to frame the statement as "I will stay dry all night."

- Make sure your child has mind/body tools at his or her command, and practice them together.

# Chapter 11

# The Healing Touch:

## *Manual Medicine for Children*

n the last chapter, we talked about mind/body medicine, or how abstract things like thoughts and feelings can affect your children's physical health in concrete ways. In this chapter we talk about therapies that rely on the physical—touch, movement, or manipulation—to improve mood, build immunity, treat disease, and create a sense of overall wellness. We categorize these therapies as manual, or body/mind medicine. Although their word order is reversed, body/mind medicine and mind/body medicine are really just two sides of the same coin. Both approaches are based on the belief that mind, body, and spirit are linked together in the creation and maintenance of good health and are all affected during times of poor health.

So what is manual (body/mind) medicine? We use the term to encompass both a complete system of medicine, such as osteopathy, and such techniques as chiropractic, massage, exercise, and various forms of body work. These modalities use physical movement and/or touch to:

- *Express caring, or transmit healing energy.* Many doctors today have become so dependent on science that they have forgotten the healing power of a hand held or a shoulder patted in a reassuring manner.

- *Relieve muscle tension.* This can reduce pain, improve circulation, boost immune function, and change unhealthy patterns of movement or behavior.

- *Restore systemic balance.* Most practitioners of manual medicine have an integrative point of view, and believe that injury or imbalance in one organ or body system implies imbalances in other systems as well.

- *Access the unconscious.* Wilhelm Reich first hypothesized that traumatic memories are stored not only in the mind, but also as patterns in muscle, collagen, organs, and other tissues. He believed that these stored experiences could be accessed and released by physical manipulation of the body, allowing habits of unhealthy physical, mental, and emotional behavior to be changed.

- *Restore energy flow that has been blocked by physical or psychological trauma.* Manual techniques from Chinese Medicine, such as acupressure, are the most common ones used for this purpose.

- *Heighten awareness of body function and increase alertness to important body cues.*

- *Encourage appreciation of the pleasure of nonsexual touch.* Body/mind therapies like massage teach children to feel comfortable with touch, and understand its healing power. If they learn to give massage as well, they have another way to exercise their compassion.

In this chapter we will introduce you to forms of manual medicine we think most useful or suitable to help prevent or treat disease in children. In our experience, children respond especially well to these therapies, because they haven't yet formed any adult biases against them. We'll tell you which forms of body/mind medicine you and your children can learn to do for yourselves. In cases where a trained practitioner must provide the treatment, we'll explain the philosophy behind the technique, the conditions for which we find it most useful, and what to expect in a typical visit. We will start with osteopathy, which is a complete system of medicine, and then deal with those body/mind tools that can be used as a complement to conventional medicine.

# Osteopathic Medicine

Many people do not know what an osteopathic physician is, and might even be surprised at the inclusion of the word "physician" in the title. But in fact we have two kinds of "approved" conventional medicine in this country—allopathic medicine and osteopathic medicine—with similar training and accreditation. Osteopathic physicians, or D.O.'s (Doctors of Osteopathy), go through college, four years of medical school, internship, and usually years of specialist training just as M.D.'s (Medical Doctors) do. They are licensed to prescribe drugs and to perform surgery, and have hospital privileges. Most provide primary care as family practitioners, internists, pediatricians, or gynecologists, but some specialize in areas such as surgery or anesthesiology. In short, they have similar training and licensure and can provide the same breadth of care as M.D.'s.

Despite these similarities, osteopathic training traditionally has an essential component that conventional medicine lacks—a holistic philosophy that encourages hands-on healing. In addition to the usual armamentarium of conventional medical doctors, osteopathic physicians are also taught how to prevent, diagnose, and treat illness with their hands, using a series of techniques called Osteopathic Manipulative Treatment (OMT). Their use of touch allows them to be more alert to asymmetry, restrictions in range of motion, and abnormalities of texture in the tissues that might indicate dysfunction, and to treat them by manipulating muscles, joints, and other tissues to restore normal function.

Andrew Taylor Still, M.D., founded osteopathy in the 1870s as a gentler alternative to the "slash-and-burn" conventional medicine of the time, which relied heavily on treatments such as purging, bleeding, and amputation. Dr. Still believed that the body was an integrated system that had a great capacity to heal itself. (Does this sound familiar?) He felt that the physician's role was to facilitate this process by encouraging healthy habits of diet and exercise, and using touch and manipulation to counterbalance any disturbances in the neuro-muscular system that were causing or reflecting ill health. He taught that a disturbance in one system of the body often impacted other systems as well, a philosophy called "wholism." Early practitioners of integrative medicine, osteopaths were labeled a "cult" by the American Medical Association in the 1940s. Now however, they are well regarded and their numbers are once again growing, especially in underserved rural areas.

As you can imagine, we find much value in the osteopathic philosophy, and we are just as comfortable recommending primary care for your child from an osteopathic physician as from a medical doctor. Our preference is for practitioners who still follow the traditional methods of osteopathic manipulation. Unfortunately, such practitioners are a bit of an endangered species right now. The majority of D.O.'s have become very allopathic in their practice, though that trend may be reversing. Only a small percentage of D.O.'s still use OMT to correct structural or functional abnormalities in addition to providing conventional care. Even fewer perform cranial osteopathy, the diagnostic and manipulative technique we find most interesting from a pediatric point of view. Those of you who have read the books of Dr. Andrew Weil will be familiar with his stories of the healing power of cranial osteopathy in the hands of his gifted mentor, the late Robert Fulford, D.O.

The concepts underlying cranial osteopathy are controversial, and little data yet exists to support them. Osteopaths believe that cerebrospinal fluid normally moves up and down within the spinal column between the sacrum ("tailbone") and the brain with a subtle pulse called cranial rhythmic impulse (CRI) that is similar to and just as important as the more obvious rhythms of blood and breath. They believe that CRI is reflected in the barely perceptible movement of the bones of the head and face, sacrum, and associated body membranes. This movement can be restricted by minor falls and accidents or trauma incurred during birth that prevent those bones and membranes from expanding and contracting freely. The resulting imbalance in the body can lead, according to practitioners of cranial osteopathy (CO) say, to a range of pediatric and adult conditions from colic to learning and behavioral problems.

A treatment with CO starts with a gentle, hands-on examination to evaluate the cranial rhythmic impulse and pinpoint any restrictions in the movement of cerebrospinal fluid. Then extremely light pressure is used to release any restrictions in the sacrum, head, or facial bones, restoring movement to the bones and balance to the body as a whole.

Even though debate about cranial osteopathy rages on, we have been impressed by the healing potential for CO that we have seen in our own practices. We refer patients to cranial osteopathy for recurrent ear infections, headaches, sinus or respiratory problems (including asthma), learning disabilities, and attention deficit disorder. Dr. Russ brought his infant son for a few sessions of CO to address any possible aftereffects of his birth. If you decide to try this therapy for your child, we recommend that you look first for an osteopathic physician, because CO is an integral part of osteopathic philosophy and training. If you cannot find an osteopathic physician who is skilled in cranial osteopathy near you, look for an M.D., dentist, or other allied health professional with pediatric experience who has been trained at a reputable school in cranial osteopathy or in a related, stand-alone, technique called craniosacral therapy (CST). Dr. Stu refers his patients to a chiropractor who is trained in pediatric craniosacral manipulation. We do not recommend taking a child to "cranial therapists" who are not licensed health professionals, as they will not have the medical training to recognize serious problems that require conventional treatment, nor are they necessarily able to see the bigger health picture.

# Chiropractors

Back pain is such a common symptom in this country that most adults are familiar with the kind of care offered by a chiropractor. We're used to lying on the special table while the chiropractor works on our spines, and many of us have found relief from these treatments. But how useful is chiropractic care for children, for whom back pain is a less common problem?

Developed in 1895 by Iowa grocer and healer Daniel David Palmer, chiropractic medicine has outgrown its humble beginnings to become the most widely used "alternative" modality in the United States. Chiropractors are now the third largest group of practitioners in the country (after medical doctors and dentists), and polls find their patients very satisfied with their care. Doctors of Chiropractic (D.C.) are licensed in all fifty states after four years of medical training, with a focus on spinal manipulation.

D. D. Palmer decided, after reportedly curing a janitor's deafness with a spinal manipulation, that the majority of all disease arose from "subluxations" (misalignments) of the spine that impeded the free flow of a life energy he called "Universal Intelligence" through the nervous system. Palmer believed that using physical manipulation to return the vertebrae to their proper place rebalanced life energy and restored optimal function to the nervous system, which in turn promoted proper function in all organs and systems. At the college he founded, Palmer taught students noninvasive, patient-centered medicine that relied heavily on physical touch and good patient-doctor communication. Chiropractors are not trained or licensed to prescribe drugs or perform surgery.

Today only a small percentage of chiropractors (dubbed "straights") still believe that spinal adjustments (manipulation) cure all disease. Another small group ("evidence-based") dismisses these broad claims and restricts their practice solely to those musculoskeletal complaints for which spinal adjustment has been scientifically proven to be effective. Most chiropractors nowadays, however, are "mixers" who acknowledge other causes of disease, and use botanicals, nutritional supplements, physical therapy, homeopathy and/or other techniques in their practice in addition to spinal adjustment. These practitioners are more likely to see themselves as offering primary care, a position we think unwarranted. Chiropractors are not trained as broadly or as deeply as D.O.'s and M.D.'s, and they are not licensed to provide conventional care (drugs, surgery, in-hospital testing, etc.) when needed.

In adults, chiropractic is now considered as effective a therapy for the treatment of acute low back pain as is available, and many people report it to be of use for neck pain as well. However, there is very little research on the use of chiropractic on children. Although chiropractors are now treating children for asthma, allergies, ear infections, colic, bedwetting, and other disorders, there are few studies yet to prove benefit (and some studies showing no benefit at all).

The chiropractic profession is currently engaged in outreach to establish themselves as "gatekeepers to the health care system," and increase the number of children under their care. While there are many compassionate healers in the chiropractic profession, we do not recommend chiropractors for primary care at any age. We have the following additional concerns about chiropractic care for children:

- Most chiropractors do not have special training in pediatric problems, which are very different from those of adults.
- Chiropractors are not trained or licensed for comprehensive care, so they may not recognize serious illness and cannot prescribe drugs when needed.
- Some chiropractors make overzealous use of X rays during diagnosis and treatment; we believe it is important to minimize exposure of children to X rays.
- A vocal element of the chiropractic profession has been very active in the debate against childhood immunizations, which we believe are essential.
- Many chiropractors make use of diagnostic tools such as applied kinesiology that are too unorthodox even for us.

That said, you should also know that Dr. Stu does refer some of his patients to a chiropractor for craniosacral manipulation, and has been pleased with the results. However, he did have to search quite a while to find a practitioner with whom he was comfortable, who had extensive experience with children. If you choose to go this route, ask your doctor for a referral to a chiropractor with whom he or she has a working relationship; this makes integrated treatment more likely. We do not recommend chiropractic care for young infants. We differ about chiropractic care for older children. Dr. Stu trusts the chiropractor he works with to treat children as young as fifteen months, because he knows that she is experienced with children, her adjustments are gentle, and she has a finely tuned sense of when conventional care is needed. Together they have treated children for asthma, coughs, recurrent ear infections, temperomandibular joint syndrome (TMJ), headaches, and gait problems, as well as musculoskeletal injuries. Dr. Russ, however, rarely recommends chiropractic therapy for children under twelve. He is far more likely to refer children to a D.O. for manipulation or cranial osteopathy, because osteopaths have been trained to treat children. Chiropractic care can stretch out for very long periods of time; we recommend a re-assessment by parents of the need for further treatment after four or five sessions. We do not believe that it is useful for healthy children to make the regular "maintenance" visits suggested by some chiropractors.

# Massage

Isn't it great when something that feels so good is good for you, too? You might not realize it, but massage is more than just some "oohs" and "ahs" and a sense of well-being. As performed by professionals, massage can be used to stimulate, relax, or rehabilitate. Studies—many of them done at the Touch Research Institute at the University of Miami—have found that therapeutic massage helps boost immune function, ease pain, improve circulation and muscle function, treat stress-related illness, and even helps premature infants gain weight faster. Some of the benefits of massage may be attributable to caring touch, but many come from actual physiological changes activated by the manipulation of skin, muscle, and joints.

Massage has been practiced for millennia by cultures around the world. Hippocrates, the ancient Greek considered to be the father of modern medicine, advised that "the physician must be experienced in many things, but most assuredly in rubbing." Our culture is not a very tactile one, by and large, but the benefits of touch are enormous. In fact, babies deprived of touch may suffer "failure to thrive," and may not bond easily with their caregivers. When we touch someone in a caring way, we activate millions of sensory receptors on the skin, which can affect breathing, heart rate, and the production of hormones, immune cells, and other chemical transmitters. Far from being an indulgence, massage (either amateur or professional) is an important way to maximize health.

Massage is a body therapy that can be enjoyed on a variety of levels, from amateur back rub to specialized professional massage therapy. Certification and licensure of massage therapists varies from state to state, but we recommend getting a referral from your child's doctor or the American Massage Therapy Association if your child needs massage for rehabilitation from injury, or has a condition that requires special care. (The bones of children with spastic neurodevelopmental disorders can be fractured accidentally with overaggressive massage.) According to studies done with children by the Touch Research Institute, therapeutic massage can not only produce quicker weight gain in premature babies, but also improve colic, reduce levels of stress hormones in children with asthma, lower blood sugar levels in children with diabetes, improve lung function in kids with cystic fibrosis, decrease restlessness in kids with ADD, and relieve sleep problems. Not bad for something so simple and pleasant.

Parents make great massage therapists, too, starting right after your baby is born. Studies have found that brief periods of gentle massage can help babies sleep better, grow faster, bond sooner, and be less irritable. We teach infant massage techniques to new parents who are at a loss as to how to handle colicky or irritable babies. Massage soothes these babies and gives their parents a positive experience with them, besides. It's not tricky: Just mix one drop of lavender oil into a palmful of moisturizing cream or vegetable oil, then gently stroke your baby's body, uncurling clenched fingers, rubbing the feet in little circles. Use some pressure, so it doesn't feel like tickling. Do this at least once a day, especially at bedtime. Keep the massage sessions short, no more than 10 minutes at a time, as too much can overstimulate an infant. If you feel all thumbs around a new baby, you can take one of the popular baby massage classes being offered all over the country or purchase an instructional videotape (see Resources).

As the baby gets older, you can continue massage, maybe adding to your repertoire of massage moves by taking a class or learning through a book or video. The most common form of massage is Swedish massage, an adaptation of ancient Chinese techniques developed by a Swede in the nineteenth century. We've listed the five techniques of Swedish therapy in the box below. Teach these techniques to your children as well, so that eventually everyone in the family knows how to give a back, shoulder, head, hand, or foot massage. Family massage is a handy stress-reduction technique, an easy way to help your children experience the sensation of truly relaxed muscles so they can better identify areas of tension, and a fine display of concern for others. Massage offers two-way satisfaction; studies show that both the giver and the receiver of massage experience a reduction in feelings of anxiety and depression. And it's simple—all you need is a firm but comfortable surface, a bottle of scented or unscented oil or lotion, and a body.

# Five Basic Techniques of Swedish Massage

*Stroking (effleurage).* A gliding stroke with the palm, much like stroking a cat. Often used to begin or end a massage session.

*Kneading (petrissage).* Squeezing, pressing, and rolling the muscles using hands, thumbs, and fingers—just like making bread.

*Friction.* Deep circular or crosswise motions with the fingers or thumbs to relax "knots" in the muscles.

*Percussion (tapotement).* Gently striking the body with cupped hands, fingers, or the edge of the hand. May feel and sound like falling rain or a light karate chop.

*Vibration.* Gentle shaking, rolling action not unlike a vibrator.

When her son was younger, our coauthor, Lynn, used to give him a 10- or 15-minute massage at bedtime to relax him. Since she had to learn to let go of her own daily tension in order to do this properly, these nightly back rubs turned out to be a form of mutual stress reduction. When he was three, Brook liked to return this kindness by walking on his parents' backs, his own form of massage. Eventually he became familiar enough with the techniques to offer massages in return. His hands were not strong enough for a really satisfying massage until he was older, but his parents appreciated the love involved and looked forward to getting massage coupons from Brook at birthdays. When Brook ran cross-country in middle school, three-way foot massages in the evening were common. By that time, he was comfortable enough with this form of touch to enjoy an occasional visit to a massage therapist for a full 1-hour session of professional massage.

We recommend a visit to a massage therapist for any member of the family who wants a real treat. In addition, professional massage may be therapeutic to children with muscle spasms and other musculoskeletal problems and other disorders such as recurrent infections; in such cases, you may want to ask your doctor for a referral or ask around to find a therapist skilled in working with children. A full professional massage generally takes place on a special padded table in a relaxing environment that is warm enough for the patient to feel comfortable. The child may be clothed if modesty is an issue, but it is preferable to have him undress to the underpants and be draped with a sheet, exposing only the areas being massaged at the time. The therapist will use oil or lotion to reduce friction; if it is scented, they may ask first if he likes the scent. Soft music is often played; be sure to let him know it's okay to ask to have the music changed if it gets in the way of his enjoyment of the therapy.

# Energy Massage

There are several forms of massage that are aimed less at relaxing the muscles and more at releasing an unseen force the Chinese call "Qi," or "chi." According to Chinese Medicine, which we will describe more fully in chapter 15, Qi is the life force ("energy") that travels freely through the body when we are healthy. Ill health comes from stagnation, blockage or loss of Qi. Chinese acupressure, Japanese shiatsu, and reflexology are all forms of massage designed to unlock energy and allow it to flow freely again.

*Acupressure* is a needleless version of acupuncture that relies on pressure from the fingers or thumbs on certain points of the body (not just the feet and hands) to unblock Qi. We will discuss this further in chapter 15. *Shiatsu* is a Japanese form of acupressure.

*Reflexology*, or zone therapy, is a fairly modern modality based on the premise that areas on the feet, hands, and ears correspond directly to various parts of the body. Pressure applied with the thumb to a specific point is believed to open up energy blockages in the related area and help heal imbalance or illness there. For instance, you might rub and press the bottoms of the four smaller toes of each foot, which are associated with the sinuses, on a child with sinus congestion in hopes of promoting drainage.

# Other Forms of Bodywork

What we collectively call bodywork are a variety of forms of therapy with many different purposes but one thing in common. Bodywork techniques may be used to repair an injury, change a structural imbalance, access buried emotions, improve range of motion, or simply to relax and enjoy oneself, but they are all based on the idea that manipulation of the body can free up any restrictions imposed by habit or muscular tension that are affecting physical and emotional health. There are too many bodywork techniques for us to be able to discuss them all, so we will refer you to Mirka Knaster's excellent book *Discovering the Body's Wisdom* (Bantam 1996) for more detail. Most forms of bodywork are aimed at adults, who have had years to develop unhealthy patterns or injuries. We do not generally refer children for bodywork, although children with scoliosis may benefit from the Feldenkrais Method or the Alexander Technique (well described in Mirka Knaster's book).

# Therapeutic Exercise

In the broad sense, exercise is a body/mind therapy, too. It is well proven that exercise affects not just your bones and muscles, but also your body systems and your emotions. Regular exercise boosts immunity; lowers the risk of cardiovascular disease, diabetes, osteoporosis, obesity, and certain cancers; and is a proven antidote to depression and anxiety. Some people even use exercise as a spiritual practice—Buddhists often engage in walking meditation, and millions of people in China perform tai chi communally every morning.

In addition to informal methods of exercise, there are schools of what might be called "integrative exercise," such as yoga and tai chi, which combine structured physical activity with a meditative element. Both yoga and tai chi are part of much broader philosophies, but can be enjoyed at a purely physical level as well. We have already touched briefly on yoga in the previous chapter. Whereas yoga springs from India, tai chi is an ancient martial art form from China. Anyone who has ever lived in an area with a concentration of Chinese people has probably seen older people in the parks in the morning performing silently the slow sweeping movements of tai chi. The graceful movements of tai chi are designed to facilitate the free flow of energy ("Qi" or "chi") through the body. Tai chi promotes awareness of the body and its movements, flexibility, and balance in both body and mind. The basic movements are simple, and can easily be done by children.

# Chapter 12

# "Herbs and Spices":

## *Botanical Medicine for Children*

america has lost much of its herbal heritage. Few of us know how or why to harvest rose hips or raspberry leaves anymore; we don't eat dandelion greens as a spring tonic or pick chamomile to brew a sleep-inducing tea. In America, twentieth-century medicine had moved so far away from the use of medicinal plants that as modern doctors we used to scoff at patients who asked about what we called "herbs and spices." Herbs were "unscientific," something for cooking, not therapy. Fortunately, our patients and experts like Dr. Andrew Weil began to open our eyes to the botanical research being done by scientists and clinicians in other countries. They passed on to us stories of their successes and failures with botanicals. Our own research was fueled by intellectual curiosity and especially by the desire to be able to give parents using herbs the proper advice and cautions. Now we see that herbal remedies potentially have an important place in the practice of integrative pediatric medicine, although we would like to see more research done on the use of medicinal herbs specifically in children.

Medicines made from the flowers, leaves, bark, roots, and other parts of plants have been the basis of medical care for millennia. Even today, about 30 percent of the prescription drugs on the market (including important drugs for pain, heart disease, and cancer treatment) were initially derived on plant sources. And pharmaceutical companies are hot on the trail of new ones, investigating the secrets of healers and shamans in traditional societies around the world. The traditional Chinese and ayurvedic medical systems are rooted in herbal medicine, but even conventional M.D.'s in countries such as Great Britain, France, Germany, and Japan prescribe many herbal remedies as a matter of course. Pharmacies in those countries stock botanical medicines, and their staffs are able to offer informed advice to customers interested in herbal approaches. We are not so lucky here in the United States, where few conventional doctors or pharmacists are well trained in the use of botanicals. As a result, too many people rely on the advice of the clerks in health food stores, an approach we do *not* recommend.

Until recently, Western medicine dismissed regional lore about botanical remedies as being backward, dangerous, and, well, dumb. Most Americans have lost—or never had—the familiarity with the use of local medicinal herbs that has been passed down through generations of local healers and "plant ladies." But the pendulum is swinging back, and plant remedies are now being used by at least a third of Americans. The nearly $4 billion annually they're spending is a market a lot of companies are eager to crack, as witness the new lines of over-the-counter botanical remedies being sold by giant pharmaceutical companies. These companies tend to treat herbs like chemical drugs, looking for the one active ingredient that they can extract, standardize, and package. On the one hand, this approach may give us botanical remedies that are made under safe, sanitary conditions and that are tested to assure that they contain just what they say they will. On the other hand, some benefits—such as reduced side effects, gentler action, and therapeutic synergy among the constituents of the herb—may be lost when medicinal herbs are no longer taken whole as foods, extracts, or teas.

This swing toward "natural" medicines comes with a few concerns. Contrary to myth, herbs are not necessarily safer than medications. Medicinal herbs are drugs, by definition, although usually less concentrated than most conventional medicines. They should be used with at least the same caution and respect given to their pharmaceutical cousins. **So we repeat: "Natural" does not mean "safe."** Some herbs are toxic with overdose, some interact adversely with prescription medication, and some are contaminated or made therapeutically worthless in processing. Dr. Stu once consulted on a fifteen-month-old girl who was taken to the emergency department of a hospital where he was lecturing. She was critically ill, with a heartbeat gone wild. Dr. Stu suspected a medication overdose, but the parents denied that there were any medications in the home. Upon further questioning, it turned out that they had been giving the little girl some "vitamins" provided by a local "nutritionist" to relieve her ear infection. The "vitamins" turned out to be an extract of the very potent herb belladonna. To make matters worse, the parents had been giving their daughter more drops than prescribed under the mistaken—and very dangerous—notion that more was better. As a result, their child spent a night in the pediatric intensive care unit, and Dr. Stu developed a dislike of herbal remedies that did not waver until he eventually realized that the case was not an illustration of the use of herbs, but of the *mis*use of herbs. Parents need to treat herbal remedies with respect, and not use an herbal remedy when the situation really calls for a visit to the doctor.

The Food and Drug Administration classifies herbal remedies as "dietary supplements" rather than over-the-counter medicines, which means that their quality and purity (and their advertising) are largely unregulated and therapeutic claims cannot be made for their use. Because the government only loosely regulates the herbal industry, consumers must educate themselves about herbs and learn to identify manufacturers who abide by recommendations for Good Manufacturing Practices. Recognizing a potentially huge market, manufacturers of herbal products are increasingly promoting them for childhood illnesses. You should know that few herbs have been tested clinically on children (or even on adults). **That's another point that bears repeating: There is very little clinical data on the safety and efficacy of herbal remedies for children.** (In all fairness, we should add that few prescription medications have been well studied in children, either.)

Despite the lack of medical research, we do think that there is a place for botanical remedies in integrative pediatric care. There are sixteen herbs that we are comfortable recommending and using with children: echinacea, astragalus, garlic, ginger, elderberry, stinging nettle, chamomile, peppermint, green tea, flax, and slippery elm (taken orally); calendula, aloe, and tea-tree oil (used topically); and eucalyptus and lavender (used as aromatherapy oils). We'll talk about these herbs, some herbal oils, and a few medicinal mushrooms in detail later in the chapter. First, however, we would like to explain how and when herbs are used.

## Using Herbs

We are not herbalists by trade, and your child's doctor is not likely to be one, either. However, thanks to an explosion in research on botanical medicines in the past few years, and a significant amount of personal experience using plant medicines in our practices, we feel comfortable making some broad recommendations regarding the use of herbs in children. We predict that doctors and pharmacists will soon be more familiar with plant remedies, and better able to educate parents about them. The United States Pharmacopoeia is now setting standards for the manufacture of some botanicals (look for the "USP" on the package), a practice that should raise the quality of herbal products on the market.

We use selected herbal remedies in treating our patients and our own children. We think that botanical remedies like the sixteen mentioned above can safely be given to children in several situations:

- *To relieve symptoms or shorten the duration of acute illnesses that generally heal on their own within a certain length of time.* The chapters in Section III dealing with these conditions—coughs, colds, flu, upset stomach, cuts and scrapes—include a number of herbal remedies.
- *To shore up immune function for the short term, especially during the cold-and-flu season.* Echinacea is the classic example of an immune-boosting herb that can be taken for short periods of

time to shorten the duration of an upper-respiratory infection, or possibly even prevent one.

- *To treat some chronic conditions.* For instance, garlic can be used for recurrent ear infections, cranberry for recurrent urinary-tract infections, and evening primrose or black currant oils for eczema.
- *To reduce the side effects of conventional medicine.* An example would be the use of ginger for chemotherapy-induced nausea.
- *To strengthen or tone the body's organs and systems, especially after an illness.* Tonics for overall health were once very popular in America, but Western medicine has since shifted its focus to drugs with specific effects on specific conditions. Eastern medicine, however, places the highest value on those drugs/herbs that have more general effects, so tonics that strengthen resistance are considered to be "superior" drugs. Tonics that might be used with children to restore health or prevent disease include the herb astralagus and the mushroom maitake.

As integrative practitioners, we tend to turn to herbs as an alternative to over-the-counter medications and as a way to support the body's healing capability. When properly used, herbs have a gentler action with fewer side effects; they are also usually less expensive. Botanical medicines are available in a variety of forms, but we recommend standardized liquid or solid extracts, tinctures, or capsules of freeze-dried herbs (in that order) for oral use. (Remember, homeopathic medicines are made and used quite differently from botanicals, even though both may be based on plant substances.) Both herbal extracts and tinctures are made by soaking whole herbs in alcohol and/or water and distilling the resulting liquids. Tinctures and liquid extracts are taken by the drop or by the dropperful. Solid (dried) extracts are swallowed in capsules. Tinctures have more alcohol and less plant matter in the finished product, but, oddly enough, they appear to work better in some cases. Some parents are concerned about giving their children alcohol-based botanicals, but a child really gets very little alcohol (a few drops) from a dose of a liquid extract or tincture. Much of the alcohol will evaporate if the extract or tincture is

# Important Terms

*Tonic.* A tonic herb is one that is taken regularly for the generalized effect of strengthening and toning the body. It helps the body respond better to physical and emotional stress, and normalizes function (both excess and deficiency). Astragalus and the maitake mushroom are tonics.

*Tincture.* The fluid that is pressed or filtered out after an herb has been soaked in alcohol and/or water or other solvent mixtures to separate out the medicinal agents.

*Extract.* A more concentrated tincture that contains less alcohol and more plant material. Solid extracts (liquid extracts with the solvents removed) are more stable and more concentrated than liquid extracts.

*Standardized extract.* An herb that has been distilled and processed to contain minimum levels of the active compound or a marker compound if the active agent is unknown. Standardized extracts may be more expensive, but they offer the best assurance of a consistent, quality product, because levels of the active compounds in medicinal plants can vary tremendously depending on individual plant makeup and growing, harvesting, and storage conditions.

*Freeze-dried extracts.* Liquid extracts that have had their solvents removed through flash evaporation. These encapsulated products are more stable than air-dried extracts and herbs.

*Herb teas.* Single herbs or herb blends dried and sold loose or in teabags to be steeped in hot water and served warm or cold. These are a less potent form of the herb because of greater exposure to air, light, and moisture during processing and storage.

*Ground or powdered herbs in capsules.* Not recommended. This form of the herbs is very unstable due to greater exposure to air, heat, light, and moisture during processing and storage. The exception is freeze-dried herbs.

*Loose or bulk herbs.* Not generally recommended. This is the least active and most unstable form.

served in a warm drink. We do not recommend vinegar- or glycerin-based extracts, as in our experience they are not as effective as alcohol-based remedies.

We prefer single-plant products from reputable manufacturers who guarantee that a certain percentage of the active or marker compounds of an herb will be present (a process called standardization). We look for whole-herb products rather than isolated factors from an herb because herbs have many constituent compounds; some produce the therapeutic effect and others act synergistically to enhance the benefit and reduce possible side effects. Truth is, we don't really have the research yet to know which compounds are truly extraneous. We do not recommend buying loose herbs or powdered herbs (with the exception of freeze-dried herbs) in capsules, as herbs deteriorate quickly when exposed to light and air. We don't recommend teas for the same reason, with the exception of chamomile and peppermint teas packed in sealed single servings.

There are a number of ways to administer herbs to children. You can add liquid extracts or tinctures to a strong-tasting juice like purple grape juice. You can put them in a mug, add hot water to evaporate the alcohol, and serve when cooled with a little sweetener (avoid honey for kids under 1). Capsules of freeze-dried herbs can be broken open and mixed into applesauce or used to make teas. (Do not sprinkle freeze-dried nettle on food as the herb retains its "sting" in this form).

# Herbs for Children

If your child is seeing an integrative practitioner, you will have a ready source of information on any botanical remedy prescribed. However, many doctors are still learning about botanical medicine, or are closed to the idea. In such cases, there are a few steps cautious parents should take before giving an herbal remedy to a child (or to themselves, for that matter).

- *Do a little research.* We recommend a number of books and Web sites in our Resources section. Make sure you clearly understand the correct diagnosis so you can look for herbs that are used for this condition. Learn their scientific names, their specific uses, their possible side effects, and any potential interactions with food or drugs.
- *Do not keep the doctor in the dark.* Your child's doctor needs to know about any herbs (or any supplements for that matter) that your child is taking, even if that physician does not appear open to their use. It's the only way the doctor can protect your child from potential adverse interactions between those herbs and medication, and he or she may know of contraindications to the use of the herb of which you are not aware.
- *Be a careful shopper.* Know what you want before you go to the store (or the catalog). Product labels cannot by law tell you an herb's specific medical effects or its side effects, and store clerks are rarely able to provide unbiased and dependable information. Look for a standardized extract or tincture from a reputable manufacturer, and check that the expiration date has not passed—you want a fresh extract made with fresh herbs.
- *Use according to package directions for children.* Remember, there is still very little data on the use of herbs in children, so any dosages suggested are approximated. A good rule of thumb for children of average size is one half the adult dose for kids six to twelve, and one quarter the adult dose for kids two to six.
- *Do not give children higher-than-recommended doses of an herb in the mistaken belief that more is better. It's not.*
- *Do not expect an herb to work immediately.* Some, such as stinging nettle, do work quickly, but with others it may take a month or two before results are seen.

- *Do not give children herbs on a long-term basis without follow-up*, because there is so little research on the long-term effects of any herb on developing bodies. Most professional herbalists recommend taking an occasional break even from tonics, which are usually taken for weeks or months at a time. You should schedule regular follow-up visits to the doctor or herbalist at whatever schedule they suggest any time you are giving a child an herbal product for longer than three weeks.
- *Try to avoid using more than one herb at a time.* We don't yet know enough about herb-herb interactions.
- *Be careful using herbs in children under two years of age.* The only herbs we regularly use in children this age are chamomile or peppermint teas. We also make short-term use of calendula for diaper rash and echinacea or garlic for colds in younger children.
- *Watch for allergic reactions.* Discontinue the herb and contact your child's doctor if symptoms such as skin rash, wheezing, tummy ache, or nausea do not clear up.
- *Discontinue the use of any herbs two weeks before any surgical procedure.* Some herbs—especially ginger, garlic, evening primrose oil, black currant oil, and flax—can increase bleeding at such times.

The sixteen herbs described below are the ones we have found to be most helpful with children's conditions. As new botanical remedies are rediscovered and researched we expect to add others. Our dosing recommendations are very conservative because of the lack of research data with children.

**Echinacea** (*Echinacea purpurea, angustifolia,* and *pallida*). Echinacea is a beautiful flowering plant known in this country as purple cone-flower. The roots, leaves, flowers, seeds, and juice of various species have been found to have some benefit in preventing the development of upper-respiratory tract infections such as colds and flu, and significant benefit in shortening the duration of these illnesses when taken at the first sign of symptoms. Echinacea may also be beneficial for ear infections, bladder infections, and perhaps as supportive therapy for recurrent vaginal yeast infections. Echinacea appears to stimulate the immune system.

Because the majority of the research has been done on the aboveground parts of *Echinacea purpurea*, that is the species we recommend, alone or combined with the roots of *E. angustifolia* (another well-researched extract). In our experience, alcohol-based extracts are the most effective, although alcohol-free forms can be found if needed. The most therapeutically effective echinacea liquid extracts and tinctures cause a tingling or numbing sensation on the tongue.

The dosage is 6 to 8 drops of liquid extract or tincture two to five times a day in water or juice for kids two to six, or 8 to 15 drops four to five times a day for kids six to twelve. If using capsules or tablets of solid extract, for children six to twelve, give 250 to 500 mg every 8 hours. Stop once the symptoms of the cold have subsided. Use no more than 5 to 7 days, at most.

There is a theoretical concern about the use of echinacea for children with autoimmune disorders or HIV or for children with an allergy to plants in the daisy family.

**Astragalus** (*Astragalus membranaceus*). Astragalus, or *huangqi*, is a member of the pea family whose sweet-tasting root is used to enhance immunity. It is a common ingredient of Traditional Chinese herbal formulas, and is just becoming better known in the United States. Astragalus appears to increase the production of white blood cells and immune mediators such as interferon. We recommend astragalus to help regain strength after flu; to build resistance in kids who have been suffering recurrent colds, flu, or bronchitis; and to support immune function during chemotherapy. (Astragalus is typically used as a preventive measure, but Dr. Russ has used it successfully for treatment, too.)

Children aged two to six can be given 4 to 8 drops of liquid standardized extract or tincture every 12 hours; give kids six to twelve years old 8 to 15 drops every 12 hours. If using capsules of standardized solid extract, use 250 to 500 mg every 12 hours for kids six to twelve. Astragalus can be taken daily as a tonic to prevent upper-respiratory infections.

As far as we know, there are no cautions for this herb.

**Ginger** (*Zingiber officinale*). Ginger is familiar to us all as an ingredient in ginger ale, gingersnaps, and some great Chinese food. This root has also long been used in Traditional Chinese Medicine as an anti-inflammatory and to relieve nausea. We use it today to treat motion sickness, nausea, tummy aches, migraines, and inflammatory conditions such as juvenile rheumatoid arthritis.

Ginger can be eaten as a food or candy (watch out, though, it's hot!), grated or sliced thinly and used to make a tea with honey, or taken as an extract. Kids six to twelve can take 250 to 500 mg of encapsulated freeze-dried extract up to three times a day. Take liquid extract at one half the recommended adult dosage listed on the package for kids six to twelve, and one quarter the adult dose for children two to six.

**Garlic** (*Allium sativum*). This familiar kitchen herb, and its relative the onion (*Allium cepa*), provide sulfur-containing compounds that appear to lower blood pressure, decrease cholesterol, fight disease-causing microbes, and improve immune function. Though data on children is scant, we have lots of experience using garlic successfully to stave off upper-respiratory infections.

Start putting lots of garlic in your kids' food from an early age and they'll grow up to be big fans of this healthy bulb. In fact, food is the best way to get garlic into children. Just chop it, let it rest for a few minutes to develop the most beneficial compounds, and use raw or lightly cooked. (Eating parsley or protein at the same time may reduce potential breath problems.) For kids who for some wild reason cannot bear the smell or taste of "the stinking herb," deodorized garlic extracts are available in solid or liquid form. Look for a product standardized for at least 1.3 percent allicin.

In our experience garlic is a very safe herb. Rarely, garlic or onion use by a breastfeeding mother may cause stomach upset in sensitive infants, though there is conflicting evidence that some babies feed better when nursing moms eat these herbs. As with ginger, discontinue use two weeks before any surgery just in case.

**Elder** (*Sambucus nigra*). The berry of the European black elder contains compounds that inhibit two most common strains of flu virus from reproducing in the body. We prescribe elderberry extract at the first sign of the flu (there is no evidence as yet that it has any effect on colds). In our experience it can stop flu nearly in its tracks in some people, and in others greatly reduce its severity and duration. The usual dose for children is 1 teaspoon 2 to 3 times a day, but more specific dosing instructions may be found on the label.

**Stinging Nettle** (*Urtica dioica*). We learned about stinging nettle for hay fever from Andrew Weil, who claims this herb has made more people believers in botanical medicine than any other. Capsules of freeze-dried stinging nettle extract can provide the symptom relief of antihistamines without the side effects. Reserve stinging nettle for children old enough to swallow capsules. When hay fever symptoms develop, give them 1 capsule every 4 hours until they feel better, which is usually by the third dose. (Nettle does not stop hay fever from occurring, but alleviates symptoms.) You can try a liquid extract of nettle, but in our experience it does not work as well.

Don't open capsules of freeze-dried stinging nettle and sprinkle the herb on or in food because it retains its sting in this form.

**Chamomile** (either *Matricaria recutita* or *Anthemis nobilis*). The daisylike flowers of this fragrant, low-growing plant have been used as a sedative and digestive aid for centuries. We use chamomile primarily in the form of a tea for the treatment of colic, anxiety, teething, upset stomach, or difficulties falling asleep. It has been shown in at least one study to limit the duration of diarrhea, when given in combination with pectin.

Steep fresh, good chamomile tea for 10 to 15 minutes and serve up to 3 or 4 ounces of the tea a day, diluted to taste, warm or cool. You can even give chamomile tea to infants at nighttime or naptime with a dropper or in a bottle.

It's unlikely, but children who are severely allergic to ragweed may be allergic to chamomile, a member of the same plant family. In such cases, a tea made from fennel seeds would work equally well for colic. Pregnant moms should not drink chamomile tea, as the herb can cause uterine contractions.

**Peppermint** (*Mentha piperita*). The lush, green, spreading herb peppermint has a long history of safe use as a digestive aid. If your little one is suffering from an upset tummy or colic, you might fix a cup of pleasant-tasting peppermint tea, following package directions. Be sure to cool to lukewarm before serving. Avoid the use of peppermint oil, which can cause choking in young children. We make an exception for enteric-coated capsules of peppermint oil, which can be used to treat irritable bowel syndrome in older children; the coating assures that the oil will not be released until the capsule reaches the intestine.

Children with reflux should avoid any form of peppermint, as it relaxes the sphincter between stomach and esophagus and can worsen their symptoms.

**Slippery elm** (*Ulmus rubra*). The inner bark of slippery elm is what herbalists call a demulcent, that is, it soothes mucous membranes. We recommend it for sore throats, coughs, and intestinal upsets. If using it for upper-respiratory infections, try lozenges, or a tea of 1 or 2 teaspoons of slippery-elm powder in hot water. For gastrointestinal problems, a thin gruel of the powder mixed with warm water or milk may be soothing.

**Calendula** (*Calendula officinalis*). Compounds in the flowers of this relative of the garden marigold act as an antiseptic and an anti-inflammatory. We use calendula lotions, creams, or gels for abrasions, burns, diaper rashes, and eczema.

**Aloe** (*Aloe vera*). Every kitchen should have an aloe plant in a pot on the windowsill. Then if little (or big) fingers get burned, all you have to do is slice off a little piece of this succulent tropical plant and open it up. Apply the sticky, soothing gel found inside the middle portion of the leaf to the burn. Aloes are undemanding, easy-to-grow plants, but you can also buy pure aloe gel at the drug or health food store. We use topical aloe not only for kitchen burns but for sunburns, canker sores, insect bites, psoriasis, and minor abrasions, as well.

We do not recommend using aloe to speed healing of surgical wounds, as it may actually slow down the healing process. We do not recommend that aloe be taken internally, as it can cause gastrointestinal cramping.

**Green tea** (*Camellia sinensis*). The potential health benefits of green tea are a hot research topic these days. We've been flooded with studies suggesting that the antioxidants and other healthful compounds in green tea can lower cholesterol, reduce the risk of heart disease and cancer, protect skin, and fight bacteria. Other research suggests that green tea, which is simply a less-processed form of the more familiar dark-brown tea, might help prevent cavities if drunk after a meal. The main reason we think it's a good idea to introduce your children to the taste of green tea while they are young is that green tea has potential long-term benefits against two of our biggest killers—heart disease and cancer.

Once found only in Asia, green tea is increasingly available at supermarkets, speciality stores, and Internet sites. To prepare, allow loose or bagged green tea to steep in hot but not boiling water for just a few minutes. Dr. Russ's kids like to spoon it out of his cup. They love the taste as is, but you can add a little sweetener if necessary. Green tea contains about as much caffeine as a cola drink, and a quarter to an eighth the caffeine of coffee (depending on your blend); decaffeinated brands are available.

Infants should not be given green tea, as there have been reports that it may interfere with their absorption of iron.

**Evening primrose and black currant oils.** Evening primrose (*Oenothera bienis*) is a common North American wild flower, and black currant (*Ribes nigrum*) is a European berry bush. EPO and BCO, the oils from these two plants, are good sources of the anti-inflammatory essential fatty acid known as GLA (gamma linolenic acid). We recommend EPO or BCO (which is more expensive) for eczema and other skin problems, and for other inflammatory disorders such as arthritis and inflammatory bowel disease.

Fairly high doses of these oils are needed, in the range of 125 mg twice a day for kids two to six and 250 mg twice a day for kids six to twelve, and it may take a month or two to see results. A blend of the two oils is also available, for which doses are ½ teaspoon a day for children fifteen months to three years, or 1 teaspoon a day for older children. These oils should not be given to children with epilepsy.

**Flax (*Linum spp.*).** The seeds of the flax plant are the greatest vegetarian source of omega-3 fatty acids. They also have a reputation for easing the symptoms of anti-inflammatory conditions and autoimmune disorders. While both ground flaxseeds (flax meal) and flaxseed oil contain omega-3 oils, flax meal is also high in fiber and the phytoestrogens called lignans. We recommend ground flax seeds for constipation and either the meal or the oil for itchy dry winter skin.

Flax seeds go rancid quickly when exposed to air, so it is essential to keep the seeds, the fresh oil, or freshly ground meal well sealed and refrigerated. We use a coffee grinder or blender to grind small batches of seeds into meal, and have found that a small, tightly sealed glass jar will keep the meal fresh for a few weeks in the refrigerator. We sprinkle a teaspoon of the pleasant-tasting meal on our kids' cereal or salad, and add it to smoothies or pancake batter. Golden flax oil can also be added to smoothies. Do not heat or cook with flax oil, or you will destroy its healthy compounds. (It's okay to bake with ground flax seeds.) Do not use any seeds, meal, or oil that smell like paint—a sign of rancidity.

Although they are heavily marketed herbs, we do not recommend either St. John's wort (*Hypericum perforatum*) or goldenseal (*Hydrastis Canadensis*) for children. St. John's wort does appear to have benefit for mild to moderate depression in adults, but we are strongly opposed to parents using this herb to treat a child. If you suspect depression, bring your child to a medical doctor. Goldenseal has been touted as an "herbal antibiotic," but there is little support for this claim. We recommend avoiding it, until it is clear whether overharvesting has made the plant endangered in some areas. Goldenseal is often packaged with echinacea in cold-and-flu herbal products, but in our opinion you would be better off using echinacea alone.

We'd also like to mention one more "herb" that might not ordinarily come to mind. Medicinal mushrooms—especially reishi (*Ganoderma lucidum*), shiitake (*Lentinus elodes*), and maitake (*Grifola frondosa*)—have been eaten in Asia for centuries as a way to boost the immune system. Today they are also an important complement to conventional cancer treatment in Japan and China and may help lower cholesterol levels as well. These mushrooms are best cooked and eaten as foods or made into teas, but they are also available as extracts. Dr.

Stu frequently uses an extract of maitake mushroom for fighting upper respiratory infections and flu.

In addition to these oral and topical uses of medicinal plants, there is a whole school of therapy based on the use of essential plant oils to influence physical and emotional well being. You are probably familiar with beauty products, room fragrances, and candles that employ aromatherapy, but may not have realized that essential oils of lavender, orange, vanilla, and other plants have therapeutic uses as well. We use aromatherapy diffusers in his office to create a more relaxed and welcoming atmosphere. These essential oils are finding their way into hospitals (scents are used to relax people having medical procedures such as magnetic-resonance imaging), massage-therapy offices, and other therapeutic locations especially because of their ability to influence mood.

Essential oils—highly concentrated plant extracts—are very strong and potentially toxic, so if they are to be used with children, special care must be taken to avoid oral use (an exception is made for enteric-coated peppermint oil for children over 44 pounds) or use of the undiluted oil directly on a child's skin. Never apply essential oils in or around the nose, mouth, or eyes of a child, but confine their use to the areas of chest and back. Keep them where children cannot reach them, as drinking them can be lethal. When buying an essential oil, make sure to get pure products and not synthetic scents. For instance, don't be fooled into buying lavendin (a synthetic) rather than oil of lavender.

We use a few essential oils, but rarely more than one or two drops. When an essential oil is to be used on a child's skin, it should always be well diluted in lotion or a vegetable or nut "carrier" oil such as almond or olive oil. With essential oils, less is more. You really only need one drop of an oil on a child's blanket or pillow, one drop in a warm bath, one or two drops in a handful of carrier oil or lotion, or a few drops in a diffuser (which warms and spreads the scent with no physical contact with the oil). The essential oils we are most comfortable using with children are the following:

**Lavender** (*Lavendula angustifolia*). The oils from this familiar purple and gray border plant were the first to be studied by René-Maurice Gattefossé, the French chemist considered the father of medical aromatherapy. Studies have found lavender oil to have both antiseptic and sedative properties. We use it mostly for relaxation—on a blanket, in bath water, in massage oil, or through a diffuser. Vanilla has a similar relaxing effect for some people. In France, bunches or bags of lavender flowers are often hung near a child's cot to promote restful sleep.

**Eucalyptus** (*Eucalyptus radiata*). The leaves of this tree from Australia contain aromatic oils that fight congestion and bacteria. We rec-

---

# *S*ummary *of Useful Herbs for Children*

Echinacea for colds and flu, and as tonic

Astragalus as a tonic, especially after or to prevent recurrent respiratory illness

Ginger for nausea, tummy troubles, and inflammation

Garlic for infections

Elderberry for flu

Stinging nettle for hay fever

Chamomile for colic, teething, anxiety, and sleeplessness

Peppermint for tummy troubles

Slippery elm for sore throat and tummy troubles

Flax for constipation, inflammatory or autoimmune disorders, and dry skin

Green tea for general good health

Evening primrose or black currant oil for skin problems

Calendula for diaper rash and other skin problems

Aloe for sunburn and burns

Lavender for relaxation (aromatherapy)

Eucalyptus for congestion (aromatherapy)

Tea tree oil for cuts and fungal infections

ommend a few drops of essential oil of eucalyptus in a cup of vegetable oil as a rub for a congested chest. A single drop of eucalyptus oil can also be put on a corner of a child's blanket to help unstuff a stuffy nose. Eucalyptus oil is poisonous, so keep out of the reach of children.

**Tea tree** (*Melaleuca alternifolia*). The aboriginal people of Australia used the leaves of the tea tree as a potent germicide to prevent infections in wounds. We recommend it in a diluted form as a natural antiseptic for cuts, scrapes, insect bites, and acne. Dr. Russ also uses it as a topical antifungal for athlete's foot and ringworm, and uses it undiluted on fungal nails (the only time that it can be used undiluted). Be cautious with use, as tea tree oil is strong and can cause a rash in sensitive people.

# Buying Botanical Medicines

Herbal products are so easily available in the marketplace, and their claims may be so expansive, that we would like to give you a few tips to make you a more informed consumer. We recommend you start with some research of your own and consultation with your child's doctor to determine the herb needed. We also recommend a visit to one of the Internet sites (see Resources) that offers information on the quality of various herbal products by brand, as some products have been found in laboratory tests to contain very little of the actual herb advertised. In addition:

- Look for products from reputable companies.
- Look for standardized extracts, which guarantee a specific amount of an active or marker compound.
- Look for products that contain the same species (Latin name) and parts of the plant used in the scientific medical research you have found.
- Look for products that use fresh herbs.
- Look for organic products when possible.
- Look for the letters NF or USP to indicate the product meets standards set by the United States Pharmacopoeia.

- Look for single herb products rather than combinations.
- To make sure the product is fresh, check the expiration date.
- Check the dosage. Two brands may charge the same dollar amount for sixty capsules, but if the daily dosage is 500 mg and the capsules in one bottle are 100 mg and the capsules in the other are 250 mg, the second bottle is obviously the better buy.
- Be wary of extravagant claims from manufacturers. Advertising for herbal products is not well regulated.

# Chapter 13

# Like Cures Like:

*Homeopathic Medicine for Children*

a t first glance, homeopathy appears to be a bit of a tough sell. After all, how likely are most people to be interested in a form of medicine that claims to cure people sick with fever and chills with a medicine that gives *healthy* people fever and chills? A form of medicine that relies on little sugar pills that may contain less than a molecule of the allegedly therapeutic agent, pills made from odd and sometimes toxic substances such as squid ink, red onions, duck's liver, daisies, arsenic, and table salt? Not likely, right? Well, truthfully, we looked at homeopathic medicine with a pretty jaundiced eye at first, too. But we kept hearing good reports from patients who were using homeopathic remedies to nip influenza in the bud, treat ear infections, ease teething pain, and take the "owie" out of bee stings. Now we no longer dismiss homeopathy as an oddball practice. Even though we cannot explain *how* it works, it often *does* work. Most conventional Western medical authorities say this is due to a placebo effect (although studies cast doubt on that theory). We say if minor injuries and minor (or some chronic) illnesses can be alleviated safely and easily, we're happy with the results.

We ourselves are still just getting acquainted with the homeopathic approach, but we feel comfortable recommending homeopathy to parents to use on their children for first aid and minor, self-limiting illnesses because the remedies are safe, inexpensive, and—when used properly—often appear to be of benefit. We would refer parents of children with chronic illnesses (such as asthma, recurrent otitis media, anxiety, or attention deficit disorder) that might benefit from an in-depth homeopathic evaluation and stronger remedies to a medical, osteopathic, or naturopathic physician who is board certified in classical homeopathy. We do not recommend homeopathic medicine for acute, life-threatening illness.

Homeopathy may well be the hardest therapy for a conventional physician to swallow. After all, if there is not even a molecule of the active agent left in some of the more potent homeopathic remedies, how can they cure anything? There are all sorts of theories as to how it might work, the acceptance of which generally depends on a willingness to suspend current medical beliefs. Some advocates of homeopathy suggest that certain steps in the preparation of a highly dilute homeopathic remedy make available the inherent "vital energy" of the active substance, perhaps by imprinting the remedy with the "memory" of this agent. (It's not hard to see why homeopathy is hard for Western science to swallow, is it?) If homeopathy is indeed a form of energy medicine (see chapter 15) as some hypothesize, Western medicine may need to change its current understanding of healing before we even have the concepts and tools to figure out how homeopathy works. However, in the case of homeopathy we think it may be less important to ask "does it make sense?" than, "does it work?" And it's only fair to say that we don't understand how many of the conventional treatments work either.

So far, there are a few solid studies published in medical journals finding homeopathic remedies effective in a few situations (diarrhea in children, influenza and vertigo in adults), and a recent survey of the literature that found homeopathy in general to be better than a placebo. In fact, many conventional physicians in Great Britain, Germany, France, India, and some parts of South America are trained in homeopathic medicine and prescribe homeopathic remedies as a matter of course. Here in the United States, where it is more difficult to find a homeopathic practitioner, many people use homeopathic remedies for self-care, and the market is booming—$250 million worth of the remedies were sold in 1996, and sales are still climbing as the

European makers of homeopathic products move into U.S. markets.

Homeopathic medicine does have a history in the United States. In the late 1800s homeopathy was the most popular form of medical care here. There were twenty-two colleges of medicine and more than a hundred hospitals based on the principles of homeopathy developed by German physician Samuel Hahnemann earlier in that century. Like the founder of osteopathic medicine, Andrew Taylor Still, Samuel Hahnemann was looking for gentler alternatives to the often brutal treatments of conventional medicine of the time. While experimenting with cinchona bark, a botanical treatment for the fever and chills of malaria, Hahnemann discovered that giving high doses of the bark to healthy people gave them fever and chills, which stopped when the bark was withdrawn. He was intrigued by this idea that "like cures like," which dates back to Hippocrates. With further research, Hahnemann found that extreme dilutions of the bark produced the greatest healing response. He performed continued experiments ("provings") with various plant, animal, and mineral substances throughout his life, producing the first hundred remedies in the homeopathic pharmacy.

Over the course of his career, Hahnemann developed the two primary principles of homeopathy:

1. *The law of similars.* Substances that cause certain symptoms in healthy people can cure those same symptoms in sick people. The word "homeopathy" comes from the Greek roots *homeo* ("the same") and *pathos* ("disease") and reflects this principle. Hahnemann dubbed conventional medicine "allopathy" (*allo* is Greek for "other"), because its treatments (antibiotics or fever suppressants, for example) act in a way that is dissimilar to the disease process.

2. *The law of infinitesimals.* The most potent remedies are those that have been diluted and vigorously shaken ("succussed") the most times—so many times, in fact, that a strong remedy may not even have a complete molecule of the therapeutic substance left in it. The letters X and C on the labels indicate how much a remedy has been diluted at each step. To make a remedy, a substance that causes certain symptoms in a healthy person is diluted in alcohol and/or purified water either one part substance to 9 parts solvent (1X) or one part sub-

stance to 99 parts solvent (1C) and shaken vigorously. They are then diluted at a ratio of 1:9 or 1:99 again (2X or 2C), and again (3X or 3C), and again, to the potency desired. Most homeopathic remedies for self-care are 6X, 12X or 30C; those prescribed by trained homeopaths may be as strong as 200C, 1M(1:999), or higher. The correct dose should match the intensity of the symptoms and achieve the desired effect, while minimizing potential reactions.

Homeopathic practitioners—much like practitioners of osteopathy, chiropractic, and Chinese medicine—believe that there is a subtle energy (homeopaths call it "vital energy," other practitioners call it "life force," or "Qi") that is the foundation of good health. Homeopaths address imbalances in the body's systems by enlisting this vital energy to restore the body's own healing power. Symptoms are seen as the body's attempts to heal itself, and this process is reinforced by medications that produce the same symptoms. This is a radically different perspective from conventional Western medicine, which is focused on suppressing symptoms.

"Classical" homeopaths treat the whole person, not just the disease. A homeopathic practitioner relies on questions and answers more than physical examination or laboratory testing. A first visit usually lasts an hour and a half to two hours (subsequent visits are much shorter). During that time, a homeopath will listen carefully and ask many questions, some of which might seem off-the-wall. The patient would of course be asked to describe the symptoms that brought him or her to the office. The homeopath will also ask the patient about the influences upon him at the time he became sick, whether he is currently cranky or worried or frightened, whether he feels better when hot or when cold, what foods he craves or cannot bear, and so on. The object of this interview is to assemble a constitutional profile of a patient that includes his or her unique combination of physical symptoms, personality, likes and dislikes, and mental and emotional state.

A classical homeopath then looks for the one specific remedy out of several thousand in the modern homeopathic pharmacy that most closely parallels the patient's profile. This is the remedy that will bring that patient back into balance. Only one remedy is given at a time. A "constitutional" remedy works at a very deep level to address physical and emotional issues and chronic conditions. Such a remedy is expected to cure not only the presenting problem, but all other symptoms as well. If it does not show effect within five weeks, another remedy may be prescribed. High-potency constitutional doses are usually available only from practitioners.

Classical homeopaths may also do what is called "acute prescribing," where they focus less on correcting your child's individual constitutional imbalances than on looking for a way to treat the problem that has brought the child to the office. In this case, the homeopathic practitioner examines the way this particular cold, say, affects this particular child physically and emotionally in order to determine which of the single cold remedies is best suited to his or her symptoms. The remedy will be less potent and taken more frequently than a constitutional remedy, should work more quickly, and will not be expected to treat anything but the presenting problem.

We have heard anecdotal evidence of excellent results from constitutional and acute remedies prescribed by homeopaths. We recommend you look for an experienced health practitioner who is board certified in homeopathy, has at least 500 to 1,000 hours of training, and is experienced in working with children. To ensure that health conditions that require conventional care are recognized, we advise homeopaths who have medical training rather than lay homeopaths. There are only a few thousand M.D.'s, osteopaths, naturopaths, and other health practitioners in this country who are well trained in homeopathic medicine (check professional organizations in the Resources for referrals), so it may well be that there is no one practicing homeopathy in your area. In that case you can consider telephone consultations with distant practitioners as a possibility, because this form of therapy relies so strongly on the interview. Be aware that there are some homeopaths who oppose childhood immunizations and suggest homeopathic alternatives; we strongly disagree with this attitude.

# Using Homeopathic Remedies

Homeopathic remedies are made from a wide variety of substances found in nature. *Allium cepa*, a common remedy for the weeping eyes and runny nose of colds, is made from red onion, which we all know makes us weepy when we cut it. *Coffea* from the coffee bean is paradoxically one of the many remedies for insomnia. *Apis*, a great remedy for bee stings, is made from the honeybee. Other remedies are made from materials as dissimilar as table salt, the venom of the bushmaster snake, windflowers, iron, St. John's wort, arsenic, and mercury. Any toxic substances used are present in such dilute amounts (if at all) that even the FDA categorizes homeopathic remedies as GRAS (generally recognized as safe). Although a number of homeopathic remedies are made from plants, homeopathy should not be confused with herbal medicine, as its principles and preparation methods are strikingly different.

It is important to underscore the individual nature of a homeopathic remedy. Because homeopathy looks at the whole person—body, mind, and emotions—two people with the same illness might respond best to different remedies because of different symptoms, different emotional states, or different conditions leading to the illness. It is also important to underscore the benign nature of homeopathic remedies, which cause no side effects or drug interactions.

The homeopathic remedies that are available over the counter at health food stores or pharmacies, or by mail order are generally low potency. Parents interested in using homeopathic remedies to care for their kids' minor illnesses can experiment with them without doing harm. Just be sure to contact your child's doctor at the first sign of something more serious brewing.

The individual or combination remedies available to laypeople are most commonly little sugar or lactose pellets or tablets or liquid formulas. Oral remedies are taken sublingually, that is, under the tongue. To take pellets or tablets, tap the suggested dosage into the cap of the bottle it came in, then pour the remedy out of the cap into the child's mouth. Have the child keep the pellets or tablets under her tongue, until they dissolve. Liquids are dropped from a dropper or the disposable container into the mouth under the tongue. Children usually like oral homeopathic remedies because they taste sweet, and so they don't fight treatment. There are also topical homeopathic products such as gels and creams for such conditions as diaper rash, itching, bruising, and muscular soreness.

Over the years, homeopaths have learned that certain foods, medications, and environmental factors can sometimes nullify the effects of a remedy. There are long and conflicting lists of these "antidotes," but we suggest that a child taking a homeopathic remedy avoid at least products containing aromatic oils such as menthol, peppermint, tea tree, camphor, and eucalyptus (hold off on the VapoRub) and coffee in any form (even ice cream). Keep remedies in a cool, dark, dry place away from strong-smelling substances.

How do you know which remedy to choose? For instance, depending on the situation, any of the remedies listed on page 231 might treat a cold.

We think it's worthwhile for parents who are interested in using homeopathic remedies for family self-care to do a little research first: take a class or a mail-order course, read a few books. (Check our Resource section for ideas.) We do recommend that you find a reference book to ground you in the philosophy and help you decide which remedies are called for in which situations. Remember that you must consider the person who *has* the illness—and not just the illness—when you are choosing a course of treatment. Ask your child questions like these: What were you doing before this started? How do you feel about this illness—are you worried or frightened? How does your whole body feel—are you hungry, thirsty, or sleepy? What are your specific symptoms? Do you feel better in warm places or cool ones? Do you feel better sitting up or lying down, on your left side or your right? Are there any foods you're craving or foods that disgust you right now? Look for the remedy that covers the widest number of symptoms.

Once you have chosen a remedy, give your child a dose per the package instructions. Remedies available over the counter are gener-

## Seven Possible Homeopathic Remedies for the Common Cold

*Allium cepa*—Sneezing, watery eyes, profuse and irritating nasal discharge

*Gelsemium*—Heavy eyelids, no thirst, dizzy, exhausted

*Bryonia*—Dry cough, irritable, thirsty, worse from motion

*Hepar Sulfuris*—Yellow mucus; congestion in chest, sinus, and ears; smells sour

*Kali bichromicum*—Thick yellow-green mucus, sinus congestion

*Natrum muriaticum*—Profuse mucus like raw egg white, sneezing, loss of taste and smell

*Pulsatilla*—Nose runs daytime only, yellowish mucus, better from sympathy

There are also remedies that are especially useful in the first stages of a cold, one for a cold that comes on suddenly (*Aconite*) and one for a cold that comes on slowly (*Ferrum phosphoricum*).

ally 6X, 12X, or 30C—all low potency. The lower the potency of the remedy (6X vs. 30C for example), the more frequently it will generally be given. Stop giving a remedy as soon as symptoms begin to abate and your child is on the path to healing. If symptoms do not improve after three doses, rethink your choice of remedy, and try once again. Call your health practitioner if symptoms persist for more than three days or worsen. Keep track of what works for each of your kids, so you know what to try first the next time a similar problem occurs.

Parents unable to deal with making a choice of single remedy may prefer to start with a combination remedy. These are broad-spectrum amalgams of two or more different remedies used to treat the condition, a disease-oriented, "something for everyone" approach that many find counter to Hahnemann's basic philosophy. Although the treatment is not as well targeted as a single remedy, it appeals to those times when we cannot decide which remedy is best. It will not work at all, however, if the correct single remedy for your child is not one of the ones included in the formula. That's one reason we lean more toward the single-remedy than the combination approach.

Once again, we suggest that parents give their children over-the-counter homeopathic remedies only for first aid (either as treatment or as a holding action while on the way to the doctor or emergency department) or for minor self-limiting illnesses—the same sorts of sit-

---

 *Homeopathic First-Aid Kit*

Ready-made kits are available, but if you want to put one together one for your family, here are a few common remedies that could come in handy when treating children:

*Chamomilla*—teething, insomnia, colic
*Arnica*—bruises and sports injuries
*Allium cepa*—colds, hay fever
*Euphrasia*—irritated eyes, conjuctivitis, hay fever
*Apis*—bee stings, burns, hives
*Hypericum*—slamming finger in a door, toothache, sinus pain
*Gelsemium*—summer colds, fever, headache
*Rhus toxicodendron*—sprains, strains, and tendinitis when worse after rest
*Ruta graveolens*—sprains, strains, and tendinitis when better with rest
*Belladonna*—sudden acute fever or pain, but no fear
*Aconite*—sudden acute inflammation when patient is frightened or anxious
*Nux vomica*—indigestion, nausea, stomachache
*Anas barbariae* (often sold as Oscillococcinum)—influenza
*Pulsatilla*—ear infections and upper respiratory infections

uations where you might turn to herbal or synthetic forms of over-the-counter medications. Books and practitioners vary in their lists of the most useful remedies for children, so we have compiled a general list at the end of this chapter to get you started.

Try not to be so free with the use of your homeopathic medicine kit that your children develop the idea that every physical and emotional condition requires some form of medication. Physical and emotional balance is a dynamic process, and typically we have the ability to right most problems ourselves, without the help of outside forces.

We want to repeat that we ourselves are just learning about homeopathy, and are in no way expert in this field. However, we do think this form of medicine provides a promising avenue both for medical research and personal experimentation (at least in the case of mild disease) without significant risk.

# Chapter 14

# A Billion People Can't Be Wrong:

*Chinese Medicine for Children*

Y ou are probably familiar with the practice of acupuncture, a therapy borrowed from Chinese medicine that relies on the relatively painless placement of thin needles into the body at precise locations to alleviate pain or restore health. However, you may not realize that acupuncture is just one of five major branches of a complex system of medicine developed over centuries that encompasses not just acupuncture, but also herbal treatments, medicinal nutrition, therapeutic massage, and meditative exercise. Studies published in Western medical journals have reported that various forms of Chinese Medicine (CM) appear to be useful for pain, asthma, ear infections, headache, eczema, irritable bowel syndrome, balance problems, high blood pressure, sports injuries, and chemotherapy-induced nausea; there is a vast amount of clinical evidence published in Chinese medical literature for other uses as well.

We ourselves are not experts in this area, but we do refer patients to practitioners of Chinese Medicine as complementary therapy for certain acute conditions and for many chronic conditions for which Western medicine has no cure or clear treatment. Although we find the philosophy behind Chinese Medicine appealing, we do not begin to understand how it works. We only know that it frequently gets results in cases that have stymied Western medical specialists. We have the most experience with acupuncture. Dr. Russ has had patients with asthma and with juvenile rheumatoid arthritis who responded well to acupuncture, with an increased sense of well-being, a decrease in symptoms, a lessening of stress, and sometimes a reduced need for medication. Dr. Stu has found acupuncture to successfully reduce pain, treat recurrent ear infections and migraines, and even improve hearing in two hearing-impaired patients. Our experiences make it clear to us that there are many useful things conventional Western practitioners could learn from this ancient way of healing.

# The Theories Behind Chinese Medicine

Over the past few millennia the Chinese have developed a system of medicine quite unlike our own, one based less on a philosophy of science than on a philosophy of nature. While Western doctors were still bleeding, purging, and otherwise mishandling the sick, the Chinese already possessed a sophisticated medical philosophy and numerous noninvasive therapies that had been tested over generations. We use the term "medical philosophy" because to the Chinese, healing was part and parcel of their Taoist philosophy of wholeness and balance. The basis of both healing practice and spiritual practice was the concept of qi (also called chi and pronounced "chee"), the invisible flow of vital energy or life force that circulates throughout the universe, and permeates the human body. In a healthy person, qi flows unimpeded, but a person who is ill is considered to have a blockage of qi that creates a deficiency or excess of energy in certain areas. The purpose of Chinese Medicine is to locate and release these obstructions, and restore good health by moving qi into areas where it is lacking. The practitioner of CM has many, many therapeutic options. Imbalances of qi can be treated with acupuncture, herbs, meditative movement, massage, and/or certain diets.

Since no one has ever seen qi, this concept has been very hard for

## Differing Philosophies

| Western | Eastern |
| --- | --- |
| Doctor as mechanic | Doctor as gardener |
| Symptoms determine treatment | Energy evaluation determines treatment |
| Condition stands alone | Condition seen in context |
| Emphasis on physical symptoms | Physical, mental, emotional, energetic, and social influences considered |
| High-tech | Low-tech |
| Disease caused by germ or abnormality | Disease caused by imbalance in body |
| Emphasis on fixing what's "broken" | Emphasis on bolstering what's "good" |
| Biochemical and biomechanical model | Bio-energetic model |
| Treatment aimed at offending part of body | |
| Independence of body systems | Treatment aimed at whole body |
| | Interdependence of body systems |

conventional Western practitioners to accept. Western medicine focuses mostly on the physical state of the body. We determine a disease state or abnormality by examination and testing of the body, and aim treatment at the part of the body found to be "diseased." Chinese Medicine is more holistic; treatment is based not just on physical symptoms, but also on the person's emotional and energetic state and relationship with the environment. Treatment attempts to improve health throughout the body, rather than just in one system, because the Chinese believe that all body systems are interconnected by the flow of qi. While sometimes the goal is just to relieve symptoms, more frequently the goal is to balance and strengthen the body so that healing can take place. The Chinese doctor compares himself to a gardener (a telling difference from the Western doctor-as-warrior or doctor-as-mechanic metaphors) whose goal is to tend so well to all the aspects of the patient that the individual can meet any challenges to his health.

The basic principles and modalities of Chinese Medicine have been adapted over the centuries to reflect various schools of thought and national differences. Although CM was revitalized during the days of Chairman Mao's "barefoot doctors," today even the Chinese health system offers the techniques of conventional Western medicine, too. In much the same way, we in the West have been incorporating traditional Chinese therapies into our own medical practice and adapting them to our own needs ever since journalist James Reston famously declared, "I have seen the past, and it works!" after receiving pain-relieving acupuncture treatment on a trip to China in the 1970s. There are now two main forms of acupuncture in the United States. Several thousand American medical doctors have received training in medical acupuncture, a westernized system of diagnosis and treatment. About 10,000 non-M.D.'s (and a small number of physicians) have received much more extensive training in traditional acupuncture at one of the fifty colleges of acupuncture and Oriental medicine in the United States or at one of the colleges in China. Herbs integral to Chinese Medicine—ginseng, ginger, and licorice, for example— have become very popular here as well. We integrative practitioners have borrowed from Chinese Medicine our foundational principles: belief in the importance of balance, the oneness of mind and body, and the ability of the body to heal itself with the proper support.

CM is a complete system of medicine, although it is more commonly used in the United States as complementary medicine. Based on the ideal of harmony and balance, CM teaches that a truly healthy person needs to be in harmony within body, family, community, and universe. We find this very poetic approach to health especially appealing as it underscores the importance of integration of mind and body and interconnection with our neighbors and our surroundings.

However, the very poetics of CM may make it difficult for Western minds to wrap around it. We are not accustomed to medical practitioners who talk about yin and yang, the Three Treasures, the Five Elements, the Eight Principles, or an invisible organ like the Triple-Burner.

The rock-bottom foundation of CM is the principle of yin and yang, universal forces of energy that must be in balance for physical and social health. The balance between yin and yang is very dynamic—it can vary by time of day, physical condition, energetic excesses or deficiency, diet, stage of life, etc. We all have both yin and yang within us, even though yin is described as "female" and yang as "male." Yin is considered to be moist, cold, dark, passive, material, and nourishing. Yang is considered to be dry, hot, light, active, energetic, and transforming. (It's no surprise that children are considered to be deficient in yin and high in yang.) The best description we have seen of this duality comes from Efrem Korngold and Harriet Beinfield, who say in their book, *Between Heaven and Earth: A Guide to Chinese Medicine*, "If Yin is a noun, then Yang is a verb, and life is a complete sentence."

CM organizes the body functionally along yin/yang lines, which is another difficult leap for people trained in Western medicine. In this system five yin/yang pairs of organs are said to rule physical and mental/emotional functions: Spleen/Stomach, Heart/Small Intestine, Liver/Gall Bladder, Lung/Large Intestine, and Kidney/Bladder (plus Pericardium and Triple-Burner, two special organs). For instance, the lung and large intestine are considered to control the body's defenses, which in CM include not only respiration, and the functions of skin and mucous membranes, but also inspiration and letting go of attachments. In diagnosing a health problem (or imbalance of qi), a practitioner of CM will try to determine whether the organ is too yin or too yang, too "dry" or too "damp," too "hot" or too "cold." Because of differences in philosophy and terminology, what we in the West call a headache, a practitioner of CM might attribute to a deficiency of spleen yang with an excess of dampness and cold. These excesses or deficiencies will then be remedied with an individualized treatment plan that makes use of acupuncture, herbal medicines, massage, meditation, and/or certain foods.

# Important Terms in CM

*Qi.* Life force or energy that flows through the universe and through the human body.

*Yin/Yang.* Dualities (damp-dry, hot-cold) that must be harmonized for good health.

*Organ networks.* Five paired organs that control the physical, mental, emotional, and spiritual functions of the body.

*Meridians.* Channels or pathways through which qi circulates in the body.

*Acupuncture.* Use of special needles inserted at points in the meridians where qi can be accessed to influence the function of organ systems.

*Moxibustion.* A form of needleless acupuncture in which the Chinese herb *moxa* (mugwort) is burned to heat acupuncture points.

*Tui na.* Medical massage techniques designed to influence the flow of qi.

CM offers very individual treatment that takes into account the full person and that person's role in family and community, looking very closely at the underlying emotional or energetic causes for symptoms, assessing the general state of health, and choosing from a wide variety of possible remedies. That is why, unlike in Western medicine, two people with the same diagnosis—indigestion, for example—may well be given different treatments. And that is why, unlike in Western medicine, two people with different symptoms may well be given the same treatment, if a practitioner feels the same underlying imbalance is at work in both cases.

# The Therapies of Chinese Medicine

Practitioners of CM use acupuncture, herbal medicine, massage, exercise/ meditation, and medicinal foods to restore balance and create an integrated and healthy system. As you can imagine, a visit to a practitioner of Chinese Medicine is very different from a visit to an M.D. The CM practitioner will take a thorough medical history, and perform a specialized physical examination, but that's where the resemblance ends. A doctor of Chinese Medicine may ask whether your child is thirsty, where and how she sweats, how connected she feels to your family, and other unusual questions. Some of the physical symptoms attended to (such as how your child smells) will be atypical, as well. The doctor will feel for not one pulse in an older child's wrist, but at least six—at different depths—to determine the state of the various organs. In infants and younger children, the veins at the base of each index finger may be examined, as will the appearance of the tongue. The child's body will be palpated at acupuncture and other points, looking for tender areas. The intention is to evaluate the life force in your child's body—how it is moving, where it is blocked, and where it is stagnant. Treatment may involve some form of acupuncture or massage to normalize or enhance the flow of qi, and/or a combination of herbs to address systemic excesses or deficiencies.

How do you find a practitioner of Chinese Medicine? Our first choice would be by referral from your child's doctor, but we know that is not often possible. So we suggest you contact one of the organizations listed in our Resource section for referrals to practitioners in your area. Be aware that the length of practitioner training can vary tremendously from weeks to years, and credentialing varies by state. Our preference is for practitioners who use the true Eastern-philosophy-based approach and have had the extensive training and clinical experience required for an O.M.D (Oriental Medical Doctor), an M.Ac.O.M. (a three-year master's degree in Acupuncture and Oriental Medicine), or L.Ac. (licensed acupuncturist). Look for someone who has trained in China, or graduated from three- to four-year training at an accredited college of Chinese Medicine. Try to find a practitioner who is certified by the National Commission for the Certification of Acupuncturists and Oriental Medicine (NCCAOM). Your insurance may cover these health-care professionals, especially if your doctor refers you.

For acupuncture alone, we would also feel comfortable referring patients to an M.D., D.O., or a naturopathic doctor (N.D.) who has been licensed and board certified in acupuncture, as long as he or she has had education and experience in caring for children. Be forewarned that even well-trained practitioners of acupuncture may not have expertise in the art of Chinese herbal medicine.

We believe that children should get their primary care from an M.D. or a D.O. trained to recognize the warning signs of serious medical illness. However, we do think CM can be very useful for preventive care or for complementary treatment of both short- or long-term conditions. Just be sure your child's pediatrician is aware of your visits to the acupuncturist or O.M.D, and that the Eastern practitioner is aware of any conventional medications your child is taking. A child should not stop important drugs, such as those for asthma or arthritis, while undergoing CM treatment, although the treatments may eventually enable your child to reduce the drug dosage with the consent of his or her physician.


**a**cupuncture. This is the form of CM we most frequently recommend and that people in the United States are most likely to use. There are a number of systems of acupuncture being practiced, but they are all based on the idea that qi flows through invisible meridians or channels that form the energy distribution network of the body. We have six distinct pairs of these meridians (yin and yang, of course) going up and down the body, and each of these energy channels is associated with a specific organ system. For instance, an acupuncturist might work on a point known as Large Intestine 20 (remember that the organ system known as Lung/Large Intestine governs the mucous membranes) to relieve nasal congestion. Many individual channels exist as well. A skilled practitioner is able to either activate or inhibit qi in organs associated with an acupuncture point by inserting very fine needles into the body at that point and letting them rest there for a period of time. This does not feel like an injection. There may be no discomfort at all besides a quick "tug," or a brief stinging sensation when a needle is inserted. Once the needles are inserted, many people report a sense of well-being and relaxation, to the point of falling asleep on the table.

Traditional Chinese acupuncture works with the whole body. There are forms developed in other countries that work only on points in the ear, hand, foot, or scalp (especially effective for cerebral palsy), but still address the whole body. In this country we also have a hybrid form of acupuncture practiced by many medical doctors that is called medical acupuncture. True to Western reductionist thinking, medical acupuncture uses those points codified as being associated with a specific conventional Western diagnosis, rather than looking at the whole person. Unlike practitioners of CM, medical acupuncturists will usually give the same treatment to all people with the same diagnosis, regardless of emotional or energetic state. Even so, it does appear to offer symptomatic relief to many patients.

Although there are studies and a great deal of anecdotal evidence that acupuncture can be effective for a number of conditions in children and adults, no one knows yet how it works. It is clearly not just a placebo effect. It appears that acupuncture can stimulate the production of pituitary hormones called endorphins that can relieve pain and affect the brain's production of chemicals and neurotransmitters as well. In recent neuroimaging studies, stimulation of distant acupuncture points traditionally associated with the eye and ear were seen to affect the portions of the brain that control those organs.

Some practitioners of Chinese medicine do not use acupuncture on children under the age of seven because they believe that the meridians of young children are not fully formed and that their qi is too changeable. Others choose to use smaller and finer needles in deference to the smaller size and more immature systems of younger patients; these needles are inserted less deeply and for only a few seconds at a time. The goal is just to give the body a subtle push that allows it to adjust itself.

If your child refuses to become a human pincushion, you might consider needleless acupuncture. Various forms include a kind of electroacupuncture that does not use needles, magnet acupuncture, moxibustion (use of heat over acupuncture points), acupressure, laser acupuncture, or Japanese systems of needleless pediatric acupuncture, such as toyo hari or Shonishin, which uses special tools to stroke or tap acupuncture points.

We feel comfortable with parents bringing their children to an acupuncturist for colds, sinusitis, chronic cough, ear infections, asthma, dental pain, constipation/diarrhea, or bedwetting. After talking with your child's doctor, you may also decide to use acupuncture for headaches, nausea, depression, and anxiety. Any child whose system appears to be out of balance (from chronic illness or severe stress, for example) is also a good candidate for acupuncture. As we said before, look for practitioners with extensive training and experience in acupuncture for children.

You cannot do acupuncture on your children at home, which is

# Useful Acupressure Points

Locate the point described, press firmly but without pain with the pad of a finger or thumb (no fingernails!), and briefly massage in tight circles.

*For pain*: Press with the thumb on the highest point of the muscle in the webbing between other thumb and forefinger (Large Intestine 4). Mothers, do not stimulate this point on yourself during pregnancy.

*For nasal congestion*: Press with the index fingers on the face just outside the edge of the nostrils (Large Intestine 20)

*For headache associated with stress*: Press with tips of middle fingers in the two depressions at the base of the skull on either side of the spine (Gall Bladder 20)

why acupressure is such a useful tool for parents and kids. Acupressure moves qi by applying firm pressure rather than needles to acupuncture points. There is currently less supportive data for acupressure, but it has been used successfully to treat headache, dental pain, nasal congestion, asthma, fatigue, stomach problems, and the nausea of chemotherapy, as well as to maintain general good health. Acupressure is often part of a pediatric program that includes self-regulation techniques and the teaching of coping skills. One example of the use of acupressure is seen in those wristbands worn to ward off nausea from motion sickness, which press on a point known as Pericardium 6.

**Chinese medical massage (tui na).** Tui na (also seen as "tuina," and meaning "pushing and pulling") is the use of soft-tissue massage and acupressure techniques to move qi in the body of a (usually clothed) patient. Sometimes substances such as ginger water or sesame oil may be applied to enhance treatment. Tui na is often offered as a form of needleless acupuncture for children. The hand movements involved are very detailed and precise, so it would best to look for a practitioner with thorough training and much clinical experience. Unlike most Western forms of massage, therapeutic tui na massage emphasizes the importance of qi.

**Chinese herbology.** In CM, herbology is used to treat specific excesses and deficiencies in the organs (too much cold in Spleen or damp in Heart). A Chinese pharmacy is a fascinating place, loaded with boxes, jars, and drawers full of interesting things that have been found over the course of three thousand years to have curative powers. Chinese Medicine makes extensive use of a wide array of plant, animal, and mineral substances, which are all categorized as herbal remedies. Western researchers are just beginning to look more closely at Chinese herbal formulas, and recent articles in major medical journals have reported some of them to be quite effective in the treatment of irritable bowel syndrome, heart disease, and eczema.

In keeping with the principles of harmony and balance, herbs are always given in combination, rather than singly. An individual herbal prescription may include both major herbs that deal directly with the problem and minor ones that work synergistically with them and prevent side effects. In a true Chinese pharmacy, these herbs are combined and then cooked or made into a tea. However, since many of these concoctions taste and smell awful, common herbal combinations are also available in tablets, capsules, pellets, or liquid extracts. We strongly advise against buying any Chinese patent remedies such as you might find in Chinese markets or grocery stores. These products are frequently adulterated with prescription drugs, heavy metals, and other unwanted substances. For safety's sake, use fresh loose herbs only if they have been prescribed and provided by a reputable practitioner. Alternatively, use preformulated products made by reputable American companies, which have been prescribed and/or dispensed by your practitioner. (Be aware that a licensed acupuncturist has not necessarily been trained in Chinese herbology as well.)

Many Chinese herbal remedies have been safely used in small doses in children for generations, so they are probably safe if the herbs have been properly identified and freshly collected, if they have been safely stored and processed, and if they are correctly prescribed. These are a lot of "ifs." Due to our own lack of expertise in this field, we are still very cautious about Chinese herbology with children. We generally recommend only the use of the Asian herbs ginger and astragalus and the medicinal mushroom maitake.

**Exercise/meditation (tai chi, qi gong).** Chinese Medicine makes use of ages-old exercises said to promote the proper flow of qi through a combination of physical action and meditation. These disciplines are considered to be "internal" martial arts because of the meditative component, and are recommended for self-care to maintain good health and prevent illness. The most familiar to Westerners is tai chi. As discussed before, the slow-moving and gentle exercises of tai chi are very useful for improving balance and flexibility and for reducing stress. Each exercise has a fascinating name—such as Waving Hands in the Clouds and White Crane Spreads Its Wings—that provides an image of how the movement should be done. Children may enjoy tai chi, especially when done with their parents.

Qi gong encompasses many systems of exercise and meditation, as well as a therapeutic practice. Exercises vary from the nearly passive to the dynamic, so some form of qi gong can be done even by the bedridden. Medical qi gong as practiced traditionally in China employs these exercises as preventive health care or as complementary therapy for chronic conditions. In China there are also expert practitioners of qi gong who have become so skilled at accumulating and strengthening their own qi that they are apparently able to transmit it to others to stimulate healing. While we have heard some fascinating stories about how this form of energy healing is used in CM hospitals there, the possibilities for fraud or misrepresentation of skills and training seem too great here in the United States, where experts are few and far between. That's why we'll stick with recommending qi gong solely for self-care and maintenance of general good health.

**Medicinal foods**. In Chinese Medicine most foods are either yin or yang, and can thus be used to balance an excess or deficiency of these elements in the body. Foods are considered able to heat or cool, increase moisture or dryness, build qi and blood, normalize function, and restore proper digestion. For instance, an O.M.D. might suggest that a person with nausea eat some warming ginger to dispel the cold in his stomach. Someone who felt tired and low on energy might be advised to eat foods such as yams and dates that supplement qi. In China there are even restaurants that combine diagnosis with food, serving dishes deliberately designed to incorporate herbs and foods that address a person's specific health problems. Our own mothers, although not Chinese, are firmly convinced that chicken soup will work for anything that ails us!

# Chapter 15

# Good Vibrations:

*Energy Medicine for Children*

t he term "energy medicine" is probably not familiar to you. It's a new field of research and practice, and frankly, we are just learning about it ourselves. We find it intriguing, but difficult to explain using conventional medical terms. The explanations of energy medicine we have seen run the gamut from unscientifically "woo-woo" to dense and abstract (with a few too many references to quantum physics). Although initially we were both extremely skeptical about the concept, we are becoming more open to the idea, now that we have watched energy healers at work and heard reports from our patients. We have begun to recognize the subtle energies at work in our own lives, from the love we receive from our families to the intuition that often helps us serve our patients better. In fact, we all use and interpret interpersonal energy on a daily basis.

Physicists define energy as the capacity to do work, to cause an action or reaction. Simply put, then, energy medicine is based on the concept that we are energetic beings in an energetic universe—that we continuously interact with the life energy of the universe and produce energy ourselves through our thoughts and actions, and that this life energy can be sensed and manipulated for health and well-being. The concept of human energy fields may seem really weird, but the fact remains that we already have the language to talk about it. Like great art, most of us recognize energy medicine when we see it. For instance, we talk of a person as having "personal magnetism," or a place as having "bad vibes." The Beach Boys had a hit song called "Good Vibrations," and everyone knew what they meant. We talk about two people being "in synch," or "on the same wave length." We refer to people or events that really "drain our energy." Most of us have experienced the "click" of instant rapport with a new acquaintance or sensed somehow when someone else was watching us. We have all, at one time or another, had our own mood influenced by the anger, anxiety, or grief of others. We may well have asked someone to "send healing energy" when we were feeling ill.

As doctors, we know the effect that a health-care worker's "energy" can have on a patient. A doctor who comes into her office hurried and distracted will not have the same therapeutic effect as a physician who greets her patient with a smile and a warm handshake. We also have seen how often the "negative" or "positive" energy of a parent affects the course of a child's illness. Our intentions then, may be a form of subtle energy passed between us. Perhaps a doctor's empathy and desire to heal and a parent's unconditional love and sense of hope are all forms of healing energy.

But what does all this talk of "energy" have to do with *medicine?* There are entire medical philosophies that are grounded in the idea that good health depends on an unimpeded flow of vital energy through the body—among them Chinese Medicine, Ayurveda, osteopathic medicine, chiropractic, and homeopathy. Practitioners of these forms of medicine use tools such as acupuncture, acupressure, physical manipulation, and energetic remedies to strengthen or redirect the flow of energy in the body. Practitioners of energy therapies such as Jin Shin Jyutsu and Reiki take a somewhat different perspective, believing that they themselves can channel "universal energy" and stimulate a patient's own healing potential by focusing their awareness on that person's health and well-being. Spiritual healing practices such as prayer, ritual, and the laying on of hands seem to us to have an energetic component too, although it is a Higher Power rather than a nonspecific "universal energy" that is being accessed.

We're on somewhat shaky ground scientifically when we talk about energy medicine, because we are talking about subtle energies that cannot be measured by currently available scientific instruments. There is no way to directly measure the power of a prayer or the blockage of qi. We can look only at the results of these actions, see that something otherwise inexplicable has happened, and theorize about the cause. There are those who look at energy medicine as the future of medicine, and others who consider it sheer poppycock. Yet some of the most important tools of Western diagnostic medicine rely on the measurement of energy produced by the human body. Electrocardiography (EKG), electroencephalography (EEG), and electromyography (EMG) record the electrical energy emitted by the heart, the brain, and the muscles, respectively. Magnetic resonance imaging (MRI) is based on electromagnetic activity in the body, thermal diagnostics measure heat production, and Doppler scanners pick up sound waves. Biofeedback programs record any of several kinds of body energy. In each case, although we can see the results of the energy, we cannot see the energy itself.

Conventional medicine also accepts the idea that energy can heal. We use ultrasound waves to reduce inflammation, laser light waves to repair or excise tissue, electricity to speed bone healing or restart a stopped heart, vibration to improve bone density, heat to ease pain, and radiation to cure cancer. By our use of these therapies we acknowledge the ability of certain forms of energy to make changes at the cellular level.

It's a big leap from MRIs and ultrasound to Reiki energy healers, though. Research in the field of energy medicine is still scanty, but these are the basic assumptions:

- There is a life force or energy in the universe that permeates everything and everyone.
- Interruption in the free flow of that force can cause or be caused by illness, emotion, or structural problems.
- Physiologically, our bodies produce subtle forms of energy, which may not yet be measurable, but which can travel beyond the body.
- Exposure to even low levels of energy (electrical, magnetic, sound, light, radioactivity) can affect body processes.

- People can intentionally transfer or conduct energy to others with or without touching them.
- A person's energy can be perceived, assessed, and influenced positively by another.
- Good intentions must be present for the transfer or conduction of healing energy.

Some fascinating research—both secular and spiritual—is being done on energy medicine. At the University of Arizona's Human Energy Research Laboratory, for example, psychologist Gary Schwartz and his co-director, Linda Russek, have been studying the unconscious ways in which we are influenced by "subtle energies." In one of their early studies they found signs of interaction between the electrical impulses from the heart of one person and those in the brain of another. Other research centers are focusing on the power of prayer and religious belief to affect healing. A number of studies have associated religious participation with lower levels of stress, greater coping skills, greater sense of well-being, and even reduced incidence of cancer and heart disease. Still other studies have focused specifically on the power of prayer, with some of them finding positive effects on healing even when subjects did not know someone was praying for them.

There are more forms of energy medicine than we can count. We have seen promising anecdotal or research evidence for some of them, and others are simply too wacky for us to consider. We think it's fine to experiment with energy medicine as long as it is only used for complementary care and not as a replacement for conventional treatment, and as long as it does not drain your pocketbook. While we don't have extensive experience with these modalities ourselves, our patients report benefit from them. Some describe the sensation of receiving healing energy from a practitioner as like being cradled in someone's arms and gently rocked. Energy therapies well done appear to help people cope with difficult times, ease stress, lessen pain, and speed healing. While some feel that distant, or energy, healing reflects a strong placebo effect, we think that something more is involved.

Ask your child's doctor or people you trust for referrals, however, as this is clearly territory where charlatans roam. There are practitioners with excellent training and credentials who have a strong desire to heal, there are "practitioners" who set up shop with little training but a strong desire to make a buck, and there are "practitioners" with good intentions but no skills or a reliance on bizarre machines. In controversial areas such as this, clearly the buyer must beware. As attitude and intention are important to energy healing, look for a practitioner who shares your values, and with whom you feel a sympathetic "click." If you cannot find one, consider learning some of these techniques yourself through books, classes, or videos.

We discuss Chinese, osteopathic, homeopathic, and chiropractic medicine elsewhere in this section of the book. In this chapter we will briefly introduce you to five intriguing forms of energy healing with which you may not be familiar, and we will discuss the therapeutic uses of one very familiar method of healing: prayer. Most of these forms of healing have some common threads. Typically the practitioner will begin by "centering" or "grounding" herself to focus her concentration, establish her intention, and either open herself to an energy source (such as God, or the universe) or strengthen her own compassionate sensitivities. She will then usually assess the energetic field of her patient, by touch or not, and evaluate the situation. Then she will transmit or manipulate energy to strengthen or balance the patient. The patient, who is clothed, may feel nothing at all during this treatment, or may feel tingling, warmth, or a sense of relaxation and well-being.

Energy healers do not have supernatural powers. They are just good people who are willing to open a space in themselves through which to transmit healing energy. Everyone naturally possesses the power to offer compassion and love to benefit others, but few make the conscious choice to do so. Maybe you will be inspired to learn how to use one of these forms of energy healing with your own loved ones.

# Forms of Energy Medicine

We're beginning our discussion of energy medicine with some we consider "secular" rather than spiritually based, partly so you can choose whether you prefer a therapy with or without a spiritual component, and partly because they operate from somewhat different assumptions. In spiritual forms of energy medicine, the energy transmitted is assumed to come not from the practitioner but from a Higher Power. In contrast, practitioners of more secular forms of energy medicine will say they tap into a universal energy, that they help unblock or strengthen a person's own internal flow of energy (Qi), or that they open or balance energy centers known as chakras. In all forms of energy medicine mentioned here, secular or otherwise, the healer is not the source of the energy, merely its conduit. We'd give a wide berth to anyone who claimed to be the source of healing energy.

For the purposes of this discussion, we are considering Therapeutic Touch/Healing Touch and external qi gong to be secular forms of energy medicine. Although qi gong sometimes has a spiritual component in Chinese culture, it is more likely to be used in this country purely as a healing tool. Therapeutic Touch is based on traditional Christian and Hindu religious practices, but was purposely separated from those spiritual traditions by its developers to make it more acceptable in the secular hospital setting. Next, we will briefly discuss three Asia-based therapies that straddle the boundary between secular and spiritual forms of energy medicine. Reiki, Johrei, and Jin Shin Jyutsu all have a spiritual component, and a spiritual commitment by the practitioner, but can be used in a secular manner. Finally, we will talk about the current attempts to understand the role of prayer in medicine. We list resources for these therapies at the back of the book.

*Therapeutic Touch.* Developed by a nurse, Dolores Kreiger, and a spiritual healer, Dora Kunz, this therapy is based on the Christian healing practice of laying on hands and the ancient Hindu practice of manipulating body energy, but is now secular in nature. Kreiger and Kunz believed that interruptions in the free flow of universal energy through the body could be perceived and modified by trained professionals and lay people. Therapeutic Touch (TT) and a related form of energy healing called Healing Touch are practiced by nurses the world over, and can be used by parents and children for self-care as well.

A session of TT lasts about 20 minutes, or less for children. The TT practitioner will first center herself to focus on the intention to heal and to become more attuned to a patient's energy fields. Then she will move her hands over and around the patient's body about 2 to 4 inches from the skin, feeling for places that are colder (energy deficient) or thicker (energy congested). She will then employ techniques to "unruffle" or "smooth" the energy field, sending intentional energy to correct imbalances.

*External Qi Gong.* We are becoming more familiar in this country with the Chinese practice of qi gong, a series of meditative and physical exercises designed to build and balance qi. This form of self-care is known as "internal" qi gong. "External" qi gong is the transmission of energy for healing from the hands of a skilled and long-time practitioner who has been able to intensify his own store of qi for this purpose. While such practitioners are common in traditional hospitals in China, they are few and far between in America.

*Reiki.* Based on ancient Tibetan practices, this form of healing was developed about a century ago by Dr. Mikao Usui, a Japanese Christian minister and educator. Reiki (ray-key) is based on the idea that practitioners can channel the energy of the universal life force for healing through the gentle use of their hands, either by touch or from a distance. Practitioners of Reiki are either lay people or medical professionals who have taken up to three brief courses of training that prepare them to work on their own energy, treat others, or train others. The training required to call oneself a "Reiki Master" is not analogous to a master's degree.

A Reiki treatment will take 60 to 90 minutes. The practitioner will usually begin at the head and assess the energy at each of the chakras, transmitting energy when appropriate for health, with the goal of balancing and toning the system. One or two sessions should be enough for relaxation, general "tune-ups," or for acute conditions; chronic problems may take longer. Practitioners say that the energy they channel can do no harm to the patient, as it goes only where it is needed.

*Jin Shin Jyutsu.* Like the other forms of energy medicine we're discussing, Jin Shin Jyutsu claims only to help balance "life energy"; practitioners neither diagnose nor treat illness *per se.* Practitioners evaluate twelve pulses in the wrist to determine which of a person's twenty-six "safety energy locks" need to be opened or adjusted by a series of gentle hand placements at trouble spots. A Jin Shin Jyutsu session with a trained practitioner will last about an hour. Certain simple positions can be learned and used by anyone—even children—as self-help.

*Johrei.* Members of the international, multifaith Johrei Fellowship are dedicated to a life of service. Through their practice of Johrei, they channel "the divine light of God" to others for their purification and healing. Those who receive this energy therapy need not be believers to reap a benefit. A Johrei session lasts about 20 minutes, and there should be no charge for it (although donations are accepted). After centering, the practitioner raises a hand and transmits energy to nine energy centers on the front and back of a person. Dr. Russ has recommended Johrei to many patients with chronic or life-threatening illness, for whom it often provides a sense of connection and kindness that brings serenity.

# The Role of Spirituality in Medicine

We combined energy medicine and spirituality/religion in one chapter because in all these healing therapies something invisible, immeasurable, and powerful appears to be at work. In addition, underneath the differences in semantics, both modalities are talking about accessing an energy or power outside ourselves. Be it God, vital force, or universal life energy, this source of healing is something larger than the individual and something not adequately explained by science.

The earliest physicians were both healers and spiritual leaders. With the advent of scientific medicine, doctors separated their professional from their shamanistic selves. They set aside their traditional spiritual role so completely that issues of spirituality are seldom brought up in conversations between doctors and patients. Few patients broach the subject for fear of appearing unscientific or unsure of the doctor's skills. We regret this split, because it divorces a doctor from an important healing tool and diminishes his or her own influence. Although it's not acknowledged, doctors still retain some shamanistic power. A visit to a doctor's office with its signs and symbols of arcane knowledge (the white coat, the stethoscope) can induce a different state of consciousness. That's why kids, for example, are more willing to accept a doctor's suggestion than the same advice from a parent. That's why the visit itself can evoke a placebo response in both children and adults.

As integrative physicians we believe strongly that spirit plays a role both in sickness and in healing and should be discussed in nearly any healing encounter. After all, in recent polling 80 percent of Americans said they believed in the power of prayer to improve the course of an illness. It makes sense to us to marshal a patient's spiritual as well as physical and emotional resources. Spirituality, in any of its forms, can help parents and children find comfort in a trying situation, increase the sense of connection to others and the world around them, and provide them with hope, meaning, and even a greater appreciation for life's magic.

Fortunately, in the past few years there's been a sea change in the attitude of the medical establishment toward spirituality, due to an increasing number of scientific studies on the topic and an increased desire on the part of patients to bring their spiritual tools into their health care. Today more than fifty medical schools offer courses in spirituality and medicine. Centers at Duke, Harvard, and other top universities are exploring the relationship between belief and health and the role of health professionals. So far, studies have linked religious faith or spirituality to greater optimism, greater coping skills, greater resilience in the face of stress, greater perceived social support, lower levels of anxiety, and a longer, healthier life. We think there may be other factors at work here as well (religious people may have a better sense of connection to the community or may just take better care of themselves), but we do believe that it is both important and healthy for children to be taught a sense of spiritual (although not necessarily religious) connection to others and to the universe, and to be given spiritual tools. We feel that personal or communal prayer can be an important complement to medical therapy, but not a substitute for it.

Although 74 percent of American adults say a doctor should address a patient's spiritual needs, no patient wants to feel pressure from a doctor to adhere to the doctor's own beliefs. You want a doctor who will support your use of your own spiritual resources. We think it is not only appropriate but even helpful to ask a patient and his parents such questions as: When things are difficult, where do you turn for comfort? What gives you strength? Is your spiritual life important to you? Do you have a regular spiritual or religious practice? How would you like me as your doctor to address these issues in your health care? The goal with these questions is to identify the spiritual tools at a patient's command so they can be mobilized for her recovery. You may think these questions are too deep for children, but in our experience, kids have spiritual values and resources, too.

How can spirituality be used for healing? We believe that most illnesses—physical, emotional, and psychological—have a spiritual component. Such spiritual conflicts as issues of trust, faith, guilt, forgiveness, and reconciliation can express themselves as physical or psychological disease. In addition, many times a disease can cause a spiritual crisis. But most importantly, spiritual rituals and tools can help with healing. Now we want to make clear the distinction between "healing" and "curing." A cure gets rid of all physical signs of an illness. Healing, on the other hand, goes beyond the physical to encompass the emotional, psychological, and spiritual aspects of an illness as well. A disease does not have to disappear for a person to feel healed. We consider that healing has occurred if a patient has come to feel whole and blessed and alive, even if the disease still exists in the body. We have both cared for exceptional patients who taught us that dying and healing are not in fact incompatible, experiences that were life-changing for us.

We believe that spiritual practice always offers healing and the possibility of something more. People of faith have different spiritual tools at their command, although they can be loosely described as personal prayer/meditation; prayer by others (intercessory prayer); ritual; or contact with a holy book, person, or place. To our minds, prayer and other spiritual tools can be exceptionally powerful therapies. Herbert Benson of Harvard's Mind/Body Medical Institute has said that he thinks prayer and meditation are effective therapy for any condition that is made worse or caused by stress, such as pain, infertility, anxiety, and depression. Prayer offers benefits both to the person praying and the person prayed for. We don't know if it will ever be scientifically proven that prayer speeds healing, but we know it gives us something positive to do when we feel powerless, and allows an outlet for our feelings of love and compassion for others. It's a gift that we can offer freely whenever someone we care about is in need of healing. And who's to say that a mother praying for her son's recovery is not transmitting healing energy that will make a difference in the course of his illness?

We don't suggest that you depend upon faith alone, however, but use it as one piece in an integrative treatment program. We haven't seen many papers on the effects of prayer alone ("miracles"), but we have certainly seen a few unexplained healings in our years of practicing medicine. There are few studies yet on the effect of spirituality on the health of children, and none on the possible negative effects of prayer as therapy (such as harm caused by the intimation that failure to cure may indicate insufficient faith).

Remember that even young children can have a sense of the spiritual, of something important that is larger than themselves. They may feel it while pondering the mystery of the stars at night, while basking in the love of their family, or during a religious ritual. We urge you to talk to your physician if you think your child's health problem has a spiritual component that is not being addressed. You may be surprised to find that she is more than happy to incorporate this element in her therapeutic plan. She can also refer you to spiritual counselors or chaplains within the community who may be able to be of help. We know that we feel honored whenever we are asked to pray for or with a patient. We both follow the Jewish faith, but we are quite willing to pray with people of any faith. It's not about religion, it's about healing.

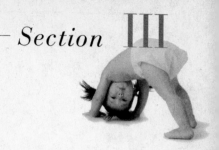

# Integrative Treatment of Common Childhood Illnesses

i t is our hope that you will already be familiar with the first two sections of this book before you dip into these last chapters. An understanding of the basic principles of integrative pediatric medicine—especially the importance of not interfering with the natural healing processes of the body—will give you the background you need to make the best use of this section of the book. We deliberately chose a narrative style rather than the "cookbook" approach of many other childcare books because we thought it was so important to ground parents first with knowledge about the importance of preventive measures such as exercise and good nutrition and the usefulness of newer medical approaches such as mind/body medicine and botanical remedies.

The next nine chapters contain advice to help you prevent and/or manage childhood complaints such as croup, flu, cough, cold, asthma, allergies, sore throat, diarrhea, constipation, and many of the other health problems parents have to deal with in the years between their children's birth and adolescence. We answer questions like: To strep test or not to strep test? Is it a cold or is it an allergy? Are decongestants the best way to go? In discussing each of the more than thirty conditions covered, we explain what's going on in your child's body, talk about strategies for prevention, and provide a list of what you can do to ease symptoms or speed healing. Don't feel that you have to follow every suggestion we make; we have purposely provided lots of ideas because what works at one time (or with one child) might not work at another.

Our goal in this section is to help you understand how to integrate conventional and alternative therapies to provide the best care for your child. We will generally start first with safe and effective methods that support your child's innate capacity for healing with few or no side effects. We do not often recommend over-the-counter medicines, for instance, because they have avoidable side effects and because they suppress symptoms rather than supporting the natural healing process. We are very cautious with antibiotics as well. That does not mean that we scorn conventional medicine. Only a foolish practitioner would neglect the benefits of conventional Western approaches. By the same token, only an arrogant one would deny the potential for healing offered by many alternative approaches.

We are both conventionally trained medical doctors, and so we have noted clearly those signs and symptoms that require a call to your child's doctor or a visit to the emergency department. Occasionally our treatment plans differ (remember, medicine is an art). In those few cases, we give our advice separately and provide an explanation of the reasons for our differences.

These chapters on preventing and treating childhood illnesses are followed by a final chapter that ties everything in the book together into one year-long program for a healthy child, and a healthy family. It contains a plan for easing gradually into changes that improve health, as well as healthy and fun activities for the whole family.

# Chapter 16

# Cold and Flu Defense:

## *Common Respiratory Illnesses*

the average young child suffers an estimated six to ten colds a year, tapering off to two to four a year as he or she nears adulthood. No wonder we associate runny noses with little kids! By the time your children are old enough to vote, you'll probably have dealt with at least a hundred runny noses, hacking coughs, and feverish flus. Our children get more colds and other respiratory illnesses than we do because their immune systems are still developing. As they grow up, their immune systems eventually learn to recognize cold viruses and organize better defenses against them.

Respiratory illnesses affect the nose, mouth, windpipe (trachea), the two airways that lead to the lobes of the lungs (bronchi), the smaller airways within the lungs (bronchioles), and/or the air-filled sacs (alveoli) that give the lung its spongy appearance (see drawing on page 264). In this chapter we briefly discuss common conditions of the upper respiratory tract (colds, croup, sinusitis) and the lower respiratory tract (bronchitis, bronchiolitis, and pneumonia), as well as one total-body flattener (influenza).

The first and most important thing to remember is that these respiratory infections are usually caused by viruses. This means that antibiotics, which do not kill viruses, cannot cure colds, flu, and most

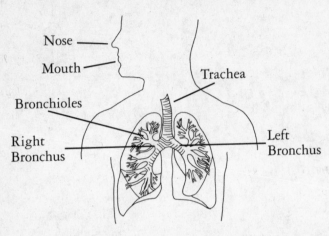

Nose

Mouth

Trachea

Bronchioles

Right
Bronchus

Left
Bronchus

cases of bronchitis. (Some cases of bronchitis, and many cases of sinusitis and pneumonia, are caused by bacteria and may require antibiotics.) Some help may be needed with symptom relief, but your child's own healing powers will resolve these mild self-limiting infections in time. Although the uselessness of antibiotics in viral illnesses has been clearly proven, parents and physicians still find it hard to resist the antibiotic "fix." It is actually counterproductive to use antibiotics in these situations, because antibiotics upset the normal healthy balance among the many bacteria that live in harmony within our bodies. In addition, misuse of antibiotic drugs fosters the development of antibiotic-resistant bacteria (see chapter 4). We are often confronted with parents and family members willing to cut any deal for that golden prescription, and we know that many physicians cave in to the pressure. We prefer to reserve antibiotics for those times when we suspect that sinusitis or pneumonia is bacterial in nature. Even then we always start by prescribing the simplest narrow-spectrum antibiotic (such as amoxicillin) in otherwise healthy children, advancing to broader-spectrum drugs only if there is no improvement. We ask you not to pressure your doctor to start with the highest potency antibiotics; this practice harms your child and your community in the long run by encouraging the development of more strains of resistant bacteria.

Immune function plays a role in colds and other respiratory illnesses. Although we are all exposed to the viruses that cause these ill-nesses, those of us who are under stress or run-down are far more likely to actually get them. (And everyone knows that moms *never* get colds and flu because they don't have time.) That's why it's so important to eat well and get enough rest during the late fall and winter months we call the cold and flu season. That's the time of year you'll want to be especially careful to keep up the immune-boosting strategies we dis-cussed in chapter 2.

However, even healthy children will get at least a few mild respi-ratory illnesses and suffer symptoms that may make both child and parent very unhappy. That's the reason more than $3 billion worth of over-the-counter cold, flu, and cough medications are sold every year. In general, we do not recommend these O-T-C medications, because they are not very effective, and they have significant side effects. We believe that the best treatment for self-limiting illnesses is to get out of the way and let the natural forces of healing do their work. Our treatment advice is therefore simple: Rest and keep the body hydrated. Encourage your child to sleep as much as possible to allow the immune system time and energy to battle the virus. Give moderate amounts of clear fluids—water, broth, juice, even juice pops—to flush the body of toxins and provide the moisture the mucosal tissues lining the respiratory tract need to repel viruses effectively.

While the common respiratory illnesses usually clear up on their own with a little time, parents should still stay alert for any worsening of symptoms, as complications can occur or what seems at first like a cold may actually be something else altogether. **Call your child's physician** if symptoms last longer than a week, if fever returns after the initial fever has wound down, if your child cannot keep fluids down, or has pain in the face or teeth. **Go to the emergency depart-ment or call 911** if a child complains of chest pains, has difficulty breathing or is breathing very rapidly, has a bluish cast to his or her skin (cyanosis), or is not behaving normally.

With that general introduction, let's move on to specifics about symptoms, prevention, and integrative treatment of the more com-mon forms of mild respiratory illness.

# Upper Respiratory Infections

**The Common Cold.** Almost all of the common respiratory infections seem to start out as a cold, which is formally defined as a viral infection of the mucous membranes of the nose, sinuses, throat, and upper airway. Someone with a cold may have a runny nose, tearing eyes, scratchy throat, cough, congestion, sneezing, poor appetite, mild fever, and may just feel "icky." The mucus (or colloquially, snot) draining from our noses that we associate with a cold is actually a defensive tactic. Early on, when a cold is at its most contagious, the clear and watery mucus is chock full of viruses being flushed out of the body. Later the mucus becomes thicker and whitish or yellowish because it is also full of dead immune cells that have fought the offending virus. Parents often worry that thick, yellowish or greenish mucus signals a bacterial infection in the sinuses, but this is not always the case. We don't worry unless we also see more serious symptoms, such as high fever and facial pain or swelling, which might indicate a bacterial sinus infection. A cold in a young child generally lasts about a week, but can last significantly longer. Most colds are uncomplicated and resolve completely.

**Prevention.** It would be nice if we had a vaccine that could prevent the common cold, but that's unlikely, because there are about 200 viruses that can cause one. Colds are very contagious, with viruses being spread through sneezing (they can travel 12 feet!) or hand-to-hand or hand-to-object contact. The best way to prevent a cold is to have all members of the family wash their hands often and well; use the methods we described at the end of chapter 4. In studies at elementary schools and child-care centers—hotbeds of respiratory illness—that one precaution alone has been found to significantly reduce the number of colds. Children should also be taught to cover their mouths when they sneeze or cough.

Very young children get more colds not only because their immune systems are still being educated, but also because they don't wash their hands often, tend to wipe their noses with their arms or a sleeve, and have a lot of physical contact with their playmates. The good news is that this exchange of common viruses provides most children with the stimulation necessary to build a healthy immune system. The bad news is that they catch half a dozen colds a year. Most children suffer more colds during their years in preschool and kindergarten than they will at any other time in their lives. Those who spend the day in overcrowded day-care centers, or are exposed to airborne pollutants like second-hand tobacco smoke, tend to get more colds. Their colds last longer, too, yet one more reason for parents to quit smoking.

You can sometimes avert or reduce the severity or duration of a cold by taking quick action in its early stages. At the first sign of a cold, you can start feeding your child foods high in vitamin C, such as orange juice or citrus fruit, kiwi, strawberries and other berries, melon, bell pepper, and broccoli. Alternatively, you can give a child a quick-loading dose of vitamin C (100 mg total per day for a toddler or 200 mg a day for an older child) when they first notice a scratchy throat or sniffle. The easiest forms of vitamin C for children to take are chewable tablets or powdered vitamin C mixed in water or juice. If your children prefer the chewables, make sure they brush their teeth or rinse out their mouths afterward to avoid any tooth damage from the ascorbic acid. Although studies have not conclusively shown that vitamin C can *prevent* colds, there is good evidence that vitamin C can reduce the duration and severity of some colds, and there is little downside to using this benign intervention.

We generally recommend the herb echinacea as a way to lessen the severity or duration of a cold, but in some people it may actually halt a cold in its tracks. As with vitamin C, there is very little data on use in children, but we are comfortable enough about their safety to give these remedies to our own children. (Children with autoimmune disorders or known allergies to plants in the ragweed family should not take echinacea until studies disprove theoretical concerns about these uses of the herb in these situations.) It is not clear yet which variety of the plant or which part of the plant is most effective for colds, although *Echinacea purpurea* flowers and berries seem to show the best results in studies. In our experience, alcohol-based tinctures of the herb are most effective, but standardized extracts or alcohol-free tinctures (for families concerned about alcoholism) can also be used. We give kids age two to six 6 to 8 drops of the liquid extract or tincture in water or juice two to five times a day. The dose is 8 to 15 drops at a time for kids aged four to six. Start at the first sign of symptoms and continue for no more than 7 days. Echinacea is definitely an acquired taste, so we usually mask it with grape, raspberry, or other strong-flavored fruit juices. There is no evidence that it is useful to take it for the full cold season as a general preventive.

There are two other herbal remedies we often recommend to kids with colds: garlic and maitake. Although clinical research data are slim, garlic appears to be an excellent antimicrobial both in laboratory studies and in our own experience. You can either feed your children plenty of fresh garlic in their food, or put ½ teaspoon of a liquid garlic extract such as Kyolic (for kids one to five, older kids can take a full teaspoon) into grape juice twice a day. Dr. Stu has also found that a special liquid extract of the Japanese medicinal mushroom maitake (called maitake d-fraction) seems to help abort a cold. The dosage for children one to five years old is 5 drops (10 drops for children six and over) three times a day. He puts it in a teaspoon of chocolate syrup, which makes the medicine go down quite well. Dr. Russ has had success treating colds with another Asian herb, astragalus, although it is more generally used as a tonic to prevent upper respiratory illnesses. The dosage is 8 to 15 drops of astragalus tincture two or three times a day for a child aged six to twelve; halve the dose for children two to six. (See chapter 12 for more on this herbal tonic.) As with the other remedies we have recommended to avert or ameliorate a cold, there is no good data yet on their safety or efficacy in children or on the optimal dosage to take.

We are split on the value of zinc lozenges to prevent a cold or reduce its symptoms. Dr. Stu has had many parents report good results when their children take zinc at the first sign of symptoms and as the package directs. The few studies done on the use of zinc lozenges by children found little benefit and some gastrointestinal side effects, so Dr. Russ is less enthusiastic about this remedy. You'll have to make your own call. A new nasal gel containing zinc may be more effective, but it has not yet been tested in children.

*Treatment of congestion.* If your child does get a cold, we do not recommend most over-the-counter cold remedies. We're not convinced they work very well at the low doses given to children (or even at higher doses in adults), and some, such as Afrin and NeoSynephrine, are actually contraindicated in children. Although decongestants generally decrease swelling in the nasal cavities and make breathing a little easier, we believe they sidetrack the natural healing process. In addition, they have many potential side effects, including irritability, increased blood pressure, and rapid heart rate. These drugs offer four to six hours of relief at most, and can cause *increased* mucus production and congestion (the "rebound" effect) if used for more than five days. We give decongestants (primarily pseudoephedrine) only when a child has severe discomfort.

Antihistamines are designed to counteract the effects of histamine, a substance released by the body during allergic responses. They are sometimes used with colds as well to dry up secretions. Unfortunately, thickening up the nasal mucus slows it from draining. Drowsiness is the usual side effect of this medication, but some children are paradoxically hyperstimulated, becoming "wired" for hours after taking one dose. We don't recommend antihistamines unless the child is extremely uncomfortable and no other options are working.

We recommend natural measures to reduce the congestion of a cold. Some of our favorites:

- Use nasal aspirators (inexpensive little rubber bulbs) to suction excess mucus from the nose of a baby with a cold.
- You or your child can use a store-bought or homemade saline spray or nose drops five or six times a day to loosen thickened nasal secretions and allow for freer breathing. (Just mix ¼ teaspoon table salt in a cup of warm water.) This is especially useful with nursing babies who cannot eat if they cannot breathe.
- Older children should be taught the fine art of gently blowing one's nose so as not to send germ-laden mucus up into the ears or sinuses. If nose blowing leads to a raw nose, use petroleum jelly, aloe gel, calendula cream, or other salve.
- Get plenty of rest.

- Drink lots of liquids. Don't forget chicken soup—studies suggest that your grandmother's favorite remedy really does improve cold symptoms.
- Use steam to soothe and moisturize nasal passages and open sinuses. A cool-mist vaporizer can moisturize the air in your child's bedroom. Or you can run a very hot shower and let your child sit in the bathroom and breathe in the steam.
- Consider experimenting with a homeopathic remedy. Refer to chapter 13 for help in choosing one that suits your child's symptoms.

We don't have a general rule about the use or avoidance of dairy products during a cold, as in our experience it all depends on the child. Clearly there are children who can tolerate dairy products during colds, and there are others who cannot. If you find that your child's congestion worsens when she eats cheese or drinks a lot of milk, avoid them at the outset of the cold. Don't worry if young children vomit up mucus; this is actually a good way to eliminate mucus that has drained and been swallowed. We don't have any proof that the old maxim

## Is It a Cold or an Allergy?

Both colds and allergies can cause sneezing, stuffy nose, scratchy throat, and reddened eyes. Colds peak in the late fall and winter and last about a week; allergies last longer, and can occur anytime, although often at the same time each year (grass or pollen allergies). Allergies can leave you more susceptible to colds. Mild fever or body aches typically signal a cold; itchy eyes or itchy skin point to allergy. White, yellow, or green mucus may accompany a cold; clear mucus is seen with allergies or the first days of a cold. (For more on allergic rhinitis, see chapter 22.)

"Feed a cold, starve a fever," has any truth to it either. Some children want to eat during a cold, others lose their appetite.

**Treatment of cough.** Like a runny nose, a cough is a defensive mechanism. It clears the throat and airways of obstructions and foreign matter to allow better breathing. Much of the cold-related coughing in children is in response to the scratchy, irritable sensation caused by mucus dripping down the back of throat. The cough caused by postnasal drip tends to flare up when the child is lying flat, causing nighttime coughing and sleeplessness for child and parent alike. Although sleep-deprived parents are frequently anxious about this symptom, it is a normal response to mucus dripping down towards the airway.

A persistent cough may be a sign of something more than a cold, such as gastroesophageal reflux, asthma, pneumonia, croup, or pertussis (whooping cough). **Call your child's physician** for any cough in an infant under three months, or for a cough in an older child that causes wheezing or other breathing problem, comes with high fever, or lasts longer than two weeks.

We do not generally advise treating the coughs that accompany colds with suppressants. A cough, after all, serves the important function of ridding the body of irritants. Furthermore, over-the-counter cough medicines do not cure a cough, but merely stifle the cough (suppressants) or cause the cough to be more "productive" (expectorants). We discourage their use because they have significant side effects and are not always effective for children. Cough suppressants are often based on compounds such as dextromethorphan (DM) or codeine. While they are safe in pediatric doses, it is easy to take an overdose. The side effects of the narcotic codeine, for example, include drowsiness, constipation, and nausea. We do occasionally prescribe codeine, but only in situations where a child older than five is just not getting any sleep because of a cough.

The active ingredient of many expectorants is guaifenesin. Although the drug does thin mucus, in our experience it often causes more profuse postnasal drip and increased coughing in kids. Once again, we rarely recommend expectorants, except for the occasional case where a child with bronchitis needs help expelling mucus from his lungs.

A cough is the body's way of getting rid of secretions and debris. Rather than suppress it, consider taking a natural approach to reducing discomfort associated with cough.

- Probably the best method for reducing cough symptoms is to encourage your child to blow his or her nose frequently (and gently) to avoid postnasal drip.
- Rest and drink lots of liquids to speed healing. Warm fluids like broths, teas, and heated juices may be best because they promote circulation, soothe the throat, and replace liquids lost in the course of illness. Dr. Russ has fond memories of the hot tea with honey that his mom always gave him when he had a cough. (Remember, though, that honey should not be given to children under a year old because of the potential for botulism.)
- A cool-mist vaporizer in your child's room can ease a cough, as can elevating the head of your child's bed or crib (or tucking a folded blanket or pillow under the head end of the crib mattress).
- Lozenges can ease the throat tickle that triggers a cough. In addition to the familiar cough drops of all sorts, we also like the cherry-flavored lozenges made of slippery elm, an herb that soothes the mucous membranes.
- Liquid extract of slippery elm is a useful herbal treatment for coughs. Give children aged two to four a ½ teaspoon twice a day, and older kids 1 teaspoon twice a day until the throat feels better. You can also mix 1 teaspoon of slippery elm powder with 1 tablespoon of sugar, a sprinkle of cinnamon, and 2 cups of boiling water for a soothing drink that can be sipped (once cooled) throughout the day.

**Treatment of fever.** Sometimes a cold is accompanied by a fever—an elevated body temperature that signals the body's attempts to fight off an infection. The fever is not itself an illness, but a natural defensive reaction. Many parents are frightened by fever, and start giving antifever medications as soon as a child's temperature goes above 98.6 F. They forget that some children normally run a little hotter or cooler than 98.6 degrees (which is just an average), and that body temperature will normally be a degree or two higher in the evening than in the morning. Besides, fever by itself is rarely harmful unless it is extremely high (106 degrees F and over) and prolonged.

We do not normally treat children over a year old with any medications for low-grade fever unless a child is uncomfortable or looks sick. Although clearly you should consult a doctor if your child's fever is prolonged or very high, the fact is that we are less concerned with numbers than with how a child looks and feels. If a child *is* uncomfortable from a fever, we suggest a dose of children's acetaminophen or ibuprofen appropriate for the child's weight. (Never give aspirin to a child who might have a viral illness because of the risk of a liver-damaging disease called Reyes Syndrome.) Be sure to use the dropper or measuring cap that came with the medicine, or a measuring spoon (not a teaspoon from your silverware drawer), and give the correct dose for the form (drops, elixir, or chewable). Do not give over-the-counter cough or cold medicines that also contain acetaminophen at the same time (check the label), as you may unwittingly give your child an overdose. You can continue giving acetaminophen until your child starts to feel better or the fever goes down. The purpose of the acetaminophen is purely to make your child more comfortable, so there's no reason to wake up a sleeping child for another dose.

When should parents worry about a fever? **Call your child's physician** for a child under three months of age who has a fever of 100 degrees F (rectal) or more, a child three to six months old who has a fever over 101 degrees (rectal), or an older child who has had a fever over 103 degrees F (oral) for more than a day or a bad headache associated with the fever. Call the doctor if your child has suffered a seizure from the fever. It is also best to have a doctor check a feverish child who shows a rash. **Call 911 or go to the emergency room** if a child suffers a febrile seizure and you cannot contact your physician, or if a feverish child has trouble breathing, turns blue, is in pain, or delirious.

It is very common for a child to spike a fever of 103 to 105 degrees for a fairly benign virus. When parents call Dr. Stu about feverish children, he always asks whether the child can still be made to smile when the fever abates. If so, he feels reasonably certain that the fever is not being caused by a serious bacterial infection. Fevers rarely go high enough to cause lasting harm except in situations where there is also interference with a child's heating and cooling mechanism, such as when a feverish child is wrapped in too many blankets or a child is left in a closed car on a hot day.

For the mild fever that may accompany colds, there are a few other remedies that may help. Rest and liquids are especially important when a child is running a temperature; juice popsicles feel especially good. Sponge a very hot child with a washcloth dipped in lukewarm water and wrung out.

**Sinus pain.** The sinus cavities are air-filled pockets in the bony structure of the skull located above the eyes, behind the cheeks and to the sides of the nasal passages. The sinuses make mucus, which is then swept into the nose by tiny hairs called cilia that line the respiratory passages. A child's cold will often be accompanied by at least mild pain in the forehead or face from an excess of mucus in the sinuses or an obstruction in the flow of mucus. To relieve these cold symptoms, you can:

- Ease mild sinus pain and speed up drainage by placing very warm washcloths on the face over the sinuses.
- Give children's acetaminophen or ibuprofen at dosages indicated on package labels to relieve more severe sinus pain.
- Massage the chest of a child over the age of three with an herbal aromatic rub made by mixing a drop of essential oil of eucalyptus in an ounce of a vegetable or nut oil such as olive or almond oil. (Do not apply essential oils undiluted to a child's skin.) Don't use the rub on the face, where it can get into the mucous membranes. If you prefer, you can rub a drop of eucalyptus oil on your child's blanket at bedtime to relieve congestion.
- Give an O-T-C decongestant such as pseudoephedrine for up to five days. This is one of the few instances when we do recommend decongestants. We may also prescribe nonsedating antihistamines if symptoms persist.
- Try acupuncture. Dr. Russ has seen some astonishing results in the treatment of acute sinusitis, with clogged sinuses starting to drain freely during a treatment.

- Cranial osteopathy (described in chapter 11) provides excellent relief of symptoms for chronic sinusitis and may prevent recurrence.

The sinus problems that accompany a cold can sometimes turn into something more serious because the mucus backed up in the sinuses creates a friendly incubator for bacteria. It can be difficult then for a physician to tell whether or not the problem is bacterial sinusitis, which should be treated with antibiotics. Fortunately, viral sinusitis is 20 to 200 times more likely than bacterial sinusitis in children. Some doctors recommend an X-ray, CT scan, or MRI to determine the presence of more severe bacterial sinusitis, but these procedures have their drawbacks: Interpretation of the images is very difficult because young children have poorly developed sinus cavities and may show abnormally fluid-filled sinuses even with routine colds or allergies. **Call your child's physician** if your child has facial or dental pain or a fever that returns after initial cold symptoms have subsided. In cases such as these, we do prescribe antibiotics, as these are symptoms that may be associated with a bacterial sinus infection. We start with the simplest form of antibiotic (amoxicillin) and advance to stronger, broad-spectrum antibiotics only if no improvement is noted in the first three days. Be sure that any child on antibiotics takes the full course, even if symptoms disappear before the prescription is finished. Antibiotics for sinusitis need to be taken longer than usual, preferably two to three weeks. We usually recommend that these patients eat lots of yogurt (fresh or frozen) with live cultures, or take a probiotic supplement, such as *Lactobacillus acidophilus* or Bifidobacteria, to re-establish the beneficial intestinal bacteria ("good bugs") killed by the medication.

**Croup.** Croup is a viral illness that usually starts with coldlike symptoms before progressing to swelling and inflammation of the vocal cords and windpipe. It can also come on without warning, with its distinctive cough the first sign. Croup occurs most often in the cold-and-flu days of winter, and is always worse at night. The most obvious symptom of croup is the notorious barking cough and restricted breathing that terrify both kids and parents at 2 A.M. The child may have significant hoarseness (laryngitis) and/or a moderate fever as well. Although it is frightening to hear your little munchkin suddenly sound like a large performing seal, there are a number of things you can do to relieve her symptoms. Among them:

- Turn the shower on to full hot, close the bathroom door, and sit with your little barking child in the steam-filled room until his cough eases. Turn the cool-mist humidifier on in his room for the rest of the night.
- Alternately, if it's cold outside, wrap your child up and carry her around outside for ten or fifteen minutes. Cold can also break the coughing spasms.
- Use relaxation techniques such as slow breathing or an imagery exercise to reduce your child's anxiety and slow his respiratory rate. Anxiety aggravates respiratory distress, so keeping your child calm is critical to relieving croup.

Generally, croup is another viral self-limiting illness that will resolve in a few days and can be treated at home with the guidance of a pediatrician. The frightening barking cough is usually followed by several days of a wet, looser, and less restrictive cough. Certain kids have a tendency toward croup, but they usually outgrow it by the age of six. **Call your child's physician or go to the emergency department** if your child is having severe difficulty with breathing that does not ease with steam or cold air. Warning signs include a high-pitched sound when breathing in (stridor), skin between the ribs being drawn in with each inhalation, or agitated behavior or confusion. Advanced cases of croup will require steroid treatment; occasionally a child is admitted to the hospital for further monitoring. Severe difficulty in breathing (the child has to sit upright to breathe) or a high fever can also be signs of the more serious bacterial condition known as epiglottitis, especially in children aged two to five. This dangerous disease may be becoming less of a threat as more children are immunized against *Haemophilus influenzae* type b (Hib), but it does still occasionally occur and should be treated by parent and doctor with the utmost urgency. Children with these symptoms should be brought to the nearest emergency room and evaluated immediately.

## Lower Respiratory Infections

**Bronchitis**. Bronchitis is the swelling or inflammation of the bronchi, the major airways in the lungs through which oxygen flows in and carbon dioxide flows out. Most cases of bronchitis are actually colds with predominant bronchial symptoms such as chest congestion, chest discomfort, cough, and, often, wheezing. Although frightening to parents, wheezing is not necessarily serious, as air is still flowing in and out of the child's lungs. It is actually more serious when a wheezing child stops wheezing but still has difficulty breathing, as it means that the airways are now so restricted that there is not enough air going through them to even cause a wheeze. Because colds and bronchitis so frequently overlap, we do not want to overtreat a child who is not uncomfortable or in respiratory distress. We advise parents to help relieve symptoms (see our approach to colds and coughs above), and keep an eye on the child to make sure the situation does not worsen.

We don't usually treat bronchitis any differently than a cold, recommending rest and plenty of liquids. If a child's wheezing or distress is significant, we may prescribe a bronchodilating agent, such as albuterol, to ease breathing; these medications come as nebulizers, metered-dose inhalers, or in liquid form. We do not hand out prescriptions for antibiotics for every child with bronchitis. Fortunately the practice of automatically prescribing broad-spectrum antibiotics for bronchitis is diminishing now that studies have found that bronchitis in children is generally a self-limiting viral illness that does not respond to antibiotics. There are exceptions, however. For instance, children with chronic lung diseases, such as cystic fibrosis, do generally require an antibiotic for bronchial symptoms due to underlying lung damage and mucus stagnation. And occasionally a bacterium will set up shop in the bronchi of an otherwise healthy child. We decide whether or not to prescribe antibiotics based on a child's history, current symptoms, physical exam, and a parent's ability to monitor the condition closely.

**Bronchiolitis**. Bronchiolitis is an inflammation of the smaller airways (bronchioles) deeper in the lungs, which can be caused by a number of viruses, among them respiratory syncytial virus (RSV). RSV is a common cause of many upper and lower respiratory infections, including colds and pneumonia. In older kids and adults RSV is just a nuisance, but in very young children bronchiolitis caused by RSV can progress to a life-threatening illness. It is a significant cause of hospitalizations of children under a year old in the winter and early spring, especially those infants considered "high risk" due to prematurity or cardiac problems. Such children may require treatment with medications only available at a hospital. **Call your child's physician or go to the emergency department** for a high-risk infant who has difficulty breathing or periodically stops breathing, turns blue, or has coughing, severe congestion, vomiting, fussiness, and an inability to eat or drink. Children with brochiolitis may look as if they are having an acute asthma attack, and the spaces between their ribs go in and out when they breathe. They need conventional Western medical treatment.

**Pertussis**. Whooping cough is another preventable bacterial infection that affects the same portion of the airway as bronchiolitis. It too may start with coldlike symptoms, but the hallmark of whooping cough is the "whoop" a child makes when gasping for air after one of the frequent, long-lasting repetitive coughing spells that characterize this disease. The so-called "staccato" coughing (five to ten coughs, one right after another) makes it so hard to take a breath that the child may turn blue from lack of oxygen. Whooping cough is caused not by cold or flu viruses, but by a bacterium (*Bordetella pertussis*). Thanks to vaccines, this potentially life-threatening infection is much less common but still cause for concern in cities or in areas where there are clusters of children unvaccinated for religious or philosophical reasons or inadequately-vaccinated immigrants. **Call your child's physician right away**, if you suspect your child has pertussis based on the symptoms described above. If distress is present, he may ask you to take your child to the emergency room of your local hospital.

**Pneumonia**. Pneumonia is the result of infected fluids accumulating in the air sacs, or alveoli, at the ends of the airways. In most cases, this infection is accompanied by cough, progressive weakness, rapid breathing, inactivity, poor food and fluid intake, high fever, and sometimes wheezing. Infants may show irritability, lack of appetite, and rapid breathing, but generally their diagnosis comes more from what doctors call in professional terms "sick-looking-kid" syndrome.

Pneumonia can be caused by a wide variety of organisms, and it is difficult but crucial to determine whether your child is suffering from a bacterial or viral illness when considering treatment possibilities. Viral pneumonias tend to develop more slowly and have less serious symptoms associated with them.

Typically the pediatrician will order a white-blood-cell count and chest X ray to help determine whether a child has viral or bacterial pneumonia; emergency physicians may prescribe antibiotics based on the X ray and symptoms alone. While antibiotics are not of use for viral pneumonias, bacterial pneumonia (while less common) is quite aggressive in children and should be treated with appropriate oral antibiotics for mild and moderate cases and systemic antibiotics for severe cases. Again, probiotic use during antibiotic treatment may be useful in preventing gastrointestinal side effects.

A few remedies that might be useful for a child with viral pneumonia or as complementary therapy for a child being treated for bacterial pneumonia:

- Rest and lots of fluids.
- Use of an herbal tonic, such as echinacea, garlic, maitake, or the Chinese herb astragalus (see chapter 12).
- Breath work to exercise the lungs.
- Mind/body exercises, especially hypnosis or guided imagery, to hasten the healing process.

## Influenza

**Influenza.** We don't need to tell you what flu is—once you've had it, you'll recognize it again. By definition, influenza is a viral illness that comes on suddenly and more severely than a cold and lasts a week to ten days. Symptoms include fever, aches, chills, cough, runny nose, sore throat, headache, nausea or vomiting, and a lack of energy or appetite. Most people with flu feel like they've been hit by a truck and just want to stay in bed.

**Prevention.** The best way to protect your children from flu is for everyone in the family to wash his or her hands frequently during flu season—from November to April. Influenza is spread easily by person-to-person contact, and hand washing breaks the chain. This is also a good time of year to be especially committed to following the suggestions we gave in chapter 2 for optimizing immune function.

We do follow the guidelines recommending annual immunization against influenza for children with chronic health conditions such as asthma, cystic fibrosis, or cardiovascular problems that could worsen with the flu. We do not at this point recommend that healthy children get annual flu shots, as the benefits to children do not yet outweigh the risks. While it is relatively rare, Dr. Stu has seen at least one case of Guillain-Barré syndrome that was likely associated with a flu shot. A reason often given for vaccinating healthy children for flu is to protect older adults who have not gotten their own immunizations, which we think puts the responsibility for the health of adults on the wrong shoulders.

**Treatment.** There is currently a big controversy in medical circles about the value of antiviral flu medicines for children. We only recommend them for children with chronic health problems that could worsen with flu. Healthy children are rarely affected severely by influenza, so we see no reason to expose them to these antiviral drugs, one of which (zanamivir) is associated with severe bronchospasm and serious respiratory deterioration in kids with asthma.

Instead of the antiviral medications, we turn to gentler ways of reducing the severity or duration of the flu. At the first sign of flu, have your child start taking ½ teaspoon of sweet, fruity-tasting elderberry (*Sambucus niger*) extract two or three times a day for five days. Elderberry extract has compounds that act much like those in the new flu drugs, preventing the influenza virus from reproducing. The homeopathic medicine Oscillococcinum (*Anas barbariae*) is another kid-friendly remedy that can avert flu if started when symptoms first occur; take according to package directions every 6 hours for the first 18 hours of flu.

For symptomatic relief, consider the following:

- Rest and plenty of fluids. See whether your child prefers warm or cool drinks, and keep them coming. Popsicles made of fruit juice are generally welcome, too; there are even new ones that include oral-rehydration therapy. You might try a smoothie as a way to pack more nutrition into those fluids.
- Children's acetaminophen or ibuprofen for fever, aches, or pain. Avoid aspirin.
- Massage with a pleasantly scented oil or lotion to relieve aching muscles and joints. (Vanilla, lavender, and chamomile are popular choices.)
- Give echinacea, maitake, and garlic as described previously.
- A cool-mist humidifier for stuffiness or sore throat.
- A little nibble on some candied ginger, or drinking tea made of minced ginger root and a little honey, can ease nausea in children over a year old.
- A cool washcloth feels great on a fevered brow.
- Favorite music, videos, or other forms of distraction.

# Chapter 17

# Is It Strep?:

## *Sore Throats*

there are many causes of sore throat, but parents are most frightened about those caused by *Streptococcus* infections. When a
child wakes up with a scratchy throat, parents often start to
worry, "Is it strep?" They know that untreated strep infections can be
dangerous, so they want to do the right thing. Suddenly all their plans
for the week shift as they try to decide if Sally needs to see a doctor,
and which parent will be able to take her. Will someone have to stay
home with her until the results of the strep culture are in, and should
they have the other kids tested, too?

A sore throat (pharyngitis) is an inflammation of the pharynx, the
muscular tube that delivers food and air from the back of the nose and
mouth to either the feeding tube (esophagus) that goes to the stomach
or the windpipe (trachea) that leads to the lungs. The pharynx, like the
nose and mouth, is lined with mucous membranes. Tucked into each
side of the pharynx at the back of the mouth (the oropharynx) are
small lymphoid tissues called the tonsils that help fight infection; the
adenoids in the upper throat at the back of the nose (the nasopharynx)
serve a similar function.

A strep infection can be mild to life-threatening, depending on its
location, the virulence of the strain of *Streptococcus*, and the quality of
the immune response. In the distant past, epidemics of virulent strains
of strep devastated communities in Europe with rheumatic disease and

death. Strep remained an ever-present threat until the advent of antibiotics; in fact, Dr. Russ's aunt died of rheumatic fever from strep in 1931 at the age of eleven and Dr. Stu's uncle suffered from the coronary aftereffects of a strep infection for thirty years. Although lethal results are rare today, strep infections can still be dangerous, and must be treated with caution. Left untreated, a strep infection can lead to damage of the heart (rheumatic fever).

We don't downplay the need to be cautious about sore throats, but we do want to relieve parents of what we call "strep phobia." Only 15 to 20 percent of sore throats in children are caused by strep. Most cases of sore throat are actually viral in origin and will cure themselves within a few days. Others are caused by environmental insults such as allergens, or pollutants such as cigarette smoke. (And a few sore throats are signs of more serious bacterial illnesses such as epiglottitis and abscesses.) Even though most cases of strep throat will resolve on their own, we treat all cases of strep throat seriously. We prescribe a full course of antibiotics in order to speed resolution of symptoms and prevent rheumatic fever and its potentially life-threatening complications.

So the million-dollar question with any sore throat is: Is it a bacteria or a virus? A child can ride out a viral sore throat with some pain and other symptomatic relief (see page 284), but a bacterial sore throat may need to be treated with antibiotics, both to treat the throat and to prevent complications. It's difficult even for a doctor to tell from symptoms alone whether a red or aching throat is caused by a strep infection, so we just regard any sore throat that has lasted for more than 24 hours as suspicious and culture it appropriately. A throat that clears up in less than 48 hours is likely to have had a viral cause, but even a quick resolution is not a guarantee.

A doctor cannot tell a viral from a bacterial sore throat just by looking at it and taking a child's history. Since a strep throat requires antibiotics, and a viral throat inflammation doesn't, it is necessary to test for the presence or absence of Group A beta-hemolytic streptococci, the strain that causes rheumatic fever and other nasty strep complications. There are still some doctors who routinely hand out antibiotic prescriptions for acutely sore throats without doing a definitive test, but we are not among them. The cheapest and, surprisingly

# Signs of a.....

**Viral Sore Throat**
Throat pain.
Fever.
Difficulty swallowing.
Enlarged lymph nodes
    in neck.
Red pharynx, beefy tonsils.
White, cheesy stuff on tonsils.
Cough or running nose.

**Strep Throat**
Throat pain.
Fever.
Difficulty swallowing.
Enlarged lymph nodes
    in neck.
Red pharynx, beefy
    tonsils.
Creamy stuff on tonsils.
Foul-smelling breath.
Headache, bellyache,
    or nausea.

There may also be a sand-papery, pink-red body rash with strep throat that is a sign of another form of strep infection known as scarletina, which is treated the same way as strep throat.

As you can see, the signs and symptoms are nearly identical, which is why a visit to the doctor will be in order.

enough, most effective test is the throat culture: A cotton swab is used to transfer bacteria from the inflamed tonsils and pharynx to a laboratory dish filled with a compound that encourages the growth of specific bacteria. Results are available within 24 hours, and the test is fairly accurate. However, if the test takes a day, and a child is still contagious for another day after beginning antibiotics, use of the culture requires the child (and parent or caregiver) to be home from school or work for at least two days. Another test was therefore developed to allow for quicker results. Although the rapid antigen-detector test (rapid strep test) gives results within minutes, it is not as accurate, missing a certain number of cases of strep. That's why it's recommended that a negative rapid strep test be backed up with a throat culture.

We treat sore throats differently because of the kind of practices we have. Dr. Stu has a stable patient base and the luxury of follow-up. In addition, the majority of the children in his practice have a parent at home to monitor their progress. He relies on throat cultures first rather than rapid strep tests, because they are more accurate and there is some evidence that it is better to let the tonsils and pharynx have the chance to build antibodies for stronger local immune protection in the future than to step in immediately with antibiotics. He does use a rapid strep test if a child is extremely uncomfortable and delay would cause unnecessary distress, or if both parents work and there are no options for sick-child care. In the presence of a positive throat culture, Dr. Stu prescribes oral amoxicillin. (If a child has a true allergy to penicillin, he prescribes another category of antibiotic instead.)

When Dr. Russ is working in the emergency department, he usually calls for a rapid strep test when a diagnosis is not clear from symptoms alone, because it gives him immediate results. It is not as accurate as a throat culture, but since Dr. Russ cannot be sure of seeing an emergency-room patient again, he needs to know right away whether or not they need antibiotics. If the rapid test is negative, he does a back-up culture in cases where follow-up with the patient is possible. Like Dr. Stu, he also suggests some of the complementary remedies listed below.

It is very important that children with strep throat take the full course of prescribed antibiotics in order to prevent complications or recurrence. We usually recommend a concurrent two- or three-week course of an over-the-counter probiotic like *Lactobaccillus GG* during treatment to protect the normal intestinal flora from being destroyed by the antibiotic medication.

# What Parents Can Do for Sore Throat

As we said earlier, most sore throats are not caused by *Streptococcus*, but by short-lived viruses, allergens, or even such environmental irritants as smog or cigarette smoke. Children who sleep with their mouths hanging open are more likely to have sore throats, because their mucous membranes there get very dry. Here are a few natural remedies to ease a sore throat, if strep has been ruled out or is already being treated.

- Liquids—both hot and cold—can soothe the mucous membranes, increase local circulation, and keep the body well hydrated. Your child can tell you which feels better—warm drinks or cold. Hot water with honey and lemon (only for children over a year in age) and chicken or miso soup are traditional favorites. Add chopped fresh garlic to the chicken broth to maximize the healing benefits of this traditional remedy. If cold feels better, offer iced noncaffeinated teas, full-strength fruit juices, juice-sicles, or Pedialyte pops, a frozen form of oral rehydration therapy.
- Food hurt going down? Try some slippery noodles with olive oil and crushed garlic (which has a reputation as an antimicrobial herb).
- To relieve pain, use children's acetaminophen or ibuprofen as directed on the package. Do not use aspirin products.
- Turn on the cool-mist vaporizer to keep mucous membranes in the throat moist.
- A gargle of one part hydrogen peroxide to three parts water can be soothing for any child old enough to know how to gargle. Dr. Stu finds that a gargle made of ½ teaspoon of table salt in an 8-ounce glass of warm water works well too.
- Immune-boosting herbs can speed healing. Use echinacea (4 to 8 drops of standardized extract in water or juice two to five times a day for kids two to six, and 8 to 15 drops for kids six to

twelve). Dr. Stu has found liquid garlic extract shortens the duration of a sore throat and prevents recurrences. The dose is ¼ to a ½ teaspoon twice a day for kids eighteen months to three years or a full teaspoon for kids three to twelve. Add to a big glass of fruit or vegetable juice or mix with a little choco-late- or fruit-flavored syrup to improve the taste. Dr. Russ prefers to crush fresh garlic and add it to salads or to hot foods during the last five minutes of cooking.

- Essential fatty acids appear to help treat and prevent sore throats. Dr. Stu likes to recommend a liquid product that com-bines black currant and evening primrose oils, which are high in gamma-linolenic fatty acids (GLA). A child eighteen months to three years old would take ¾ to 1 teaspoon once a day for prevention and twice a day for treatment. The dose is doubled for kids three to twelve. Dr. Russ prefers to give his patients essential fatty acids in the form of food—salmon or flax seed, either ground fresh and sprinkled on cereal or apple-sauce or as a golden oil added to a fruit smoothie.
- Choose a homeopathic remedy that suits your child's symp-toms, say, *Apis* for a very red throat that feels better with cold drinks. (See chapter 13.)
- Throat lozenges can relieve pain for a short time, and there's a wide variety to try.
- Massage the outside of the throat with an aromatic herbal rub, perhaps an ounce of nut or vegetable oil with a drop or two of eucalyptus essential oil in it, but only for kids over three.
- Do the Lion, a yoga exercise designed to increase circulation in the throat, as described in chapter 10.

**Call your child's physician** if in addition to a sore throat your child has a fever and swollen glands, a barking cough, a change in his or her voice, or difficulty in swallowing or keeping fluids down. **Go to the emergency department** if your child has difficulty breathing or assumes the "sniffing position" (head and neck extended to ease breathing), or appears abnormally lethargic or confused.

# Listen Up!:

*Ear Infections*

ost parents are familiar with ear infections (otitis media), because two thirds of all children experience at least one before they're two years old. In the days before antibiotic drugs, kids' earaches were handled at home with a variety of natural remedies. Most of the time the earaches went away on their own after a few days. But occasionally earaches progressed to very serious infections, so eventually parents started bringing children to the doctor for antibiotics to prevent these complications. Within twenty years, the number of office visits for earache nearly tripled, from 9 million in 1975 to more than 25 million in the 1990s. Given our national love affair with antibiotics over this period, it's no surprise that the number of prescriptions rose in a startling fashion as well. In 1980, 12 million prescriptions were written for antibiotics to treat ear infections in the United States; by 1992, the number of prescriptions had leapt to 23.6 million. Ear infections are now the most common reason for antibiotic prescription in children. Part of that rise is due to the increasing number of young children in day care (who are at greater risk for these sorts of infections), but much of it was due to a cavalier attitude toward antibiotics by both doctors and parents. Now the bacteria responsible for ear infections are becoming resistant to antibiotics, limiting their usefulness. So what should you do with a kid with an earache?

We're not surprised that parents are confused, because, frankly, many doctors are confused, too. The issue of antibiotic resistance has caused the medical profession to look much more closely at the way we have been treating ear infections, and to make changes. Doctors haven't all agreed on *which* changes yet, but we can help you understand the issues and recommend an integrative approach to the common earache.

Let's start with a little basic ear anatomy. You are probably already familiar with what is called the outer ear: the shaped cartilage on the side of the head and the ear canal that leads to the eardrum, a tight membrane that transmits sound. The inner ear, which is important to balance, is the portion of the ear located most deeply inside the head, closest to the brain. Between the eardrum and inner ear lies the middle ear, an air-filled cavity that contains three tiny bones (the anvil, stirrup, and hammer) that are important to hearing. The middle ear is connected to the back of the nasal cavity (the nasopharynx) by the eustachian tube, which provides the air to equalize pressure on both sides of the eardrum. The eustachian tube also allows any fluid produced in the middle ear to drain freely.

You may have already spotted the weak point in this system. Obviously a tube that leads from the back of the nose to the inner ear goes both ways. Not only can fluid drain out of it, but mucus and bacteria from the nose or throat can travel up it. Any obstruction in the tube—from a plug of dried mucus, for example—can trap fluid in the middle ear, providing an excellent incubator for stray bacteria. In addition, the eustachian tubes of children under two are more nearly horizontal and more collapsible, so fluid that gets into them cannot easily drain out. (These tubes become more vertical as children get older, one reason why older children and adults have fewer ear infections.)

The important thing to determine about a middle-ear problem, then, is whether or not an infectious process is at work in any trapped fluid. A child with fluid behind the eardrum but no sign of infection has otitis media with effusion (fluid), which generally does not require antibiotics. A child with acute otitis media, which is what parents usually mean by the term "ear infection," will have fluid in the middle

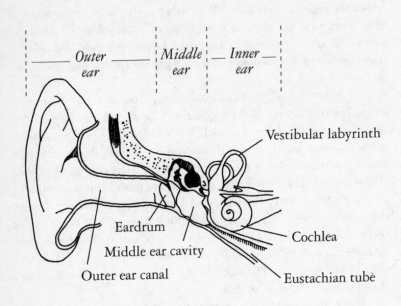

_Outer ear_ _Middle ear_ _Inner ear_

Vestibular labyrinth

Eardrum

Middle ear cavity

Outer ear canal

Cochlea

Eustachian tube

## Structures of the Ear

ear plus additional symptoms that may signal the need for antibiotics. As doctors, we want to be very sure which of these two conditions a child has before forming a plan of treatment.

Let's take a minute to talk about the various forms of otitis.

**Otitis media with effusion (OME).** OME is the term we use for situations where fluid is present in the middle ear but there is no infection. The term "serous otitis media" may also be used. Symptoms of OME might be a temporary reduction in hearing, a "popping" of the ears, or a feeling of fullness in the ears. Many people—even doctors—

confuse fluid in the ear with an ear infection, which is unfortunate, because it leads to 8 million unnecessary courses of antibiotics a year. The middle ear, like the nose and the sinuses, can collect fluid when a child has a cold or an allergy. Fluid can also be present in the middle ear because of blockage of the eustachian tubes by mucus or enlarged adenoids. In infants, small children, and people with eustachian tube abnormalities, fluid may be present for weeks or even months after a previous ear infection because of inefficient drainage.

We no longer routinely issue antibiotic prescriptions in these situations, but prefer a policy of "watchful waiting." We monitor kids with OME intermittently with a physical exam and a look at the mobility of the eardrum using an instrument called a tympanometer. We want to know whether fluid is starting to drain or getting thicker, and whether hearing is improving or getting worse. We may issue a short course of antibiotics if a child suffers a sudden hearing loss. If OME persists for more than 3 to 4 months, we refer the child to an ear, nose, and throat doctor who specializes in pediatrics to determine the cause of the fluid and to check for the presence of a benign ear tumor called a cholesteatoma. If the OME is especially thick and persistent ("glue ear"), the specialist may recommend the surgical insertion of pediatric ear tubes (discussed in more detail below) to drain the ear.

**Acute otitis media (AOM).** AOM is what parents typically mean when they talk about an ear infection. It is often distinguished from OME by signs of infection such as fever and reddened eardrums. Older kids may complain of pain or a sensation of fullness in an ear, typically after a cold. Infants who cannot verbalize their pain will be fussy, lack appetite, and may pull or tug at an ear. However, some children with AOM have no fever or pain, and there are many reasons (crying and fever among them) why eardrums might be red. To nail down the diagnosis of AOM your child's doctor needs to use an instrument called an otoscope to examine your child's eardrum. The eardrum of a child with OME is in a neutral position, or perhaps tending slightly inward. The eardrum of a child with AOM bulges outward. It is opaque (red or yellow), and immobile when air is puffed into the ear canal through a rubber bulb attached to the otoscope.

A bulge in the eardrum is a sign that something nasty is growing in your child's inner ear. Most likely that something is a bacteria (usually *Streptococcus pneumonia, Haemophilus influenzae, or Moraxella catarralis*). That doesn't mean that antibiotics are necessarily required, a lesson the medical establishment is just learning in this country. A quarter of ear infections are caused by viruses, which we know do not respond to antibiotics. And many of the bacterial cases will get better without any antibiotic drugs. Recent studies have found that 80 percent of cases of AOM caused by *M. catarralis* and 50 percent of those caused by *H. influenzae* resolve by themselves within one to seven days. However, only 15 to 20 percent of cases caused by S. *pneumonia* resolve spontaneously.

So how do we know when to treat? We would prescribe antibiotics from the get-go for a child with an ear infection who was in severe pain, feverish, or fussy for whom more serious diseases like meningitis have been ruled out. We might also offer antibiotics from the start to children in day care, children of smokers, and children with cleft palate. In most cases of simple AOM where the child is active and alert, however, we prefer a policy of watchful waiting. That is, we treat a child over two for pain with children's acetaminophen and/or eardrops containing benzocaine (if there is no eardrum rupture). We might possibly suggest a nasal decongestant as well. We ask the parents of children under eighteen months to give us a phone report in 24 hours; parents of older children check back with us if the child's fever or pain persists for more than three days. If there is no sign of improvement after three days, or symptoms worsen, we then prescribe a narrow-spectrum, inexpensive antibiotic drug that can be taken orally, such as amoxicillin. Sometimes we give a parent a prescription for their child at the first visit and ask them to fill it only if it is still needed after three days. We do not prescribe the newer broad-spectrum antibiotics as a first line of defense, but save them for use if amoxicillin does not do the job. These new antibiotics are more expensive, have more side effects, and lead to greater bacterial resistance. When we do prescribe antibiotics, we make sure parents understand that it is important for their child to take these drugs as often and for as long as prescribed. To reduce the risk of diarrhea and other antibiotic side effects, we also suggest that a child eat live-culture yogurt or take a probiotic supplement during the course of treatment.

This policy of watchful waiting is gaining support with conventional practitioners as a strategy to slow the rise of resistant bacteria. Up to 58 percent of the bacteria most often responsible for ear infections are now resistant to first-line drug treatment; if doctors focus on saving antibiotics for use only when they are appropriate, drug-susceptible strains of these bacteria may be restored. Dr. Stu has reduced the use of antibiotics in his practice by 60 to 70 percent with no harm—and probable benefit—to the health of his patients. He is now seeing far fewer cases of recurrent AOM, which is more difficult to cure. And he has the satisfaction of knowing that he is not unnecessarily giving his patients drugs that alter the normal balance of bacteria in the body, or cause troublesome side effects.

There were once concerns that delaying use of antibiotics for ear infections would lead to serious complications such as the spread of infection to the mastoid area (a spongy bone directly behind the external ear), brain, or blood. However, studies in The Netherlands, one of the few developed countries where antibiotics are not routinely used for ear infections, found this not to be true. In the extremely rare cases when these complications did occur, they were easily treated with drugs. Parental fears are often eased by hearing that another Dutch study found that antibiotics were eventually required in fewer than 3 percent of children with untreated ear infections. This Dutch practice of watchful waiting has led to a large decline in resistant bacteria in that country.

Sometimes the eardrum bursts spontaneously with sudden pain and discharge of yellowish fluid that may be streaked with red. This relieves pressure (and pain), drains fluid, and allows healing to begin; the eardrum will repair itself naturally. We handle perforated eardrums differently because of the differences in our practices. Dr. Russ always prescribes antibiotics to any child with pus coming out of a ruptured eardrum that he sees in the emergency department, because he cannot insure adequate follow-up. Dr. Stu, on the other hand, can monitor his patients' progress and prescribe antibiotics only if necessary. We do not recommend in-office intentional perforation of the eardrum; we think it's too aggressive and too difficult to do safely on a pint-sized moving target.

**Recurrent AOM.** About a quarter of visits to the doctor for ear infection are for recurrent AOM—acute ear infections that occur three separate times in 6 months or four or more separate times in a year. (Any AOM that occurs within 30 days of another is considered to be a continuation of the first case rather than a separate case.) We're fairly certain of some of the risk factors for recurrent AOM: Recent antibiotic use, age under two years, attendance at a day-care center, exposure to tobacco smoke, use of a pacifier, and formula (not breast) feeding all factor in. Underlying conditions such as gastroesophageal reflux, food allergies, and enlarged adenoids that serve as a reservoir for bacteria may also play a role and must be treated.

Recurrent cases of AOM are usually treated with higher-dose or wider-spectrum antibiotics. We would also try to determine and address the underlying problem. We might refer a child to an osteopath or other skilled practitioner for cranial osteopathy or craniosacral manipulation, or we might suggest consulting a practioner of Chinese Medicine. We might refer the child to a specialist for an evaluation for gastroesophageal reflux (GERD). We would certainly recommend trying a dairy-free diet or other strategies against allergy. We would make sure immune-supportive measures like drinking fluids and getting enough rest were in place, and we might suggest a daily tonic of the Chinese herb astragalus.

We do not recommend putting children with recurrent AOM on long-term low-dose antibiotics as a preventive measure as this use strongly supports the development of resistant bacteria. If other measures have not been effective and ear infections keep recurring frequently, we would consider surgical insertion of pediatric ventilation ear tubes instead. Although this invasive procedure requires general anesthesia, it is usually quite safe, even for infants. We think it is much less troublesome than months of antibiotic use. A child with tubes will have to wear earplugs for swimming afterward, but the middle ear will be able to drain more freely, and there will be less scarring than from repeated rupture. Eventually your child will outgrow the need for tubes, which usually fall out naturally on their own within a year, allowing the eardrum to heal over.

Parents of children with recurrent AOM can now consider having their child vaccinated with the new multivalent pneumonococcal vaccine. *Streptococcus pneumoniae* is at work in about 20 percent of AOM cases. Since these cases are the least likely to resolve themselves, and *S. pneumoniae* is rapidly becoming resistant to antibiotics, immunization would both provide protection and reduce the need for antibiotics. Flu vaccines, currently not recommended for otherwise healthy children, also reduce the number of ear infections suffered. The new nasal flu vaccine has been found in one study to cut the risk of middle ear infection by 30 percent.

**Otitis externa ("swimmer's ear").** Otitis externa is an inflammation of the external ear canal. It is not caused by the same bacteria as acute otitis media, but can be caused by inflammatory conditions of the skin, trauma, or by organisms such as *Pseudomonas, Staphylococcus aureus,* and various fungi that get too comfy in the moist environment of the ear canal. Otitis externa in children is a moderate local inflammation with no serious complications, although it can cause itching, discharge, and pain. (As the same symptoms present when your child has put a bean in his ear, check for foreign objects first.)

We take a two-pronged approach to otitis externa. We prescribe eardrops to treat infecting organisms and we try to restore the acid pH of the ear canal to prevent their return. Preventive drops can be made simply by mixing together equal parts alcohol and white vinegar. Put a few drops of this solution into each ear, especially after swimming. If a child has a tendency toward swimmer's ear, we might recommend the use of earplugs when swimming.

As a final note on earaches, keep in mind that not all earaches are caused by one of the forms of otitis. Your child can also suffer ear pain from an abscessed tooth, a sinus infection, a pharyngeal infection, and temperomandibular joint syndrome (TMJ), and these conditions will need to be ruled out.

# What Parents Can Do to Prevent Earache

- Avoid exposing your child to tobacco smoke. Children of smokers have more ear infections.
- Breast-feed your child if possible. Infants who have been breast-fed at least three or four months have fewer ear infections. Do not feed infants in a flat position, or give a baby a bottle to take into the crib.
- Limit the use of a pacifier to just a few minutes at bedtime.
- Encourage frequent hand washing, especially before snacks or meals.
- Teach your child to blow her nose gently and without pinching her nostrils together to avoid shooting that gunk up into her middle ear.
- Consider a smaller day-care situation if your child has recurrent ear infections.
- Try eliminating dairy products from your child's diet for a month or two if he has recurrent ear infections. (Be sure to provide adequate calcium from other foods or supplements.) Children who are sensitive to milk proteins can develop increased irritation and inflammation.
- Consider dietary supplements that might help prevent recurrent infections. Dr. Stu has seen good results from both essential fatty acids and garlic extract.
- Consider having your child vaccinated against *Streptococcus pneumoniae*, which causes 20 percent of ear infections and accounts for many of the cases of recurrent AOM.
- Consider cranial osteopathy. Birth trauma and minor childhood accidents may increase susceptibility to ear infections by restricting the free flow of fluids in the head. Dr. Russ has heard many reports of recurrent ear infections resolving from this treatment.

# What Parents Can Do to Treat Earache

- Use children's acetaminophen and anesthetic eardrops for pain relief.
- Use antibiotics properly if your child's physician determines they are appropriate. Make sure your child takes all the pills or liquid prescribed.
- Apply gentle heat to the ear with a warm compress.
- Put two or three drops of garlic oil or garlic-mullein oil in the ear several times a day and plug loosely with a little cotton. (You can make garlic oil by letting crushed garlic steep in some olive oil for a day or two. Keep refrigerated until needed; warm to room temperature before using.) Do not put drops in any ear with discharge or a suspected rupture of the eardrum. You may supplement this topical treatment with garlic taken orally as food or supplement.
- Acupuncture can be a helpful preventive and therapeutic intervention in some cases of recurrent AOM.
- Echinacea can sometimes be helpful at the start of an ear infection.
- Try a homeopathic remedy that suits your child's symptoms, preferences, and temperament. Some possibilities: Aconite, Apis, Belladonna, Capsicum, Chamomilla, Kali bichromate, Mercurius, Silica, and Pulsatilla.

# Chapter 19

# Cry Babies, Cry Parents:

*Colic and Reflux*

t's the middle of the night, and six-week-old Amanda has been screaming at the top of her lungs for hours. Her exhausted parents are nearly in tears themselves from their inability to comfort their tightly wound child. They look at the red-faced Amanda and exchange a glance, then her dad throws a coat over his pajamas, wraps up Amanda, and heads for the car. He'll drive his little girl around for a few hours, the only thing that ever seems to soothe her.

Dramas like this are played out in households around the country, though the makeshift solutions to a colicky child vary. We've heard of kids soothed by driving, by the sound of a washer/dryer, and by the touch of massage. We know how exhausting and stressful colic can be for both parents and child. And we know how difficult it can be to build that essential parent-child bond when parents feel helpless and frustrated by their inability to provide comfort. We'd like to offer some suggestions to help you through this rite of passage that has brought even the most stable parents to their knees.

When dealing with an irritable baby, *colic* is the diagnosis we make when more serious problems have been ruled out. Colic is not a specific disease with a set cause, but rather a group of behaviors that occur in about 20 percent of infants in their first few months of life. Babies are considered to have colic if they cry intensely for three or more hours a day at least three days a week and do not have any obvious physical reason for the crying. A child with colic screams for longer periods of time than average children, and is more difficult to console. Colicky children are irritable and frequently have difficulty relaxing. Infantile colic seems to occur most often in the evening. It usually appears at about two weeks of age, peaks at six weeks, and disappears when the child is three to four months old. If "colic" continues for longer or involves vomiting, it is probably actually reflux, which we'll discuss below. Colic has no adverse long-term effects. **Call your child's physician** if your child has persistent or rapid-fire vomiting, fever, lethargy, refusal to feed, or is inconsolable.

Despite any number of theories, medical research has not identified the cause of colic, which may in fact be caused by different factors in different children. Food allergies or intolerances, abdominal pain, intestinal gas, and difficult parent-child relationships have been studied and dismissed as overall causes, although each can contribute to the symptoms of colic. Current research leans toward colic being either a neurodevelopmental stage in certain children who are extremely sensitive to their environments or an immaturity of the gastrointestinal tract that only time can cure.

While we don't know much about the cause of colic, we do know that infantile colic *will* go away with time. In the meanwhile, parents need to experiment until they find a few comfortable positions or soothing behaviors that calm their child. Once you have a few trusty tools, plan to use them as soon as possible after crying starts, as it is easier to relax a child who is not yet totally wound up. Take care of yourselves, too, as colic can give parents an extremely stressful few months. Make sure you have some release valve, a good friend or an emergency child-care site, to which you can turn if sleep deprivation and frustration lead you to think about shaking or hurting your child. There's no shame in asking for help when you and your child need it. Colicky babies can wear out even the most durable parents over time, if parents do not take the time-outs they need to regroup.

# What Parents Can Do for Colic

Since there is no disease process to arrest with colic, we target our treatment to the symptoms. There are over-the-counter medications containing simethicone for colic, but we have not found them to be effective. Below are nine strategies that we—and our patients' parents—have found to be helpful. Because every child is unique, we cannot predict what strategies will work for your child. One of our children was soothed by dancing to Paul Simon's "Kodachrome," one by the sound of the dryer, and another found comfort only in the video of *Top Gun*. Be reassured that every baby has an "off" switch; you just have to find what activates your child's. We suggest experimenting with various levels of stimulation. Some babies are soothed by the stimulation of sound, motion, or touch. Others need calm, quiet surroundings, and a lack of stimulation. Only experimentation can determine which your own child prefers.

1. *Massage your infant.* Gentle massage is a simple and effective way to reduce the pain and tension of both colicky baby and parents. We recommend massaging your infant for up to 15 minutes once or twice a day. Use a palmful of moisturizing baby cream or lotion or vegetable oil. For additional sedative action, add a drop of lavender oil; make sure to blend well.
2. *Try an herbal remedy.* Chamomile tea is a wonderful thing to give an irritable child. A bottle containing up to four ounces a day of the warm (not hot) herbal tea can soothe an irritable baby for several hours. Fennel tea can be substituted for chamomile.
3. *Relax the parent.* A vicious cycle can be created between an irritable baby and an overstressed parent. That's why it's especially important for you to find time for whatever form of stress reduction works best for you. Nervous or agitated parents aggravate regurgitation in babies, so try to lower your own

anxiety level. Don't feel guilty or incompetent. Remember, this too shall pass.

4. *Try some lavender aromatherapy.* In addition to lavender-scented massages, you can use a little sedative lavender oil in a diffuser in baby's room.

5. *Keep that baby moving.* Rock or roll your baby in a rhythmic and relaxed manner. Put him in a front- or backpack and go for a walk. Drive aimlessly around in the car.

6. *Try white noise.* Turn on the washer/dryer or the vacuum cleaner. Put on a tape of a mother's heartbeat, ocean waves, or lullabies.

7. *Assume the position.* Some positions are better than others at soothing a colicky child. One of the classics is the "flying baby" or "sack of potatoes" pose, with infant draped, stomach down, along a parent's forearm.

8. *Swaddle the baby.* Some babies like to have their bodies wrapped snugly (face free) in a sheet or blanket.

9. *Experiment with an alternative.* Some parents swear by cranial osteopathy for colic, others say homeopathic remedies have done the trick.

But what if it's not just colic? There is another condition that is often confused with colic in young children: *gastroesophageal reflux,* or *reflux.* Reflux is most familiar to adults as the "heartburn" caused by acidic stomach contents backing up the esophagus. Infants may experience heartburn and abdominal pain with reflux as well, but their primary symptom is often frequent or recurrent spitting up. In some cases the stomach secretions rise high enough to irritate and inflame the upper and lower airways (nose, throat, and bronchial tubes), and may even lead to chronic respiratory infections, cough, sinusitis, ear infections, or congestion, or the wheezing of reactive airways.

How can you tell colic from reflux? A baby more likely has reflux if she spits up frequently or if her symptoms last longer than three months. Some infants with reflux (known as "happy spitters") eat well and spit up without pain, others have pain associated with their vomiting. Some of the sickest and most uncomfortable babies with reflux, however, never spit up at all.

That's why doctors and parents should pay attention to feeding patterns. Usually, healthy babies look forward to and enjoy feeding times. Babies with colic may initially resist feeding, but eventually will relax and feed. Most babies with reflux, however, find it difficult to relax with feeding, and often refuse to feed because doing so aggravates the burning sensation ("heartburn") in the esophagus. They arch their backs in a certain way, and appear uncomfortable in their own skin. Babies with reflux may exhibit pain for one or two hours after feeding, and some may develop an anticipatory prefeeding pain. **Take your child to the emergency department** if reflux is accompanied by breathing difficulties, wheezing, frequent coughing, turning blue, or brief periods of not breathing (apnea).

Although older children with reflux may also have heartburn or stomachache, reflux is more likely to present in kids over three as frequent upper respiratory infections, reactive airway disease, hoarseness, or ear infections. In our experience, treating the underlying problem of reflux can eradicate these persistent conditions. Successful treatment of reflux may also eliminate the need for long-term antibiotics to treat recurrent ear and sinus infections.

Babies outgrow colic in a few months, so our approach to colic focuses on symptomatic relief. Simple reflux tends to clear up on its own by the time a child is walking (twelve to fifteen months). But untreated chronic reflux (gastroesophageal reflux disease, or GERD) can cause serious and long-lasting damage, so we try to diagnose and treat it in a timely manner.

# What Doctors and Parents Can Do for Reflux

Once your child's doctor has diagnosed reflux, there are remedies that can be employed by both parent and physician. Among them:

- *Look at the child's diet.* Since food sensitivities can play a role in reflux, usually the first element removed from the diet of a child with reflux is cow's milk. Babies being fed formula based on cow's milk should be switched to a hydrolyzed casein or soy-based formula. If these are ineffective, a very hypoallergenic amino-acid-based artificial formula such as Neocate may be tried. Sensitivity to breast milk is extremely rare, so we strongly recommend breast-feeding for babies with reflux. If reflux continues, mother may need to eliminate cow's milk from her own diet. If that doesn't do the trick, then she should try an elimination diet (see chapter 22) to identify possible dietary allergens.

Older children with reflux should avoid chocolate, caffeine, peppermint, and carbonated beverages, any of which can trigger esophageal reflux because they relax the muscle that seals the stomach off from the esophagus.

- *Consider how the child sleeps.* Babies with reflux often sleep better in a prone position (on their tummies). However, the supine position (on their backs) is recommended to prevent sudden infant death syndrome. Therefore, it is essential to take other steps to prevent SIDS: If a baby with reflux is sleeping on his tummy, be sure to remove from the crib heavy blankets, pillows, toys, and any other stuff that has the potential to suffocate him. Putting your child to sleep in a car seat or other infant seat does not relieve reflux, according to studies, although parents frequently tell us otherwise.

- *Thicken feedings.* Add a tablespoon of rice cereal to each ounce of formula to reduce regurgitation in bottle-fed babies. In families where weight gain is an issue, be advised that this increases the calories per ounce from 20 to 30. You would be better off looking for special prethickened formulas that deliver just the desired 20 calories per ounce.

- *Try a prescription medication.* When a child is in significant pain—especially while feeding—and not eating an adequate number of calories, we often prescribe the acid-reducing agent ranitidine (Zantac) to neutralize stomach acid, reduce burning, and allow the esophagus to heal. This medication can produce dramatic results, cutting pain within days. For children with more severe or complicated disease, we may prescribe one of the newer classes of proton-pump inhibitors (such as omeprazole) to reduce acid secretion.

- *Don't smoke tobacco.* Exposure to tobacco smoke worsens reflux in babies.
- *Focus on relaxing yourselves.* Like colic, reflux is aggravated by parental anxiety. Take time-outs when you need them, and practice deep breathing or some other stress-busting technique.

If reflux does not get better with dietary changes or medication, we refer the child to a pediatric gastroenterologist for a test known as a pH probe. We save this test for the most intractable cases, because it is invasive and can be hard on a child. A tiny wire with an acid-measuring tip is inserted by a pediatric gastroenterologist through the nose and into the esophagus of the child being tested, where it remains, recording levels of acid there, for 24 hours. The results are evaluated with an eye for choosing the proper higher-level medications and dosages for more effective treatment.

# Chapter 20

# Tummy Troubles:

## *Abdominal Complaints*

t he abdomen seems to be the focus of many pediatric complaints. We see lots of kids with abdominal problems from recurrent early-morning school-day tummy caused by anxiety, to uncomfortable constipation due to poor bathroom habits to diarrhea from stomach flu or contaminated food. One reason why the belly is the site of so much trouble is that it's where children tend to carry any stress from worrying or unresolved conflicts. Adults display stress more often with headache or painful muscle tension, but to kids, the belly is where it's at. Even so, parents should not jump to the conclusion that tummy trouble is always stress-related. As physicians, we know the need to sort through about a hundred possible causes of abdominal pain, from self-limiting illnesses to problems requiring surgery, to come up with the right diagnosis. In the following pages, we'll discuss some of the most common causes of tummy troubles we see in children and our recommendations for treatment.

**Appendicitis.** Whenever a child has persistent abdominal pain, it is important to rule out appendicitis—an acute inflammation of an appendage of the large intestine known as the appendix—because it can become a life-threatening condition. If an untreated "hot" appendix is not surgically removed in time, it can burst, spreading infection throughout the abdominal cavity. So whenever we see a child with abdominal pain we do a thorough physical exam, some basic lab tests if they are clinically indicated, and possibly a follow-up sonogram, because we want to be very careful not to miss a case of appendicitis. Most children with appendicitis will have vomiting and loss of appetite in addition to the abdominal pain. They may not eat for two or three days. Very young children cannot describe their pain verbally, but in older children, pain starts around the belly button, and gradually localizes in the lower right part of the abdomen over the first one or two days. The cure for appendicitis is strictly surgical—remove the inflamed appendix—and recovery is generally uneventful.

**Constipation.** A child is considered constipated if she is moving her bowels less frequently than normal, is straining or having painful voiding, or is passing hard, dry stools. Many children have problems with constipation at some time in their young lives, most often from lack of fluids, poor diet, or withholding of stool for psychological reasons. Kids may hold stool when they are being toilet trained or if they are uncomfortable using a bathroom that is not their own. We've seen plenty of cases of "school bathroom phobia" over the years; having visited a few school bathrooms where cleanliness and privacy were sorely lacking, we can't say we blame them.

In our experience, parents have a tendency to get worked up about a possibly constipated child, so we counsel you to try to project a more relaxed attitude. You don't want this to become a battle of wills. Among the suggestions below, you will find a number of dietary and other strategies for relieving constipation that can be instituted without a child's really being conscious of them. We do not generally use artificial laxatives for children with constipation, preferring gentler, more natural methods. In cases of long-term constipation, we may resort to a pediatric enema.

# What Parents Can Do for Constipation

- *Assess your child's milk consumption.* We often see problems with constipation in toddlers who drink more than two cups of cow's milk a day. If cow's milk is identified as a problem after a period of elimination from the diet, switch to calcium-fortified soy milk.

- *Make sure your child is drinking enough fluids.* Children should drink a cup of water a day for every 10 pounds of weight (up to 80 pounds).

- *Increase physical activity.* Regular exercise helps keep things moving along, intestinally speaking.

- *Increase fiber consumption.* A low-fiber diet is associated with constipation. Make sure your child eats plenty of high-fiber foods such as fruits, vegetables, whole-wheat bread, bran flakes, beans, and brown rice.

- *Try some prunes.* Grandma was right! Nearly everyone likes the natural sweetness of what we are now supposed to call "dried plums." A few tablespoons a day of stewed prunes for babies, or three to four stewed or dried prunes a day for toddlers can help keep them regular.

- *Add probiotics.* Beneficial bacteria, such as *Lactobacillus* or *Bifidobacteria*, may help, either in the form of yogurt with live cultures, fortified milk, or supplements. These "good buggies" certainly help with digestion, and some studies have found benefit for constipation as well.

- *Get friendly with flax.* Ground flaxseed meal is an excellent natural laxative due to its high fiber content, with the added benefit of omega-3 fatty acids. Kids like its mild nutty flavor, too. Keep flax seeds or meal frozen or refrigerated, as flax products turn rancid quickly when exposed to air and light. (Discard any flax product that smells like paint, a sure sign of rancidity.) Dr. Stu recommends a teaspoon a day of flax meal sprinkled over food for his patients over two; adjust the dose up or down as needed. Dr. Russ prefers using either a teaspoon of powdered psyllium seed husks (*Plantago psyllium*) a day or a mix of the powdered husks and flax meal. The plain, high-fiber psyllium should be stirred into a large glass of juice or water and drunk. A child taking either of these natural laxatives should be sure to drink plenty of water and other fluids throughout the day, otherwise these so-called "bulking agents" will just plug things up worse.

- *Check out emotional issues.* Withholding stool can be a form of control, or a sign of stress. You may need to explore with your child the reasons for this problem. Be sure not to be punitive during toilet training or to reprimand a child for bowel accidents or constipation; you'll only worsen the situation. Allow for a relaxed regular "sit down" period for your child. Self-hypnosis, meditation, or breathing exercises may be helpful with general stress reduction.

**Diarrhea.** Diarrhea is a condition of loose, frequent stools, often accompanied by a feeling of urgency. While diarrheal illness is one of the leading causes of infant death in developing countries, in industrialized countries diarrhea is usually a mild, self-limiting viral or bacterial infection. When your child has diarrhea, focus on making her comfortable and ensuring that she does not become dehydrated. Water—and in more severe cases, liquid or frozen (Popsicle-style) pediatric rehydration solutions become the primary therapy. Do not give a child with diarrhea fruit juice or soda, as these liquids contain sugars that are not absorbed well by the gut and can worsen or prolong diarrhea. Familiar remedies such as chicken broth and even sports drinks do not have the proper balance of electrolytes that only oral rehydration solutions can provide.

Diarrhea has hundreds of causes, but the most common are infectious viruses, bacteria, or parasites picked up from other kids, contaminated water, or food that has not been prepared safely. One good preventive strategy then, is to reduce exposure to these infectious agents by teaching your children to wash their hands carefully after going the bathroom and before preparing or eating food. When traveling, do not let them drink or brush their teeth with any water that is not guaranteed to be sterile, or eat food from street vendors. Failure to follow these simple rules can lead to a vacation-spoiling case of "travelers' diarrhea." At home, "food poisoning" caused by such microbes as *Salmonella* and *E. coli,* can often be quite severe, so be sure to handle, prepare, and store food safely. Do not let your child eat any foods containing undercooked meat or eggs—this means no raw cookie dough either.

So-called antibiotic-associated diarrhea is the frequent result of treatment with antibiotics that wipe out beneficial bowel bacteria as a side effect. Use of probiotics should prevent this.

**Call your child's physician** if diarrhea is accompanied by cramping pain, fever, or bloody stools; if a nonpainful case of diarrhea continues for more than five days; or if persistent diarrhea follows a camping trip or travel in a developing country. A child exhibiting signs of dehydration such as sunken eyes or "doughy" skin needs to see a doctor immediately or be taken to the emergency department.

# What Parents Can Do About Diarrhea

- *Give your child plenty of water.* Do not rely on fruit juice or soda for fluids.
- *Give a probiotic supplement,* preferably one containing *Lactobacillus GG*, which has been found in a number of studies to both prevent and treat diarrhea. We recommend that any child who has had diarrhea for more than two or three days be given supplemental probiotics for seven to ten days. If a child is too young to swallow an enteric-coated probiotic capsule, you can sprinkle probiotic powder or the contents of a capsule of *Lactobacillus GG* on food or put it in formula; this variety resists break-down by stomach acid or bile even out of the capsule.
- *If diarrhea persists, consider reducing or eliminating milk products from your child's diet.* Many children—especially those of African American, Asian, or Mediterranean heritage—lack the enzyme lactase, which is necessary to digest the milk sugar lactose. There are lactose-free dairy products available for those who are lactose-intolerant, but in our experience the problem sometimes lies in an intolerance of the protein casein instead.

Even children who normally can digest milk well may experience a temporary lactase deficiency while ill.

• *A bland diet allows the intestines time to regroup.* Aptly called BRAT, the conventional diet includes Bananas, Rice, Applesauce, and dry Toast. We add yogurt as well after the first day of a diarrheal illness.

We discourage the use of over-the-counter diarrhea remedies as they slow down the peristaltic activity of the gut so that it takes longer for a child's body to get rid of the pathogen. This is especially important with bacterial causes of diarrhea.

**Inflammatory Bowel Disease.** Whenever a child has persistent abdominal pain, unexplained recurrent fever, and bloody diarrhea, we need to consider inflammatory bowel disease, or IBD. The term IBD encompasses both Crohn's disease and ulcerative colitis, conditions that are sometimes difficult to distinguish from one another. (IBD should not be confused with irritable bowel syndrome, or IBS, which is not characterized as an inflammatory disease.) A diagnosis of IBD is made after an extensive history and physical exam, tests for inflammation or infection (such as blood test of sedimentation rate), and perhaps a barium X ray or a visual scan of the bowel through sigmoidoscopy or colonoscopy.

IBD is usually treated with an anti-inflammatory drug based on salicylic acid (aspirin) and with oral steroids—medications that have significant side effects. We have had great success with drug-free strategies, which, although they do require a great commitment from child and parents, can stop diarrhea, pain, and bleeding and help a child regain lost weight.

The foundation of Dr. Stu's IBD treatment is a dietary program designed by nutritionist Elaine Gottschall (see Resources), which has allowed many of Dr. Stu's patients to avoid immuno-suppressive therapy after a period of close monitoring. Gottschall's program focuses on reducing the presence of the undigested or unabsorbed carbohydrates that she believes create carbohydrate overload and excessive fermentation in the intestines. Although her IBD diet is quite restrictive—eliminating all cereal grains and milk—highly motivated children and families have found it well worth the inconvenience to be free of their disabling symptoms. Dr. Stu allows some modifications to the Gottschall program, but, in his experience, it works best when followed strictly.

Dr. Russ takes a more individualized tack with his patients, using an elimination diet to help them pinpoint their unique IBD triggers. He has found that this approach provides symptomatic relief while minimizing dietary restrictions.

The cause of IBD is not really known, though we do know that stress is an important factor. Therefore, both of us rely heavily on mind/body therapies as well, including relaxation techniques, biofeedback, and imagery.

# What Parents Can Do for IBD

- *Try an elimination diet* to pinpoint foods that worsen your child's symptoms, and should be avoided.
- *Work with your child on a suitable stress-reduction technique.*
- *Boost your child's intake of anti-inflammatory omega-3 fatty acids* in food (cold-water fish or flax) or supplements (black currant or evening primrose oil). One simple approach is 1 teaspoon of flaxseed oil every few days for children age two to six (2 teaspoons for kids older than six).
- *Try acupuncture.* A number of Dr. Russ's patients have experienced good results from this complementary approach.
- *Discourage your child from drinking caffeinated soft drinks.*
- *Consider enteric-coated peppermint oil capsules* for children old enough to swallow. Do not substitute any other form of peppermint oil, which in its raw form can cause young children to choke.

**Functional Abdominal Pain.** "Functional abdominal pain" is how we describe belly pain with no known organic cause. The fact that there is no physical reason for the pain does not mean that the pain is not real, and even debilitating. As we all know, stress can play a lot of nasty tricks on us. But once all the serious diseases have been ruled out, it's almost a relief to know that the kind of pain the child is suffering can be controlled or eliminated without drugs or surgery.

Most parents are familiar with the kind of belly pain we're talking about. This is the before school or bedtime pain, the pain that appears at school or in the doctor's office, or wherever a stressful situation can be found. It's the pain of fear and anxiety and conflicted feelings. It's a pain that goes away when a child is having a good time or feeling relaxed and comforted. And don't underestimate the power of parental comfort and reassurance. In our experience, kids with functional abdominal pain will not be themselves relieved until their parents are reassured that this is a correct diagnosis.

In order to provide this reassurance, we do a complete work-up to rule out serious disorders, which are more likely if fever, nausea, vomiting, painful urination, weight loss, or bloody stools are involved. We put the emphasis on talking to the child and to his parents about his social circumstances—his relationships with school, friends, and family—looking for sources of stress. Sometimes an apprehensive child simply needs to know that all tests are normal for the pain to disappear. Other times we will need to have an open discussion with child and parents about the connection between their stress and their pain and work together to create a program to manage and eliminate the source of stress.

*H. pylori* infection. The bacteria *Helicobacter pylori* has been associated with gastritis (inflammation of the lining of the stomach) and ulcers in adults, but such problems are not very common in children. That's why it's so mystifying to us that *H. pylori* infection has become such a trendy diagnosis for children. Many young children with recurrent abdominal pain are being tested (with blood or breath tests) for the presence of *H. pylori*, and if they test positive for the bacterium, they are treated with antibiotics and other medications. Unfortunately, research does not support such aggressive treatment in children. A majority of children carry this bug in their stomachs, apparently without problem, and so far there is little evidence that the adult protocol is even very effective in kids. We now reserve this full-court press for those cases of *H. pylori* infection that cause symptoms that are resistant to more integrative treatment.

While most gastric and duodenal ulcers in children are indeed caused by *H. pylori*, only a small percentage of kids carrying the bacterium develop either condition. However, lifestyle factors such as stress, poor diet, or weakened immunity may render a child more vulnerable to the bacterium's effects. In such cases, the following strategies may help prevent or ease problems.

# What Parents Can Do for Ulcers

- *Have your child practice a mind/body therapy for stress reduction.* Studies have tied an inability to cope with stress to an increase in stomach acid secretions and a worsening of ulcer symptoms.
- *Try an herbal extract called deglycyrrhizinated licorice (DGL)* to soothe a child's stomach and duodenum and support his natural defenses. It's available in tablets that can be chewed and swallowed whenever the child feels discomfort. The only catch is this—he has to like the taste of licorice. (Most candies do not contain real licorice and will not do the trick. In any case, you do not want to give a child extracts or other forms of licorice containing glycyrrhizin, as the compound raises blood pressure.)
- *Avoid soft drinks, especially caffeinated ones.* Try warm or iced chamomile or peppermint tea instead. (Peppermint tea should not be used by a child with reflux, as it can worsen that condition.)
- *Reduce inflammation naturally.* Dr. Stu, as you may have noticed, is a big fan of ginger, so he suggests experimenting to see if taking (or eating) ginger eases symptoms. Ginger also contains some compounds specifically effective against ulcer.

# It's Not All
# in Your Head:

## *Headaches*

a pounding head might seem to be an adult problem, but kids get headaches, too. In fact, 40 percent of children suffer at least one headache before the age of seven. Try to keep this statistic in mind when your son says his head hurts and your thoughts turn to brain tumors. Tragically, some kids do get brain tumors—just one reason to make sure any child with frequent or disabling headaches gets a complete diagnostic workup—but your child's headaches are far more likely to be due to one of the many other, much more common, causes of head pain.

A child's headaches can stem from a wide array of causes: dehydration, noise, glaring light, a skipped meal, exposure to chemicals, vision problems, stress, head injuries, and such medical conditions as fever, strep throat, sinus infection, meningitis, misalignment of the jaw, and yes, brain tumor. In order to treat a headache, and prevent future headaches, you and your child's physician need to figure out what factor or combination of factors is behind your child's headaches. In this chapter, we talk about the two most common forms of headache in children, tension and migraine, and briefly touch on temporomandibular joint syndrome (TMJ), which can also cause head pain.

See your child's physician or take your child to the emergency department if a headache lasts for several days or worsens, if it was caused by a fall or head injury, or if it involves seizure, lethargy, vomiting, clumsiness, or personality changes. Parents often think that a child who has sustained a fall should not be allowed to go to sleep, for fear they'll lapse into a coma. In fact, a little nap can help ease the trauma; just wake the child up in an hour. Be aware that carbon monoxide poisoning is a serious and common cause of headache and flulike symptoms, especially in the winter months when gas furnaces and space heaters are in greater use. Make sure heated areas are well-ventilated and that heaters are in good working order. Do not let children run car, lawn mower, or go-cart engines in a closed garage.

**Tension Headaches.** The main symptom of tension headache is a dull pain that affects the whole head. It can feel like a tight band around the skull or a generalized achiness. The cause of this common headache is usually physical or mental stress, which tightens up the muscles of the head, neck, and shoulders. The best approach to stress-related problems is two-fold: ease the symptoms (short-term relief) and try to get at the root of the problem (long-term relief). Take, for example, Joshua, an eight-year-old boy who was having three or four headaches a week. His mother was worried that the headaches were a sign of some disastrous medical problem. Joshua's neurological exam was normal, however, and Dr. Stu diagnosed the symptoms as being consistent with tension-type headache. In further conversation with Joshua and his mother about possible stressors, it was discovered that the boy had recently lost a friend to leukemia. Although neither parent nor child thought this event had caused the headaches, Dr. Stu suggested they talk more about it at home. Not long after, Joshua's mom reported that they had had a long, loving, and tearful conversation about the fate of her son's friend. Once Joshua had a chance to grieve openly for his friend and his parents were able to allay his fears for his friend's well-being after death, his recurrent headaches disappeared. His parents were surprised, because they hadn't believed that grief could have such a strong physical effect on a child. They were pleased, too, because they had been so worried that Joshua's persistent headaches were caused by something unthinkable. Their family discussion removed two stressors involved in Joshua's headaches—his own unexpressed grief and the anxiety he picked up from his parents.

If your child is experiencing recurrent tension-type headaches, a gentle exploratory conversation may be in order. Often children will try to hide concerns or emotions that they—rightly or wrongly—believe will add to their parents' own stress levels. Speaking freely about what's bothering them can go a long way toward easing stress-related headaches. In addition, parents would be wise to pay attention to their own tension headaches. Note when and why they occur, and what therapies or lifestyle changes make them disappear. Then, if you see similar signs of tension headaches in your children, you will have some useful tips to pass along for preventing or treating this kind of headache. Teach them that a tension headache is a message, a signal from the body that it's time to stop and take care of yourself.

# What Parents Can Do for a Tension Headache

As we said before, there are many possible causes of headache, so first make sure your child has had enough sleep, enough food, and enough water that day. Ask about any minor accidents that involved the head and check for the presence of fever or infection (call a doctor if appropriate). If you've ruled out these causes, consider strategies that address tension.

- *Figure out the cause of tension.* Has your child had an argument with her best friend? Did something happen at school today? Is she anxious about an upcoming test or performance? Are her parents stressed or anxious? Is there tension within the family that needs to be addressed? Are her muscles tight from hours spent at the computer? Talk with your child about what's going on in her life. If the problem is either severe or long-standing, and does not respond to treatment, your child's doctor may suggest a visit to a psychologist or therapist for further help.

- *Use a relaxation exercise* or some self-hypnosis to help your child reduce body tension. See the sample exercise in the box on page 318.
- *Try an acupressure technique.* A child can be taught to press gently with the tips of the middle fingers in the two depressions at the base of the skull on either side of the spine for a few minutes, or you can do it for her. Pressing with one thumb on the the highest point of the muscle in the webbing between the other thumb and forefinger may also help with headache pain. Once a complete examination by your child's doctor has ruled out other physical causes for persistent headaches, you could consult a licensed acupuncturist.
- *Keep a headache diary* if headaches become frequent, making note of the activities of the day, foods eaten, worries, etc. See if you can detect a pattern that helps unlock the cause. If the headaches seem to be tied to certain foods or food additives, use the elimination diet explained in chapter 22 to pinpoint food allergies or sensitivities.
- *Gently massage your child's head, shoulders, and neck*, with special attention to the areas above and in front of the ears.
- *Take your child on a walk* or suggest some other exercise to release tension.
- *Encourage your child to do something he loves*, for distraction and stress relief.
- *Try a homeopathic remedy*, such as *Gelsemium* or *Natrum muriaticum*.
- *Apply heat or cold*. Either heat or cold can ease a headache, depending on personal preference. You can use ice or a bag of frozen corn wrapped in a light towel, or use either warm (test it on your own skin first) or cold compresses.
- *Give your child an over-the-counter pain reliever*, such as acetaminophen or ibuprofen.

**Temporomandibular Joint Syndrome (TMJ).** Misalignment of the jaw where it meets the skull (the temporomandibular joint) is a common cause for head pain in both children and adults. TMJ can have its roots in an accident or sports injury, in misaligned teeth, or in tension or spasm that pulls the muscles and other structures of the temporomandibular joint out of place. We consider this stress-related form of TMJ as a more severe form of tension headache with slightly different symptoms. A child with TMJ might have pain radiating to one ear, difficulty chewing, loss of appetite, and/or headache. She might grind her teeth at night (bruxism). Mind/body techniques or a nighttime dental appliance can relax the muscles and stabilize the joint. There may be benefit from osteopathic cranial manipulation or acupuncture as well. Any therapies should be coordinated with orthodontic work.

**Migraine headaches.** Many parents are surprised to discover that infants as young as six months of age can get these disabling headaches, but up to 10 percent of children suffer from migraines. In fact, migraine is the most common type of headache in children. Migraines come in many forms. A migraine can give a child the throb-

---

# A Visualization Exercise for Headache Pain

Breathe slowly, deeply, and evenly. In your mind's eye, imagine that a magic wand is coursing over your head, bathing it in healing energy. As you inhale, pretend that you are bringing in warm goodness and healing energy. Hold your incoming breath longer than usual, and during that time imagine that you are squeezing and tightening the painful blood vessels in your head. Then imagine that all that blood is flowing from your head, where all this pressure is, to your fingertips. As you exhale, imagine that pain, tension, and poisons are flushed out with your breath.

[*Adapted from* Headache Help, *by Lawrence Robbins and Susan Lang, Houghton Mifflin (Boston 1995), p. 24.*]

bing headache, dizziness, and sensitivity to light and noise typical to adult sufferers, although headaches are more likely in children to be bilateral rather than one-sided. In children, oddly, a migraine is even more associated with gastrointestinal symptoms such as nausea, vomiting, and abdominal pain. Migraines can also present in bizarre ways, such as confusion, temporary memory loss, and strokelike symptoms. The migraines of children are generally shorter in duration than those of adults, lasting from 10 to 15 minutes to a few hours rather than lingering for days. They may worsen during puberty as a result of hormonal changes.

There is a genetic component to migraine that gives some people sensitive nervous systems that react more strongly to stimulation; 45 percent of kids with one parent who gets migraines will have them, too. The exact sequence of events in migraine is still a mystery, but it is clear that certain foods, activities, odors, and environmental changes can trigger a migraine. These triggers vary from person to person, but common ones include hot dogs, aged cheese, chocolate, bananas, caffeine, foods containing MSG or nitrites, stress, glaring light, hunger, noise, weather changes, and lack of sleep. Some people may react to just one trigger, others will need to have several of these factors occur at once to suffer a migraine. A kid with a history of migraines who stays up late, sloshes down several cola drinks and skips breakfast in the morning may be setting herself up for a migraine attack.

Migraine headaches are divided into two categories based on the absence or presence of a warning stage called the aura. Most people have what is called a migraine without aura, or common migraine, but some experience migraine with aura, or classical migraine. Migraine aura is a period of up to an hour in which a child experiences visual disturbances like flashing lights or zigzags, as well as fatigue, pallor, and irritability. This can be upsetting to a child who does not understand what is going on. The aura fades as the typical migraine headache kicks in. Children may also show physical or emotional symptoms (prodrome) of an impending migraine attack up to two days before the actual headache begins. Clues of a pending attack include pale skin, fatigue, food cravings, irritability, or hyperactivity. Once you and your child are aware of the meaning of these symptoms, you can use them as a cue to start preventive measures to abort or lessen an attack.

There are some migraine drugs for adults that might be of use in children with severe migraines, although they have not been tested in children and have significant side effects. So rather than prescribe dihydroergotamine, beta blockers, or sumatriptan alone for migraine, we prefer to start with noninvasive approaches, such as elimination of triggers and mind/body techniques for symptom control. Underlying issues of stress and environmental exposures are especially important in migraine and must be addressed.

# What Parents Can Do for Migraine Headaches

- *Keep a migraine diary.* The best approach for reducing the frequency of migraines is to identify your child's triggers. We suggest keeping track of weather, diet, and other factors in a migraine diary, analyzing this information yourself or with your child's doctor, and avoiding, eliminating, or preparing for those factors that seem to be potential triggers. We see the best outcomes when a child takes an active role, so let your child take the lead here.
- *Make sure your child gets enough sleep and does not miss a meal.* Missing a meal is a trigger for 25 percent of kids with migraine. Not drinking enough water can be a trigger, especially in active toddlers.
- *Teach your child a mind/body technique for self-regulation.* In Dr. Russ's experience, mind/body therapies such as biofeedback and self-hypnosis are among the most effective interventions for children with headaches. In one well-done study, hypnosis was found to be more effective than a commonly used drug (the beta-blocker propanol). A few sessions with a specialist and some practice will prepare your child ahead of time to deal with the symptoms of migraine. Older kids might benefit from

exposure to mindfulness meditation and yoga (no inverted postures), with a special emphasis on breathing exercises.

- *Allow the child to rest in a dark, quiet room.* Most children will react to the sudden onset of a migraine by wanting to go to bed. Let them follow their instincts here—rest or sleep can completely relieve a migraine attack. Talk to your child's teacher about allowing him to put his head down and rest if a migraine starts in school.

- *Use heat or cold.* Microwaved hot packs or freezer cold packs may help relieve symptoms. See which one your child prefers. Test hot packs on yourself first, and put a cloth between a cold pack and your child's skin.

- *Eliminate artificial ingredients.* Migraine attacks can be triggered by processed foods with such additives as preservatives, nitrites, MSG, aspartame (Nutrasweet), or caffeine.

- *Cut saturated fats and increase anti-inflammatory omega-3 fatty acids* in your child's diet through intake of cold-water fish or flax.

- *Relieve pain with children's acetaminophen or ibuprofen.* Use as directed on the bottle for up to two days. If symptoms persist longer, consult your child's doctor, as too much acetaminophen can be toxic to the liver. Stronger prescription pain relievers are available, but they have not been tested in children and do have side effects.

- *Consider a visit to a homeopath* for an acute or constitutional remedy to reduce migraines. Homeopathic (not herbal) *Belladonna, Iris,* and *Sanguinaria* are common remedies for migraine, based on specific characteristics.

- *Give acupuncture or cranial osteopathy a trial.* Dr. Russ has witnessed excellent results from these two therapies in children who have already been through conventional Western medical evaluation (to rule out more serious conditions).

- *Try a botanical remedy.* The natural anti-inflammatory ginger has an excellent safety profile, and Dr. Stu almost always recommends this herb to children and teens with chronic migraines to reduce the frequency of migraine episodes. Dose is one half the adult dose for kids six to twelve of either a ginger-root extract twice a day or a combination ginger/turmeric/bromelain extract once a day. Remember that long-term use of ginger can promote bleeding to some degree.

Freeze-dried stinging nettle may be useful if your child's migraines are tied to allergies. Dr. Stu has had some success with a migraine program for older children that includes a standardized extract of the herb feverfew (*Chrysanthemeum parthenium*), but because his program has a number of components, it is hard to tease out how much of its efficacy stems from the feverfew. There is some evidence that this herb is useful for preventing migraine attacks (it does not relieve symptoms of an attack), but because there are questions about which species and compounds are effective, and no trials have been done with children, we aren't yet able to recommend it whole-heartedly.

- *Massage with herbal oils.* Try massaging the head, neck, and shoulders with a few ounces of olive or almond oil with a drop or two of either peppermint or arnica essential oil mixed in. Encourage slow, deep breathing during the massage. Be careful not to get essential oils onto the mucous membranes of the nose or mouth.
- *Try caffeine.* Paradoxically, the caffeine in a flat cola drink or a cup of green tea can sometimes abort a migraine attack, but this only works in children who do not normally drink caffeinated beverages. In fact, too many caffeinated beverages can trigger migraine.

# Chapter 22

# Sneezes and Wheezes:

*Allergies and Asthma*

C hildren with allergies or asthma have been a mainstay of our practices over the years. On almost any day we can count on seeing kids suffering from some form of allergy or another, whether obvious or disguised. We see such typical manifestations of asthma and allergic reaction as recurrent wheezing, chronic cough, swelling or rashes from bee stings or medications, gastrointestinal upset related to food sensitivities, behavioral disorders, or the classic congestion, runny nose, sneezing, and itchy eyes of hay fever. And that doesn't even count visits for associated conditions like eczema or recurrent sinus and ear infections. In recent years, however, we've noticed an alarming increase in the number of patients coming through our doors with these complaints, and we have discovered that our practices reflect some sobering national statistics:

- The childhood prevalence of asthma has increased 232 percent in the past thirty years.
- Asthma and allergies account for more than 10 million and 2 million missed school days per year, respectively, and are responsible for over 600,000 visits to emergency departments.

These are double the figures seen for any other chronic afflic-
tion of childhood.
- Asthma is the number one reason for hospitalization in children age five and under.

While it is well known that genetics plays a significant role in the
development of allergy and asthma, clearly something more than
genes is responsible for the rapid increase in the incidence of these disorders. Genetic changes significant enough to cause this meteoric rise
just do not occur on such a broad scale and over so short a period of
time. So the question remains: What's causing this epidemic of atopic
(allergy-related) disease?

A number of factors are involved, and we are only just teasing out
their roles. Air quality is, not surprisingly, an issue. While there used
to be controversy about the role of air pollution in the rise of childhood asthma and allergic disorders, it has now been found that higher
levels of nitrogen dioxide, sulfur dioxide, particulate matter, and
ozone each individually contribute to an increase in childhood wheezing and emergency department visits for asthma. And it's not just the
air outdoors that's at fault. As we've pointed out repeatedly, children
today are less active than in previous generations. They spend their
days in enclosed schoolrooms, and once home they are fixed to the television or computer, often in rooms with poor ventilation. Such prolonged indoor inactivity exposes them to high levels of indoor
allergens, such as dust mites, animal dander, cockroaches, and cigarette smoke.

While these various indoor and outdoor allergens can trigger the
onset of symptoms, they do not *cause* the allergy or asthma. In fact, no
one knows for certain just what does cause asthma, although theories
abound. We lean toward the fascinating theory nicknamed the
"hygiene hypothesis," which is finding increased acceptance. More and
more studies suggest that infants who are exposed to the great outdoors and all its "dirt," to a dog or cat early in life, or to the common
childhood infections picked up at day-care centers or from older siblings
have a smaller incidence of asthma and allergy than those who have
less exposure. We think it's quite possible that in our well-intentioned

efforts to protect children from germs, we Americans have gone "clean crazy" to the point that our obsession with hygiene may be doing our children more harm than good. Our overuse of antibiotics also may leave children's immune systems in an unfit, "unexercised" state, and make them more susceptible to allergy and asthma. Although the jury is still out on the hygiene hypothesis, wouldn't it be ironic if it turned out that getting dirty in the park or playing with a friend with a runny nose actually helped prevent asthma and allergies?

While the reason for the increase in childhood allergy and asthma still puzzles medical science, we do understand what happens in an allergic reaction, and can offer an integrative approach to preventing the development of allergy and asthma in your child, or at least controlling the symptoms associated with these conditions.

# What Is an Allergic Reaction?

As we discussed in chapter two, the primary role of the immune system is to protect the body from invasion by foreign material. Typically, immune cells recognize an "intruder" and remove it without notice. Sometimes, however, the immune system overreacts to an otherwise harmless particle. We call this an allergic reaction. Cells release chemicals that cause localized or widespread inflammatory changes in the lungs, the gastrointestinal tract, the skin, and other body systems. The resulting symptoms can be mild or severe, ranging from a bothersome swollen lip or runny nose, to the sudden onset of urticaria (itchy skin wheals or bumps, also called hives) or wheezing, to the life-threatening anaphylactic reaction, when a person's airways start to swell shut and blood pressure drops precipitously. People who have severe allergies, or who have experienced anaphylaxis, are usually prescribed medication (Epi-Pen or Ana-Kit) that can be self-administered in the earliest stages of an allergic reaction to forestall a more serious attack.

An allergic reaction can be frightening for child and parent alike, regardless of its severity. We are well acquainted with the wide-eyed looks and concerned faces of child and parent during even mild allergic reactions, and we have seen too many anaphylactic reactions in our careers. Patients and their parents may also be intimidated by the variety of medications a child may need to take to address allergies or asthma. The key then, as with all aspects of integrative pediatrics, is prevention and patient education.

You might be asking yourself how you can prevent your child from developing allergies or asthma when medical science has not yet determined their cause. Although we don't yet have a complete picture of allergy and asthma, we *do* know that certain interventions during pregnancy and the first months of life are associated with a lesser incidence of allergy. Among the strategies:

- *Breast-feed your baby for the first four to six months of life.* Breast-feeding has been shown to lessen the incidence of asthma and allergic disorders. One possible exception: Recent research suggests that infants of mothers who are themselves asthmatic appear to be *more* likely to develop asthma if breast-fed. We're waiting for further studies that might clarify this point. In the meantime, we have seen preliminary studies suggesting that breast-feeding mothers can reduce their childrens' sensitization to common allergens by limiting the amount of cow's milk and saturated fats in their own diets.

- *Introduce new foods slowly.* As we've mentioned before, we think it's best to wait to introduce solid foods until a formula-fed baby is four to six months old or a breast-fed baby six or seven months old. Since the introduction of certain foods before a child's immune system is properly up and running can lead to a higher incidence of allergy, we recommend waiting until a child is at least twelve months old before offering potentially allergenic foods such as whole cow's milk, whole eggs, peanuts, strawberries, chocolate, and shellfish. This is especially important if there is a history of allergy in the family. Experts now recommend that in families where allergies are present, breast-feeding mothers should avoid eating peanuts, and their children should not be given peanuts or even peanut butter for the first three years of their lives.

- *Don't allow smoking in the house.* Infant exposure to second-hand smoke has been associated with an increased incidence of asthma (as well as sudden infant death syndrome).
- *Don't be afraid to expose your six-month old to other children, especially older children.* While consensus is still lacking on this point, it appears that experiencing the common, mild infections of childhood early in life helps prevent the subsequent development of allergic disease.

In the following pages we discuss the three most common types of childhood allergic disorders: food allergies, allergic rhinitis, and asthma. While we have divided these conditions into separate categories, it is important to realize that they overlap and are interrelated; a person with asthma is likely to experience hay fever, a person with food allergies has a high likelihood of having hay fever, certain foods may bring on an episode of asthma, etc. We start with food allergies, however, because the treatment for it is so clear—identify and avoid the offending food.

## Food Allergies

Parents often confuse true food allergies with food sensitivities or intolerances. In a true food allergy the immune system mistakenly sees a particular food as a foreign invader and mounts an immune response that causes such symptoms in children as bloating, nausea, diarrhea, vomiting, wheezing, flushing, and skin rashes, and may even lead to fatal anaphylaxis. Food allergies are most common during the first two years of life—while only 1 percent of the total U.S. population experiences true food allergy, between 6 and 8 percent of all young children have them. The higher incidence of food allergies in youngsters may well be due to their relatively immature immune and gastrointestinal systems. Fortunately, most children outgrow their food allergies.

The foods most commonly implicated in childhood food allergies include cow's milk, soy products, wheat, eggs, and nuts. Children tend to outgrow allergies to milk and egg, but tend to retain as adults allergy to nuts, fish, or shellfish. Generally the allergy is caused by a specific protein in the food. Adverse reactions (either allergies or sensitivities) to food additives like monosodium glutamate (MSG), tartrazine (FD & C Yellow Dye #5), benzoic acid, and sulfites are also common during childhood.

Skin or blood (RAST) testing performed by a physician can identify substances to which your child is allergic. Your child may have to avoid this food or foods entirely, as increased exposure to the food can increase the severity of the reaction to it. Children with serious food allergies should carry preventive medications in case of life-threatening anaphylactic reactions. To protect your child, you will have to become a careful reader of food and vitamin labels to make sure a potential allergen is not lurking far down the ingredient list. Eating out at restaurants can prove especially problematic. There are books and Internet sites listed in the Resource section that can help you protect your child from food allergens.

Food sensitivities and intolerances, though not real allergies, are often confused with true food allergy. Your child may have an intolerance or sensitivity if there are certain foods that just don't "sit right" with her stomach, or if she feels tired or "heavy" a few hours after eating certain foods. A food *intolerance* is not an immune problem, but arises when a child lacks the proper enzyme to break down a particular food in the gut. For instance, a child who is lactose intolerant lacks enough of the enzyme lactase, which breaks down milk sugar (lactose). The symptoms of food intolerance—bloating, gas, and diarrhea—are solely digestive. Common trouble foods are dairy foods, wheat, and the sweeteners fructose and sorbitol. People who are intolerant to a certain food may still be able to eat it if they supplement with the enzyme, or eat the food less often or in smaller amounts.

Food *sensitivity,* on the other hand, may actually cause some of the same symptoms as food allergy, but a different immune mechanism is at work. Sometimes these inflammatory reactions may be delayed as much as 12 to 48 hours, making diagnosis more difficult. Common triggers for food sensitivities are milk, wheat, corn, aged cheese, and food additives. Food sensitivities may be expressed as digestive difficulties, joint pain, skin rash, fatigue, difficulty concentrating, or breathing problems. Some experts believe that food sensitivities play a role in the development of recurrent ear infections, headaches, behavioral problems like attention deficit disorder, and even chronic diseases like rheumatoid arthritis.

If you believe a food sensitivity or intolerance is making your child uncomfortable or even sick, you can play an important role in helping your child's doctor uncover the culprit using two powerful tools: the food diary and the elimination diet. In the food diary you'll record every food your child eats each day, and any changes you see in his physical, mental, or emotional state. Use the diary to look for patterns, and try to pinpoint problem foods. An elimination diet, or food challenge, is designed to identify foods that may be causing symptoms. The easiest way to do an elimination diet is to pick a food to which your child appears to be sensitive, like nuts or eggs, and then eliminate it completely from his diet for two weeks. Notice how he is feeling and acting at that time. At the end of two weeks, gently reintroduce the food into his diet. If there is a significant change, such as bloating or headaches, he may indeed be sensitive to that particular food. Many people start by eliminating dairy products, but in this case parents must be certain their child is getting enough calcium from other sources.

If your child is found to be sensitive to or intolerant of a certain food, it does not mean that she cannot ever eat that food. She may just need to eat it in smaller amounts or less often. In fact, one way to minimize the chances of developing a food allergy or sensitivity is to vary your child's diet as much as possible. While kids do go through periods when they only want to eat a few foods, too much of certain foods at a young age may increase sensitivity to it. For instance, some researchers believe the rise in peanut allergies is due to the American overreliance on peanut butter sandwiches for toddlers.

As an aside, we have seen a number of people who were advised not to eat a broad array of foods, including some of the foods they enjoyed most, after blood tests reportedly revealed a possible food sensitivity. We see no reason to avoid a favorite food solely because of a test result if your child has not experienced any unpleasant symptoms when eating the food. By the same token, if your child continues to experience adverse reactions to a food that did not show up as allergenic in testing, trust the evidence of your eyes and limit the food. The idea is to treat the patient, not the test result.

There are two allergic conditions that have much in common: **allergic rhinitis** and **asthma**. We begin with five general steps you can take to modify your child's susceptibility to these conditions and follow up with recommendations more specific to allergic rhinitis and asthma later in the chapter. While the conventional approach is to cover up the symptoms associated with these disorders, the integrative pediatrician takes aim at the cause of those symptoms. As with any intervention, it is important to keep your pediatrician apprised of what you are using for your children. None of the following recommendations is a substitute for conventional medical therapy, but individually or in combination these five strategies may help your child experience allergic or asthmatic symptoms with greater ease and a sense of control over the situation, and may enable your doctor to minimize medications previously felt necessary. The treatment of any childhood illness is successful only when entered into in partnership with the child, the parent, and the physician, and this is especially true in the setting of the allergic conditions.

# What Parents Can Do to Reduce Allergic Response

1. *Stop smoking.* It has been estimated that half to three quarters of U.S. children live with at least one person who smokes. Exposure to passive tobacco smoke worsens coughing and wheezing, and makes children more susceptible to viral respiratory tract

infections. If you've not been able to quit yet, please smoke outside the home so your child is not exposed.

2. *Serve more fruits and vegetables.* Numerous studies have suggested that the high antioxidant content of a diet rich in fruits and vegetables might minimize susceptibility to irritants and allergens. We much prefer that your children get their antioxidants through proper eating, but if that is not possible, a few studies do suggest that supplementation with vitamin C may be of short-term benefit.

3. *Serve foods containing anti-inflammatory fats and oils.* Since allergy and asthma are primarily inflammatory disorders, eating foods that contain high levels of anti-inflammatory omega-3 fatty acids could prove helpful. Experiment with salmon and sardines once or twice a week to help your children develop a taste for these fish. If they turn their noses up every time and refuse to eat, try sprinkling some freshly ground flaxseeds on their cereal or salad. (Remember to keep the flaxseeds refrigerated.) Avoid pro-inflammatory polyunsaturated oils and foods cooked in them.

4. *Keep an eye on dairy products.* Dairy products may increase mucus secretion and worsen symptoms in certain allergic and asthmatic patients. It is worthwhile to give your child a trial period free of dairy products, as with an elimination diet, to see if this improves the condition. Be sure to provide enough calcium from other sources if you choose to remove dairy products from your child's diet. One dairy product to consider *adding* to the family diet is yogurt that contains live cultures. This is an easy and enjoyable way to get probiotics into your child that may decrease production of IgE, the antibody most closely associated with allergic reactions.

5. *Reduce exposure to potential environmental triggers.* This includes such factors as pollen, molds, dust-mite or cockroach waste, and air pollution. More detailed suggestions on how to do this appear a little later in the chapter.

# Allergic Rhinitis

Allergic rhinitis (an allergic inflammation of the mucous membranes of the nose) is the single most common chronic disease of childhood, affecting about 6 to 10 percent of all kids, and accounting for 2 million missed school days a year. You may well be familiar with the symptoms of seasonal allergic rhinitis (more commonly called hay fever) with its coughing, sneezing, congested nose, and watery, itchy eyes. These symptoms rise and fall with the appearance of various plant and tree pollens, with spring and summer being the worst times of the year for many people. In contrast, the similar symptoms of perennial allergic rhinitis occur year-round, because of chronic exposure to animal dander, dust mites, or the airborne spores of mold. Like allergic asthma, allergic rhinitis is a chronic inflammatory disorder of the respiratory tract. Rhinitis affects the upper airways, and asthma affects the lower respiratory system. Allergic rhinitis may be an unrecognized factor in recurrent sinus and ear infections, sleep disorders, postnasal drip, chronic cough, mouth breathing, eye blinking, fatigue, and difficulties in concentration.

In addition to the general suggestions above, we recommend seven more specific actions to take against allergic rhinitis to help reduce your child's exposure to triggers, relieve symptoms, and decrease reliance on over-the-counter or prescription drugs.

# What Parents Can Do to Relieve Allergic Rhinitis

1. *Clean off pollen.* Have your child shower or bathe after playing outside to get pollen off skin and hair.
2. *Reduce exposure to other allergens.* Take precautions against dust mites and cockroaches (see pages 337–38). Keep humidity in the house low to discourage molds and mites. Keep pets outdoors if possible, and definitely out of your child's bedroom.

3. *Take off your shoes*. If everyone takes shoes off at the door, fewer pollens will be tracked into the house.

4. *Filter the air*. Watch the news for pollen counts, and keep your child indoors with the windows closed when counts are high. Consider adding a HEPA (High Efficiency Particulate Air) filter to central ductwork to clean the air indoors during the season, and change the filters often. Clean the house frequently with a vacuum fitted with a HEPA filter. Do not use an ozone generator to clean the air; these machines make asthma worse by increasing air levels of toxic ozone gas.

5. *Give more liquids*. Mucous membranes that are appropriately moist are able to perform their immune functions more competently.

6. *Try a homeopathic remedy*. You run the risk of inducing high blood pressure in your doctor with the mere mention of this form of medical care, but Dr. Russ has seen a number of patients improve markedly when the proper constitutional remedy was prescribed. Even over-the-counter single homeopathic remedies aimed only at relieving symptoms, such as *Allium* for runny nose and *Euphrasia* for itchy eyes, may be helpful. Recently a needleless homeopathic version of conventional "allergy shots" was found to be effective in reducing hay fever symptoms in clinical trials.

7. *Try a supplement*. Stinging nettle, either in freeze-dried capsule form or as a tea made from the capsule's contents, has the reputation of rapidly controlling the symptoms of hay fever. Do not sprinkle the dried contents of capsules on food to get it into children too young to swallow pills—the name is *stinging* nettle for a reason. Early research suggests a three-week course of vitamin B-12 may help ease the symptoms of hay fever, too, although it's too soon for us to make a recommendation.

If these natural approaches don't give your child relief, you may have to consider over-the-counter and prescription drugs to try to control symptoms. Among the most common:

- *Antihistamines.* Antihistamines block histamine receptors in the body, short-circuiting the biochemical histamine reaction that causes most of the symptoms of an allergic response. Older varieties of antihistamine, such as diphenhydramine (Benadryl) and especially hydroxyzine (Atarax), produce significant side effects including either sedation or hyperactivity, impaired learning in children, and drying of the mucous membranes. The newer prescription antihistamines, like loratadine (Claritin), fexofenadine (Allegra), and cetirizine hydrochloride (Zyrtec) have a better side-effect profile, although Dr Stu has seen several patients develop incontinence on Claritin that resolved as soon as the medication was stopped. Some of the new combination antihistamine/decongestant drugs also look promising.
- *Decongestants.* Medications like pseudoephedrine (Sudafed) lessen swelling of the mucous membranes by lowering blood flow to the sinuses and nose. Unfortunately, these drugs commonly cause side effects like insomnia and agitation when they are taken orally. We reserve their use for times when a child is extremely uncomfortable due to stopped-up breathing.
- *Preventives.* The nasal spray cromolyn helps prevent allergic symptoms by blocking the release of histamine. When started before allergy season, it can really reduce seasonal suffering. While effective as a preventive measure, this inhaled drug must be taken three to four times a day (a problem for a child at school or in day care), and does not treat acute episodes. It is safe, however, even for young children. Other options for prevention include immunotherapy (allergy shots), a highly effective therapy—though not a popular one with children—that must be continued for months or years to eradicate hay fever. Newer therapies that target IgE antibodies have great promise.
- *Steroids.* Steroid drugs can be an important part of preventive care for kids, but we prefer to use other means of treating allergic rhinitis when possible. Although steroid nasal sprays can be very effective against the symptoms of allergic rhinitis, they have many side effects. We are most concerned about steroid-induced suppression of both immune response and growth, and

so we are somewhat reassured that the latest research suggests that the growth-inhibiting effects of these drugs may not be permanent. We do prescribe short courses of steroids for severe situations or when a child has not responded to conventional medications. We try to use the least potent steroid at the smallest possible dosage that obtains a beneficial effect.

# Asthma

Until recently, asthma was considered to be a problem caused by the constriction of overly reactive airways. We now know that many young children with reactive airways never go on to develop asthma. Asthma is now defined as a chronic inflammatory condition of the lower airways that leads to recurrent airway obstruction. The airways narrow when the muscles of the breathing tube contract and when swelling, mucus, and cellular debris build up in response to an inflammatory stimulus. If not recognized early and treated adequately, recurrent inflammation of the airways can cause long-term changes within the bronchi that lead to impaired lung function in adulthood. But diagnosing asthma in an infant or toddler can prove to be very tricky.

Not all children who wheeze have asthma. Most children will outgrow this tendency toward reactive airways after the toddler years. Children who have families with a history of wheezing in adulthood are more likely to develop asthma that they will not outgrow.

Asthma can be divided into two broad categories: allergic and nonallergic. Allergic asthma is triggered by many of the same things that initiate hay fever. Nonallergic asthma is most often triggered by cold or polluted air, vigorous play or exercise, emotional upset or upper respiratory infection. (Most children who develop airway obstruction in response to a viral infection do grow out of the condition.) While we separate the two classes of asthma, almost all children have some component of allergy to their asthma that causes their lungs to react as they do.

The sight of a child with an acute episode of asthma is not quickly forgotten. She complains of shortness of breath and may be audibly wheezing. A frequent dry cough is almost always present, and symptoms are often worse at night. She may say that her chest feels tight or heavy. If the episode is a severe one, her nostrils may be flaring, the muscles between her ribs may retract during inhalation, and she may not be moving enough air to even produce a wheeze. In the worst of situations, the airways are so closed off that insufficient gas exchange takes place, the child turns blue, and ultimately becomes so tired from the work of breathing that she stops breathing on her own. Every year hundreds of children die from asthma, despite the plethora of drugs available to treat the condition. Is it any wonder we take asthma seriously?

Any child who wheezes should see a doctor for evaluation. Currently, conventional asthma treatment for the 5 million children with asthma in this country rests on two prescription drugs, a daily one for prevention of attacks and another one that is used as needed to treat attacks. However, we have both successfully treated children with asthma with minimal use of the usual prescription drugs. Our individualized integrative asthma programs focus on giving children and their parents the tools to prevent or control asthma episodes with both natural approaches and, as necessary, prescription medications.

# What Parents Can Do for Asthma

1. *Follow our general allergy program above.* Be especially careful to feed your child a healthy diet, as asthma has been linked to a lack of fresh fruits and vegetables and an excess of processed and fast foods. Make a special effort to limit *trans* (hydrogenated) fats from family meals. Treat allergic rhinitis, which can trigger asthma episodes. Do not smoke tobacco in your house; better yet, don't smoke at all.

2. *Make the child a partner in his asthma program.* It is extremely important for your child to take her medication as directed,

whether for the acute treatment of an episode of asthma or for the prevention of recurrence. Inadequate treatment of asthma in childhood can lead to more frequent trips to the emergency department and long-standing problems in adulthood. The best way to instill compliance is to make sure your child understands the importance of the various elements in her treatment program, and give her some sense of control over the program.

Your child's doctor should take the time to make sure both you and your child really understand the process at work in asthma, and (when possible) give you written materials that reinforce oral instructions for prevention and treatment of asthmatic episodes. Your child should be taught by the doctor or nurse the proper use of an inhaler—the device that distributes asthma medication into the airways—or much of the medication may end up sprayed onto the back of the throat instead of into the lungs. (Young children almost always need a spacer attached to the inhaler, such as a Babyhaler or Aerochamber.) You and your child should also be taught how to use a device called a peak-flow meter if your child's respiratory function is to be monitored at home. Your child's doctor may also recommend the use of a home nebulizer, a clever device that aerosolizes medications that open airways (usually albuterol). The nebulizer can provide both preventive and acute care for asthma, and cut back on visits to the doctor or the emergency department.

3. *Reduce exposure to dust mites and cockroaches.* Don't let it freak you out, but microscopic insects called dust mites that eat flakes of human skin live on and all around us, even though we can't see them. Though perfectly natural, the mites and their waste products can be allergenic; in fact, up to half of all asthmatic children may be sensitive to dust mites. To limit your child's exposure to dust mites—especially in the bedroom, where they are most often found—enclose her pillows and mattress in airtight polyurethane covers, or use fiberfill products instead of down or foam pillows; remove carpeting

(hardwoods or linoleum are better) and curtains; wash sheets and stuffed toys in hot water every week; and clean the room frequently with a vacuum with an added HEPA filter. Cockroaches and their feces are another trigger for asthma, so don't leave food around to attract them, and wash floors and counters frequently to eliminate their debris.

4. *Provide training in a mind/body technique.* Numerous studies suggest that stress can bring on or worsen an episode of asthma, and that relaxation techniques can improve the efficiency of breathing as well as the perception of changes within the lungs. Studies examining the use of imagery and storytelling have shown fewer missed school days and fewer ER visits. Other techniques, such as massage therapy, have been shown beneficial for young children with asthma, and yoga practice has likewise resulted in a reduction in stress, an enhanced sense of well-being, improved results on some tests of breathing function, and in some cases a reduced need for medication. Even the simple activity of keeping a journal may help older children minimize systemic inflammation associated with asthma. Such techniques not only provide coping skills for the children, but also provide stress reduction for the parents. This is not just important for you the parent, but research suggests that caregiver stress is picked up by children, who become stressed themselves.

5. *Get rid of mold.* Find and repair leaks and other sources of excess moisture in the house. Use a dehumidifier in damp rooms like basements, and remove any mold that collects in showers, sinks, and garbage cans.

6. *Keep pets out of the bedroom, and if possible, out of the house.* While exposure to pets early in infancy may be protective, their dander may be another trigger for kids with existing asthma. Wash your pets at least once a week.

7. *Speak with your child's teacher.* Many schoolrooms contain triggers such as pets or plants that can induce reactions in children. Make certain the teacher understands your child's

condition, and the need to keep an inhaler on hand (not in the nurse's office) in case of difficulty.

8. *Maintain healthy body weight.* Recent studies have found that obesity doubles the risk of new-onset asthma in children.

9. *Try an herbal helper.* Little research data exists, but garlic and onions eaten as foods, and maitake mushroom or astragalus taken as supplements, may boost the immune system and help prevent upper respiratory tract infections, which may lead to wheezing. Ginkgo biloba, better known for its effects on the adult brain, may also help prevent allergic episodes. A conservative dosage recommendation for botanical supplements would be one quarter of the adult daily dose for children two to six years of age, and one half of the adult daily dose for children six to twelve. Ginkgo should be taken in two or three divided doses spaced through the day. Remember, as with all botanicals, little research data exists to support the use of these remedies in children.

The herbal remedy ephedra has been in the news a lot lately. When used correctly, *Ephedra sinica*, also known as ma huang, may be beneficial to select patients with allergies and asthma. However, because potentially dangerous side effects are associated with even mild overdosage of this herbal stimulant, **we do not recommend the use of ephedra in children.**

10. *Sign up for flu shots.* If your child has moderately severe asthma, ask your doctor if an annual flu shot is recommended.

11. *Rule out reflux.* Have your child evaluated for reflux if his condition is not responding to treatment.

12. *Promote vigorous play.* A number of studies have shown a decrease in frequency of asthma episodes, a reduced need for medication, and an increased sense of well-being and self-confidence in people who exercise on a regular basis. Swimming is a particularly good exercise for kids with asthma, as witness the number of Olympic champions who carry

inhalers. Be aware that exercise can trigger symptoms in some kids with allergic asthma, who may need to take a hit of the inhaler (usually cromolyn) five or ten minutes before engaging in physical activity.

13. *Give Chinese Medicine a try.* While the research data is contradictory, Dr. Russ has seen the conditions of a number of patients with asthma improve significantly after acupuncture and/or Chinese herbs. The emotional aspects of allergies and asthma are emphasized in the CM approach to allergies and asthma.

14. *Try manual medicine.* Although hands cannot reach into the thoracic cavity and massage the lungs to make them work better, they can address the external mechanical aspects of breathing. A practitioner can work on the muscles surrounding the chest wall to allow more efficient movement of the rib cage, which may translate into more efficient air exchange. Dr. Russ has witnessed marked improvements in patients with asthma who have had this kind of treatment.

15. *Make sure your child drinks enough water.* It is especially important to keep your child drinking frequent sips of water during asthma flares, as she can easily become dehydrated while working so hard at breathing.

# Medications Commonly Used in the Treatment of Asthma

Medical science has certainly come a long way since the time when epinephrine (adrenaline) shots were given for the treatment of asthma and even mild allergies. Now there is a wide array of prescription and over-the-counter drugs available to help children with asthma (although OTC asthma drugs are not safe for children). In general, we use steroid drugs to minimize the inflammation that can trigger an asthmatic episode and drugs called beta agonists to relax the airways during an acute attack. Most of these drugs are quite beneficial, but they have significant side effects, so our goal is to use them at the lowest possible dosage and frequency that gives a child the desired improvement.

- *Steroids*. Anti-inflammatory steroids are very effective at reducing inflammation, but they come with a price: Studies have shown that chronic use of steroids (especially when taken orally, but even when inhaled) can result in mood disturbances, loss of calcium from bones, and growth inhibition. Oral steroids also suppress adrenal function, so a child who has been taking these drugs for more than seven days must be sure to taper off the dosage rather than quitting suddenly, in order to allow the adrenal glands time to resume ordinary function. Although steroids do appear to retard growth to some degree, some new studies suggest that growth rates later normalize and there is no permanent loss of potential height.
- *Inhaled beta agonists*. The mainstay of treatment for acute asthma, most of these medications help relax and open up the airways. (The exception, a beta agonist called salmeterol, is actually a preventive and is not used for acute situations.) Both short-acting and long-acting forms are available. If your child relies on short-acting inhaled beta agonists frequently, you should pay more attention to adequately controlling the condition with preventive drugs and natural measures.
- *Leukotriene inhibitors*. These relatively new agents, such as montelukast (Singulair), inhibit the production of inflammatory mediators of allergy and asthma. They have recently been approved for use in children over four, and look quite promising.

# Chapter 23

# A Rash of Complaints:

## Skin Problems

i s there anything that feels softer and smells better than a baby's neck? As parents, we know intimately the sweet fragrance and silky feel of our own infant's skin. Yet the very perfection and innocence of a baby's skin signal its vulnerability. You'll see problems like prickly heat and diaper rash in your babies, and as they grow, rashes, bumps, pimples, welts, and other signs of trouble are likely to show on their skin. These dermatological symptoms may be caused by systemic problems like chicken pox or food allergy, or by conditions more specific to the skin, such as ringworm or contact dermatitis. In this chapter we describe an integrative pediatric approach to some of the common skin conditions of childhood.

But first, we'd like to tell you a little about the care and feeding of newborn skin. Babies are born with a protective waxy coating called the vernix over their immature skin. As they make the adjustment to an air environment after all that time floating in amniotic fluid, their skin may peel. (Don't rush to apply creams and lotions, as this is a natural process.) Newborn skin has not yet evolved its full defenses. At this age, the best protection a baby has to keep germs out and fluids in is a thin layer of natural oils. Since soaps are designed to dissolve grease and oil, we don't recommend using soap on babies under six months of age. After the age of six months, it's fine to use a mild nondrying soap or cleanser with the bath. If a cleaning product causes a skin reaction, switch to another.

If you want to use a baby skin moisturizer, be sure to choose one with the shortest list of chemical additives. Many of these cosmetic products—even some of the ones meant for babies—contain fragrances and other chemicals that, while not a problem for adults, may irritate baby's more permeable skin.

We'd like to talk now about seven common conditions of the skin and hair that affect infants and children.

**Cradle cap**. Infantile seborrheic dermatitis, or cradle cap, is a common occurrence in newborns. It's a malfunction of the young sebaceous (oil) glands in the middle layer of the skin that causes flakes of skin to be welded together by excess oil into thick, yellowish scales. While cradle cap does not bother baby and will eventually go away on its own, many parents are bothered because it looks like an industrial-sized case of dandruff. You can speed along the healing of cradle cap by massaging your baby's head gently with room-temperature extra-virgin olive oil two or three times a week. The olive oil will moisturize the skin and loosen scalp scales. Breast-feeding moms might want to add more flax and cold-water fish to their diet to get more compounds known to be anti-inflammatory (and good for hair and skin) into their milk.

**Prickly heat**. The automatic heating and cooling system of babies is a work in progress for their first few months of life, so babies can easily overheat. At their age, the sweat ducts are still immature, so sweat gets trapped under the skin and can cause a red, itchy rash known as miliaria, or more familiarly, prickly heat. While the rash usually occurs on the face, it may also occur on the body, especially if a baby has been heavily swaddled.

You can *prevent* prickly heat by dressing your baby in layers easily adjustable to changes in temperature, by avoiding the use of heavy oil-based skin creams, and by leaning more toward cotton and other natural fibers, which allow skin to breathe.

You can *treat* prickly heat by cooling your child down with a lukewarm (not cold) bath and a change to lighter-weight clothing.

Since scratching can cause infections, you also want to *relieve the itching* of this skin rash. Cold compresses and a tepid bath with a colloidal oatmeal bath product or plain old baking soda added can ease the itching. A light application of baby corn starch or anti-inflammatory calendula lotion might also be beneficial.

**Diaper rash**. Most parents are familiar with diaper rash, the irritation and redness that will at some time or another appear in the area covered by a diaper of any child wearing one. Diaper rash can be caused by a number of different factors, including prolonged contact with urine or stool, excess heat and humidity caused by restricted air circulation, friction, and allergic reaction to diapers, lotions, wipes, or even the detergents used to launder cloth diapers. Incidentally, breast-fed babies get less diaper rash, apparently because their stool is less alkaline.

You can *prevent* diaper rash by taking steps to keep your baby's skin dry.

- Change diapers frequently to reduce the length of time a child's skin is exposed to urine and stool. Very young babies need to have their diapers changed eight to ten times a day. The new superabsorbent disposable diapers can keep baby drier, though they cost more (and may contain materials to which your child is sensitive).
- Experiment to see whether your baby's skin does better with cloth or disposable diapers. If you choose disposables, you will need to experiment again to find styles or brands that are soft enough and fit well not to cause friction and which do not contain any materials that cause skin reaction in your baby.
- Be sure to avoid tight-fitting diapers and plastic pants. You want air to circulate in there. Watch for new breathable disposables, and limit the amount of time your child wears plastic pants.
- Don't use wipes or other bottom-cleaners that contain alcohol, fragrance, or other chemicals that can be irritating. Just use a cotton washcloth or soft gauze and warm water to wash the diaper area, and be sure to dry thoroughly.

- Don't overdo baby powders. Try not to spread the powder all around or near baby's face, as inhalation of powders or talc can cause respiratory problems in babies (and adults). Cornstarch-based powders may be less problematic.

You can *treat* diaper rash by following all the above suggestions, plus the following:

- Give baby's bottom a chance to breathe. Put your child down for a nap without a diaper on a waterproof sheet or let her have some time bottomless out in the fresh warm air.
- Apply a thick layer of a barrier cream every time you change your baby's diaper until dermatitis is healed. Wash baby's bottom gently with lukewarm water only, and slather on a cream or ointment that contains zinc oxide and a gentle moisturizer. Try not to remove all the barrier cream next time you clean baby's bottom, but leave a thin layer. This is especially important if a baby has persistent diarrhea that has burned the upper layers of skin and left some of the skin in the area raw. Scrubbing away all the barrier cream can slough off healing new skin. Some parents prefer to apply egg white or a blend of oatmeal and flaxseed oil intermittently, and these natural methods work fine too, especially for older children. We don't recommend over-the-counter ointments that contain corticosteroids in simple cases of diaper dermatitis, and suggest you use them only if your baby's doctor has prescribed them. These drugs are more easily absorbed in infants, who may therefore be more vulnerable to their negative side effects.
- If a child's bottom becomes raw after each bowel movement, you should also consider dietary factors. Eliminate new foods that raise your suspicions and see if the problem clears up.

If diaper rash persists or worsens, a visit to the doctor is in order, because your child may have a fungal or bacterial skin infection. Most commonly, the cause is an overgrowth of *Candida*, a yeast that typically lives on the human body in harmony with other organisms.

Sometimes changes in the usual environment, such as increased dampness or alkalinity, upset the normal balance of skin flora, and excessive *Candida* growth will cause a bumpy red rash, usually concentrated in the skin folds and sometimes accompanied by peeling. There may be additional red bumps at a distance from the main rash (satellite lesions).

If yeast is the problem, your child's doctor will probably recommend a light application of an over-the-counter or prescription antifungal cream such as clotrimazole or nystatin. If the diaper area is quite inflamed, a pediatrician may suggest that you alternate applications of the antifungal with a low-potency (1% or less hydrocortisone), nonprescription steroid cream. More potent antifungal skin creams are also available and highly effective, but we think they carry unnecessary risks to a young child. We do not usually recommend oral antifungals for diaper candidiasis (although we may prescribe them occasionally for cases of the yeast overgrowth of the mouth known as thrush). We often supplement antifungal therapy with a probiotic, either for the mother if the child is breast-fed or for the child herself, to maintain beneficial flora in the intestinal tract, mouth, and other areas lined with mucous membranes.

Bacterial infections of the diaper area are also common, typically showing oozing and blisters. A swab culture will identify the culprit and allow your child's doctor to prescribe the proper antibiotic.

**Atopic dermatitis/eczema.** Atopic dermatitis, often called eczema, is an increasingly common allergic condition of both infants and children. It is frequently accompanied by allergic rhinitis or asthma. About 10 percent of children suffer from this skin condition, a percentage that has doubled since the 1950s and 1960s. The cause of the increase is not clear. Fortunately, at least half of children with chronic atopic dermatitis grow out of it by their teens.

The hallmark of this chronic condition is severe itching and inflammation that eventually results in blisters, scales, and other lesions on the skin, especially of the face and the folds of the elbows and knees. While there is some degree of inherited susceptibility involved, atopic dermatitis appears to be driven more by environmental factors such as diet, chemical irritants, and stress.

An integrative program for atopic dermatitis would include not only the suggestions for reducing allergy severity and frequency found in the previous chapter, but the following additional suggestions as well:

- Consider the child's diet. A breast-feeding mom should eliminate potential allergens such as nuts and dairy. Babies who are bottle-fed should be using a formula fortified with omega-3 fatty acids or switched to a hypoallergenic formula to reduce sensitization to dairy. You might consider a food challenge for older children.

- Examine the physical environment for potential allergens, looking at the things a child touches, breathes in, or eats for potential triggers.

- Keep the skin hydrated. It appears that the skin's ability to act as a barrier is compromised in kids with atopic dermatitis, so you want to do what you can to help it hold water. This means not only making sure your child of any age drinks enough liquids, but also avoiding hot baths, which dissolve away natural skin oils. Children should bathe or shower briefly every day in warm water, using a mild soap (based on oatmeal, aloe, or calendula) if the child is dirty. Do not use bubble-bath solutions, which contain a lot of chemicals, and be sure to shampoo hair at the end of a bath so the child does not linger in shampoo.

- Use a moisturizer with as few synthetic ingredients as possible immediately after bathing to seal in moisture. Re-apply moisturizer several times a day. Do not use lotions, creams, or other toiletries that contain alcohol, which is very drying to the skin.

- Dress your child in soft, breathable natural fabrics as much as possible; cotton clothing is ideal.

- Ease itchy skin with oatmeal or baking soda baths. Just add a handful of either to the bath, and be sure to rinse the child in clean water afterward. You can also soothe the itch with warm tea-bag compresses of chamomile tea, or make a moisturizing oatmeal pack. Just mix oatmeal and distilled water in a blender to a pastelike consistency, add a tablespoon or so of flaxseed or evening primrose oil, blend again, and apply. Do not apply herbal tea bags or oatmeal packs to open, weeping skin because of the risk of infection.

- To decrease the risk of itches turning into scratches turning into infections, put cotton socks on your child's hands at night.
- Increase your child's intake of essential fatty acids. We have seen dramatic improvement in children given evening primrose oil at a dose of ½ teaspoon a day for children two to six and 1 teaspoon a day for children aged six and above. Or try 1 teaspoon (measuring spoon, not silverware) of natural organic flaxseed oil every few days until the problem clears up. We're cautious about the long-term use of this oil because it may possibly have estrogenic effects.
- Try calendula skin cream. This herbal remedy both soothes the skin and reduces inflammation. It has been used in many cultures as a topical anti-infective agent for generations. Pure aloe vera gel may also be soothing.
- Switch laundry soaps, or run clothes through two rinses. Allergy to ingredients in popular detergents is not uncommon, even in those with babies pictured on the package.
- Consider probiotics. Breast-feeding moms can supplement with products like *Lactobaccilus GG* and Bifidobacteria. Older kids can also take the supplements, or small amounts of the probiotic can be added to formula or food. Both moms and kids can eat yogurt with active bacteria. In probiotic products, look always for those that contain at least a billion cfus (colony-forming units), added after dairy products are homogenized— and keep them refrigerated.
- Mind/body techniques that help manage stress should be a mainstay of treatment in kids older than five or six.

If itching and scaling worsens, we might consider using a low-potency (1% hydrocortisone or less) cortisone cream with limits on the amount and duration of treatment. We are very cautious with these admittedly useful drugs, because their side effects can be serious, especially in babies. There are many documented case reports of central nervous system depression and low blood sugar in newborns exposed to these topical drugs. The armpits, groin, and face are particularly absorbent areas of the skin on an infant, so steroid creams should never be applied in those places unless your doctor has ordered it (and even then, use them minimally and cautiously).

Sometimes a severe case of atopic dermatitis may require treatment with antibiotics if repeated scratching leads to infection by *Staphylococcus aureus* or other bacteria. If the typical red, scaly, oozing rash of eczema becomes fiery red or develops pustules, bring your child to the doctor to see if an antibiotic is necessary.

**Hives**. Hives are a pretty common allergic reaction in children. These fast-rising patches or wheals, also called urticaria, usually occur in response to an immunological reaction to a food, chemical, drug, or other allergen; to a bacterial or viral infection; or to stress. They are usually, although not always, itchy. Hives often resolve without their cause ever being known. If hives are persistent, a visit to your child's doctor is in order to track down the cause. Nonsedating antihistamines or oral steroids may be prescribed to control symptoms if your child's hives are severe. Once a raging case of hives gets going, it may take two to three weeks to cool it down, as the immune system must go through its full cycle of response to the offending agent. **Take your child to the emergency department** if hives are accompanied by any signs of respiratory distress.

**Ringworm**. Despite its name, ringworm has nothing to do with worms. It is a fungus infection that typically strikes children on the scalp (Tinea capitis) or the body (Tinea corporis). It starts as a small scaly spot, which enlarges to form a ring with raised red edges with a clearing in the middle. When it occurs on the scalp, hair within the ring breaks off or falls out, leaving a bald spot. Ringworm can be itchy.

Ringworm is very contagious, which is one reason why children should be taught never to share combs, barrettes, hair scrunchies, hats, or pillows. Ringworm on the body can be cured by applications of 1½ tablespoons of 5 to 10 percent tea-tree oil diluted in a cup of water three or four times a day for two weeks, or by application of over-the-counter antifungal creams such as Lotrimin. However, ringworm of the scalp can only be cured by prescription oral antifungal drugs. Your child's doctor will probably monitor liver function, as oral antifungal drugs can temporarily impair liver function. Hair loss from scalp ringworm can become permanent if the infection is not treated appropriately. A shampoo containing selenium sulfide may also be recommended to kill the fungus.

**Head lice.** This tiny blood-sucking insect can be the cause of great embarrassment the first time your child's school or day-care center calls to ask you to come pick up your child because she has head lice. "Not my child," you stoutly retort, but when you look more closely, sure enough, she does have little nits (louse eggs) that look like rice firmly attached to some of her hairs. This observation triggers a frenzy of cleaning and disinfection of both child and environment to assuage a shameful sense that child and family are somehow "dirty."

While cleaning sheets, blankets, pillows, pajamas, combs and other personal items in very hot water (over 130 degrees) is definitely part of the louse-protection program, the sense of shame is unwarranted. Head lice do not carry disease, but they are very contagious, and children of all degrees of general cleanliness catch them (as do their parents—another nasty surprise). The usual recommendation for getting rid of *Pediculus humanus capitis* is a shampoo containing either a chemical pesticide such as lindane or malathion, an extract of chrysanthemum called pyrethin, or its synthetic analogue, permethrin. We do not recommend shampoos based on chemical pesticides, and we prefer to save pyrethrin-based shampoo for stubborn cases that do not resolve with less toxic approaches, because lice worldwide appear to be developing resistance to it.

Dr. Stu likes to smother lice to death by applying a heavy coating of margarine (mayonnaise or Vaseline will also do) to a child's hair and scalp. Cover with a shower cap or plastic wrap and leave on several hours or overnight before washing it out. It's a messy therapy, but it has shown good results. Dr. Russ prefers a remedy passed on to him by Dr. Andrew Weil: Mix 2 ounces of olive or coconut oil with 20 drops of tea-tree oil and 10 drops of either rosemary, lavender, or lemon essential oil and rub it into the scalp and hair. Cover with a towel or shower cap for one hour (no longer). In either case, wash hair thoroughly to remove these oily substances and comb, comb, comb with one of those fine-toothed combs designed to remove tiny lice and their nits. A hand-held magnifying glass is very helpful in this process. We'll tell you up front that, depending on the length and thickness of your child's hair, this may be a very time-consuming process and it may have to be repeated. Be very careful to look especially hard for the pearly nits behind the ears and along the nape of the neck. Since it can take two weeks for a nit to hatch, we suggest doing followup checks on your child's clean dry hair occasionally throughout that period to reduce the risk of recurrence.

# Chapter 24

# "What Did You Say?":

*Problems of Attention*

C hildren are active and full of energy by nature. That's what makes it so tricky to tell the difference between a child who is naturally active and one who is *hyper*active. It could be that someone—a teacher, perhaps—has already suggested that the son who always seems to be in motion or the daughter who lives in a dream world may have attention deficit disorder (ADD). So what does ADD mean, does the term really apply to your child, and what do you do if it does?

Various medical, educational, and psychological groups use the terms ADD and ADHD differently. For purposes of this chapter, we use ADD as an umbrella term covering all three attention disorders—attention deficit *without* hyperactivity (ADD), attention deficit *with* hyperactivity (ADHD), and undifferentiated attention deficit. These three neurobehavioral disorders of attention represent a spectrum of activity featuring various degrees of inattention, hyperactivity, and impulsivity. The form more common in young boys—hyperactivity disorder—tends to appear as an inability to sit still, compulsive talking, and impulsive or aggressive behavior. The impulsivity can—in some cases—be both dramatic and dangerous. The form common in girls—presents more often as daydreaming, absentmindedness, and difficulty in concentrating.

A child with ADD may fidget a lot, have difficulty organizing himself well enough to start or finish a project properly, and have trouble getting along with his peers. Dressing, meals, and bedtimes can become battle zones for parent and child. Someone with true ADD has a greater chance of also having depression, anxiety, or a conduct disorder, especially if peer relationships suffer. A diagnosis of ADD is easiest when impulsivity or hyperactivity accompanies attention problems. Unfortunately, a child with an attention disorder who lacks these two active symptoms may be mistakenly labeled lazy, unintelligent, or spacey or accused of being unmotivated by both school personnel and family members. This is both unfair and unfortunate, as many children with ADD are extremely creative.

Most experts agree that ADD is not simply a behavioral quirk but rather a complex disorder of brain chemistry and function. It does not appear that there is any one cause of ADD. Evidence suggests that attention problems run in families, thereby implying a genetic component. Other research suggests environmental factors may come into play as well. There may even be important prenatal influences; studies have found that women who smoke during their pregnancy are more likely to have children with ADD. Clearly ADD has a multifactorial etioligy, so much so that there has not even been complete agreement on the *definition* of ADD.

It is estimated that 3 to 10 percent of school-age kids have some form of ADD, but we are concerned that many more are being incorrectly diagnosed with the condition. Unfortunately, there are no laboratory tests that can determine ADD. Medical guidelines for the diagnosis of ADD have varied by specialty, and the diagnosis is often informally made by parents, day-care providers, teachers, principals, and other educational professionals as well. As a result, many kids who do not really have ADD have been under drug treatment for the disorder, and many kids who have less recognizable forms of the problem have not been treated at all. Many children thought to have ADD have actually been found to have previously undiagnosed learning disabilities that respond dramatically to individualized educational approaches. One recent long-term study of children being treated with the most commonly prescribed drug for ADHD found that more than half of the kids taking the drug did not even have the disorder.

The restlessness, inattention, and impulsivity that are the hallmarks of ADD can be due to or worsened by other causes as well, so it is important to rule them out before deciding upon a diagnosis of ADD. For instance, difficulties with schoolwork or behavior can also be caused by emotional, social, or medical problems, including hearing or vision impairment, stresses at home, lead poisoning, thyroid disease, hunger, recurrent ear infections, disturbed sleep, a disorganized home environment, epilepsy, a learning disorder, anemia, pinworms, food allergies or sensitivities, head trauma, or the side effects of certain medications. In addition, definitions of what constitutes hyperactivity can be pretty subjective—one teacher's energetic and creative student can be another's irritating interrupter. Children can act out or tune out because they're bored (many kids diagnosed with ADD are very bright), don't get along with the teacher, have different learning styles, or are too immature for the amount of discipline required. That's why many doctors—ourselves included—are not completely comfortable prescribing prescription drugs for attention disorders to children under the age of five, and that's why we always explore the child's behavior in a variety of settings. Dr. Stu sends his patients to a developmental pediatrician or an educational psychologist for a thorough evaluation that includes an extensive battery of educational and behavioral testing, interviews and assessments with parents and teachers, and sometimes observation of the child in the classroom. Such a complete analysis is more likely to insure the correct diagnosis and prevent overuse of the drug methylphenidate (the most commonly used form of which is Ritalin).

There is a lot of concern about the supposed "epidemic" of ADD in kids today. Prescriptions for Ritalin doubled or tripled in the five years from 1991 to 1995 in both children less than five years of age (despite warnings on the label against its use in children under six), and those five to fourteen. A recent report found that 10 percent of American kids age six to fourteen were taking Ritalin in 1998. In the

1980s, boys on the drug 10:1 outnumbered girls; by 1998, girls had closed the gap to 3:1. Is this astonishing increase proof of an epidemic, evidence of environmental toxicity, a sign of changing societal expectations, or a trend in diagnosis?

Currently the guidelines of the American Academy of Pediatrics (AAP) require that a child exhibit impulsivity or inattention—with or without hyperactivity—severe enough to cause functional impairment in two or more settings (say, home and school) over a period of at least six months before a diagnosis of ADD can be reached. Because of the multifactorial nature of ADD and its possible confusion and coexistence with other conditions, the AAP suggests a pediatrician make this diagnosis only after several visits with the child and discussions with the child's parents, teachers, school counselors, coaches, or other appropriate sources of information concerning the child's behavior at home, in school, or on the playing fields.

The treatment plan for kids with ADD should include a multidisciplinary approach able to address a number of elements: education of parents and child, teaching of coping and self-regulatory skills, partnership with educators on learning strategies and tools, modification of the environment, and—if needed in more severe cases—medication. However, in our opinion—and both studies and experience tend to bear us out—too many practitioners are not taking the time to make a reliable diagnosis, and too many families are just being offered the "quick fix" of stimulant drugs. This trend is propelled by school systems that press for stimulant drugs as a form of behavior management. Administrators may even refuse to pass a child on to the next grade unless the child is given Ritalin, taking diagnostic power out of the hands of the pediatrician or outside educational evaluators. We don't think any parent should seek out medications for their child—especially psychotropic drugs—without the child first going through the kind of rigorous diagnostic process we have described.

The drugs most commonly used for ADHD are central-nervous-system stimulants, most often Ritalin (methylphenidate) or its longer-acting forms, although Dexedrine (dextroamphetamine) or Adderal (mixed amphetamine salts) may be prescribed. Though it seems paradoxical, these central-nervous-system stimulants actually allow children with ADD to focus and gain some control over their actions. Use of one of the stimulants usually does reduce hyperactivity and inattention—though it may just be a temporary solution. While the drugs appear to improve organizational skills and handwriting, they seldom improve academic accomplishments or social skills. We think that Ritalin should be used only as part of a home and school program that also encompasses behavioral and educational approaches.

We have a number of issues with the routine prescription of Ritalin to children, and the lack of routine followup by prescribing doctors. First are concerns about the drug itself. Although Ritalin has been used for years and appears to have a good safety profile, it does have known short-term side effects, such as depression, lethargy, insomnia, decreased appetite, motor tics, moodiness, irritability, headaches, stomachaches, and slower growth. We are also concerned about its potential long-term effects, especially now that it is being used so commonly in children under the age of six. What are the long-term effects of drugs that affect behavior and brain chemistry? In those early preschool years the developing brain is very plastic and easily influenced. The stimulant drugs could theoretically affect brain development and function, especially in the area of serotonin production. We also have no information on Ritalin's long-term effects on conditions such as conduct disorder, depression, and anxiety that often accompany ADD. The increasing number of children taking stimulants and other psychotropic drugs are actually participating in a large-scale experiment, because we will really only more about the long-term effects of these drugs by monitoring the growth and development of the children now taking them.

Second, we have concerns about the misuse of the drug. Ritalin is often the first choice of treatment in even mild cases of ADD, and is apparently often improperly prescribed to children who do not even have ADD. The diagnosis is still so subjective that we are concerned that many children are being medicated who do not have to be.

And finally, we echo some of the concerns of parents who wonder if the medical establishment is not medicalizing typical childhood misbehavior. Is it our children that need to be changed or our attitudes toward them? Should they be medicated because it's the easiest thing to do when no one has the time to look more deeply into the reasons for their behavior? Should a child be medicated because a teacher prefers a more compliant, conforming child, when the child might only be bored senseless in an unstimulating day care or classroom environment?

# An Integrative Program for ADD

Our own experience has convinced us of the importance of an integrative approach to ADD. Dr. Stu has a caseload of several thousand patients, but he can count on his fingers (no need to use toes) the number who are taking stimulant medications like Ritalin. This is because of the rigorous diagnostic process and strong support from parents in making nutritional, behavioral, environmental, and other changes to support their children's educational success. Among the components in his treatment approach:

1. *Be confident of the diagnosis.* Make sure you, your child, her teachers, coaches, and others have provided feedback to your child's doctor, so the doctor can get a true picture of your child's behavior and function. Insist on documentation of your child's observed functional impairment over a period of time. Consider any other medical conditions that could be causing difficulties at school. Take a frank look at any stresses in her life (and your own) or aspects of your own parenting style that might be affecting her behavior.

2. *Save medication till later.* We reserve the use of stimulant drugs for the more difficult cases of ADD, as in our experience most cases can be significantly improved without the use of prescription drugs. On rare occasions we initiate drug therapy as a bridge treatment until the best alternative for an individual child has been identified.

3. *Set up consistent routines at home.* Children with ADD often do dramatically better in an environment that is more predictable to them. You can create more peaceful surroundings by turning the TV off, playing soft music, organizing a household routine, setting age-appropriate guidelines for behavior, establishing routines, making mealtimes and bedtimes more relaxed and pleasant. Make sure your child gets regular time each day to blow off some steam through physical activity. Look in the Resource section for materials on strategies that can help parents of children with ADD.

4. *Modify the learning environment.* Extensive educational testing is an important part of the diagnostic process with ADD. An educational professional can identify coexistent learning disabilities and recommend specific learning behaviors or strategies that help kids with ADD stay on task and succeed better in school. Armed with a diagnosis, you may also be able to negotiate modifications in the classroom and obtain additional education support services that make it easier for your child to focus his thoughts and energy.

5. *Reinforce desired behavior with praise and small rewards.*

6. *Teach self-regulatory skills.* Techniques such as biofeedback, guided imagery, or clinical hypnosis can help children reduce anxiety, improve self-control, manage sleep problems, and change attitudes about school.

7. *Teach relaxation techniques.* Kids with ADD often have problems with sleep and relaxation. A physical form of relaxation, such as yoga or walking meditation, may be more appealing.

8. *Add essential fatty acids to your child's diet.* Children with ADD, especially those who also have dry skin or eczema, appear to have lower blood levels of essential fatty acids, which are important constituents of brain cells. While not a cure, additional omega-3 fatty acids in the diet could have a positive impact. Make sure your child is getting an adequate amount of these fatty acids through foods such as cold-water fish, flaxseed meal or flax oil, or through supplements such as evening primrose oil (EPO) and black currant oil.

9. *Test for food sensitivities.* A significant percentage of children with ADD appear to have their condition exacerbated by certain additives and foods. Try a two-week elimination diet that cuts out all foods that might be problems (studies have identified food colorings like tantrazine, preservatives, and foods such as wheat, corn, and milk as problematic for some children). Although sugar may not be the issue it once was thought to be, a diet high in low-quality carbohydrates (white flour, white sugar, and fructose) may be associated with behavioral problems; provide a more nutrient-dense diet with some protein to balance the carbohydrates.

10. *Visit a homeopathic practitioner.* We have heard some powerful stories of children with ADD who have been helped by constitutional remedies prescribed by a homeopath. If you are interested in this approach, see the Resources section for more information.

11. *Try an herbal remedy.* Data are slim and we are just beginning to experiment with these herbs ourselves for ADD, but it might be worth occasionally trying one of the sedative herbs, such as valerian, kava, or lemon balm (*Melissa officinalis*), to help your child's anxiety or sleep problems. We do not recommend any of these herbs for long-term use.

12. *Consider another modality.* Dr. Russ has heard some positive feedback for both cranial osteopathic manipulation and acupuncture. Recent research suggests that regular massage—from a professional or a parent—can significantly improve the symptoms of ADD.

13. *Limit exposure to environmental toxins.* (See chapter 8.)

Despite these helpful strategies, there is clearly a subset of kids—generally the most impulsive and hyperactive—who will need stimulant medications. We encourage you to make a strong effort with the above alternate approaches first. Even if it is decided that your child does need prescription stimulants, these natural approaches may reduce the dosage of drug required. Parents should make it clear to children with ADD that their difference is not a bad thing—that in fact they may be more creative or gifted in other ways than their classmates.

Don't forget to take care of yourself. A child with ADD can be quite a handful—lovable, but very, very stimulating. Take time to recharge your batteries so you can continue to deal with your child with love and patience.

# Chapter 25

# The Healthy Child, Healthy Family Program

Y ou may well be wondering how you can *ever* incorporate all our ideas for raising healthy kids into your current lives. We know it takes time to change habits, so we're going to make it easy for you. In this chapter we've outlined a year-long program to help you and your family make lifestyle and attitude changes at the pace that's comfortable for you. Each month we focus on a different aspect of preventive health care, while building on the months that have gone before. We offer activities for both parents and children, because involving your children as active partners in this enterprise is key to its success. You'll enhance the sense of this being a parent-child partnership if you try to do as many as possible of the suggested activities together, even the ones aimed at the kids. If you want more information or support, just flip back to the appropriate chapter in this book, or check out the books, retailers, organizations, Internet sites, and other resources listed at the back.

Don't stress yourself out trying to follow this program "perfectly." Just pick up and use what you can this year. By easing yourself into healthy behaviors, we think you'll find that you and your children can make a great start on the road to wellness in just twelve months. If it takes longer to put more of these changes into place, so be it. There's no way to fail this program. *Any* change your family makes toward healthier attitudes and behaviors is for the good.

# Month One

THEME: *Integrative Medicine.* Start talking with your family about integrative health, using the ideas presented in the first chapter of this book. Explain that good health requires healthy habits of living. Introduce the idea that your thoughts, emotions, and relationships with others and the world around you can all influence how you feel physically. Talk to your family doctors (both your children's and your own) about your interest in integrative medicine, and develop guidelines for how you can best work together. Expand your knowledge by checking out some of the books on integrative medicine listed in the Resources section.

ACTIVITY: *What Makes a Body Healthy?* Ask your children to draw pictures that illustrate what good health looks and feels like to them. (Don't forget to do your own picture.) Display them around the house. Use them as the starting point for discussions about what things—foods, activities, thoughts, emotions—make them feel especially alive and healthy, and what things make them feel low-energy or unwell. You can point out how quickly their cuts and scrapes heal, how good they feel after a full night's sleep, or how alive they feel after a little exercise. The goal is to help your children understand that their bodies are strong and able to heal themselves much of the time.

# Month Two

THEME: *Physical Activity.* Brainstorm ways to sneak a little more physical activity into your lives. Maybe you can park the car a little farther away from the place where you work, or get off the bus a stop early and walk the rest of the way. Maybe you can take the stairs instead of the escalator or elevator at the mall or the office. Maybe the kids can do homework later and play outside for a while after school. Maybe everyone can do a few exercises or yoga poses while watching TV or listening to music. Maybe the whole family can play catch after dinner or do something physical together every weekend. Once you get started, we're sure you'll think of lots of ways to up your daily physical activity.

ACTIVITY: *Add Up Your Exercise Minutes*. Have every member of the family keep track of how many minutes they are physically active on one day near the beginning of the month. Kids can count PE or sports practice time only for the amount of time they are actually moving. Set a goal—for both kids and parents—of a total of at least 30 to 45 minutes of physical activity a day by the end of the month. Assign one family member each week to be the "Coach"—the person in charge of motivating the whole family and keeping track of everyone's activity level. At the end of the month check your records (which may be as simple as colored-in squares on graph paper—one square for every 15 minutes). Celebrate your improvement with some special family exercise activity you all love—a favorite hike, ice-skating, a day trip to the slopes, or a visit to a pool with water slides.

# Month Three

THEME: *Optimize Immunity*. Before the next cold and flu season, talk with your family about the immune system and how to keep it strong. Emphasize that the best defense against getting sick is a healthy body, mind, and spirit. Try to implement some of the suggestions found in chapter 2 for optimizing immunity. At the very least, everyone should wash his or her hands regularly with plain old soap and water and get enough sleep. How to tell if you and the kids get enough? If you sleep more than two hours past your usual wake-up time on the weekends, you're in sleep debt and not going to bed early enough during the week.

The family should continue to try to sneak more exercise into their day.

ACTIVITY: *My Defense System*. Using some Lego or other toy figures to represent the various parts of the immune system, act out the immune system process for your kids. For instance, little blue blocks can be the germs; bigger red blocks can be built into the "walls" that protect the body from these "invaders"; big yellow blocks can come along and snap up any germs that make it past the initial defenses. Or have kids paint a picture of how they think their bodies deal with "bad buggies." Emphasize the idea that their immune systems are strong and protective. Have younger children practice washing their hands using the artist's or happy birthday methods given at the end of chapter 4.

# Month Four

THEME: *Good Nutrition*. This month, pass on to your kids the basics of good nutrition. Make an effort to incorporate a few changes in your usual diet—replace white bread with whole-grain bread, eat more fish or bean-based dishes, add yogurt, or switch from full-fat to low-fat (or nonfat) dairy products. Put a stronger emphasis on fruits and vegetables; it's time to stop sticking them like an afterthought on the edge of the plate. Explain to the children why you buy the foods you do for the family, and the reasons why certain foods are better for our bodies than others. When you shop, enlist older kids in reading nutrition labels to help find healthy foods to taste-test. Cruise the refrigerator and pantry shelves and see what—in the interests of health—shouldn't be there.

The family should continue to try to sneak more exercise into their day, wash hands regularly, and get enough sleep.

ACTIVITY: *Build Your Own Food Pyramid*. Show your kids our version of the healthy food pyramid in chapter 5, get out the art supplies and a stack of old magazines with pictures of food in them, and let the kids customize the pyramid to reflect their own favorite healthy choices for each food category. Stick them up on the refrigerator door to remind the kids what foods they like in each category and how many servings they should eat daily. Even grown-ups can benefit from this artistic exercise.

# Month Five

THEME: *Getting Regular Exercise*. Regular exercise is essential to good health. The best way to insure that you and your family exercise regularly is to pick favorite physical activities and make them a habit. Both how and when you exercise are individual choices; some in your family may only be able to get in the exercise groove if they do it first thing in the morning, others at lunchtime, or even in the evening. Do whatever you can as a family to support each member's exercise program, even if it's a little inconvenient for you.

Building on what was started in the second month of the program, all family members should continue to try to sneak more physical activity into their day, wash their hands regularly, get enough sleep, and eat more whole grains and other nutrient-dense foods.

ACTIVITY: *My Body Likes to Move*. An ideal program of exercise includes aerobic, stretching, and strength-training activities. Ask your kids for their favorite ways of moving their bodies, and try to come up with at least two for each of the three categories. Have them make a chart with pictures of these activities and choose a different kind of sticker or different color star for each of the three kinds of activities. Let them put the appropriate sticker or star on the chart for every 15 minutes of activity. The goal: 30 stars or stickers a week, with some in each category. Kids should get to dole out the stickers for their parents.

# Month Six

THEME: *Stress Management*. Parents and kids both need to know ways to reduce unhealthy stress. Explain to your children what stress is, and how it can affect their young bodies. Try out a few stress management techniques to see what feels the most comfortable for each of you. Practice the breathing or imagery exercises in chapter 10, follow a yoga tape or take a yoga class together as a family, paint or play music together, or give meditation a try. Consider family massage. Try a variety of techniques until you find some that offer the members of your family the feeling of complete and utter relaxation. Don't forget to point out that exercise is a great stress buster.

The family should continue to try to sneak more physical activity into their day, wash their hands regularly, get enough sleep, eat more whole grains and other nutrient-dense foods, and stick with a regular exercise regimen.

ACTIVITY: *Learning to Relax.* Here's a brief exercise (three minutes or less) called Floating on a Cloud to get you started. If your child doesn't like heights, the cloud can stay at ground-level, or you can use the image of a fluffy feather bed instead. Tell your child:

Lie down on your back with your arms at your sides, your legs slightly open, and your feet falling out to the sides. Relax your face and relax behind your eyes. Let your muscles go loose. Imagine that you are soft as a warm marshmallow. Now imagine a cloud floating down from the sky to pick you up. As you lie there, see the cloud gently collect around you and lovingly pick you up. The cloud is so full and fluffy you feel as cozy and comfortable as if you were safely riding on a big overstuffed pillow. As you drift lazily in the calm blue sky among clouds of many different shapes and sizes, look at all the colors around you. Notice how light your body feels as you float around in this beautiful place feeling peaceful and happy. Now imagine your cloud drifting back to earth. See the cloud gently place you on the ground without your having to move a muscle. Notice yourself lying on the ground, and allow yourself to feel heavier again. Take a deep breath and stretch your arms and legs, and then your face. Slowly bend your knees to your chest and roll to the left. Rest for a minute, then roll to the right and sit up. Take a deep breath. Don't you feel great?

[Adapted with permission from Thia Luby's *Children's Book of Yoga* (Clear Light Publishers, Santa Fe, 1998*)*.]

# Month Seven

THEME: *Fruits and Vegetables.* Fruits and vegetables are full of vitamins, minerals, fiber, and a host of beneficial phytochemical compounds, yet few of us manage to eat the five to nine recommended servings a day. One reason is lack of familiarity with the many kinds of produce available. Spend a little time with the kids checking out the fresh, frozen, and dried fruits at the supermarket, or take the whole family to the farmers' market or a U-pick farm on the weekend. Sample any fruit or vegetable that looks interesting. In fact, you might invest in or borrow from the library a good book on cooking with vegetables and fruits to give you inspiration. There might be a free class on vegetarian cooking at your hospital or local adult-education program. Offer fruits and vegetables as snacks or fruit for dessert instead of less healthy fare. Famished kids have a hard time resisting a plate of fresh fruits and vegetables after school or play. In order to give your family the benefit of the greatest variety of nutrients, offer them a wide array of colors (phytochemicals such as carotenes determine the color of the produce, with different beneficial compounds producing different colors).

The family should continue to try to sneak more physical activity into their day, wash their hands regularly, get enough sleep, eat more whole grains and other nutrient-dense foods, stick with a regular exercise regimen, and practice a relaxation technique.

ACTIVITY: *Shopping Cart Color Wheel.* Fruits and vegetables come in all colors, shapes, and sizes. Divide a paper circle into eight "pieces of pie" and write the name of a color in each one: red, orange, yellow, green, blue, white, brown, purple/black. Challenge your kids to find at least two fruits and vegetables for each box (give them a "pass" for blue vegetables). They might have to do some exploring at the farmers' market or supermarket to fill some of the spaces. Help them pick out favorites in as many color categories as possible, and try to include them in the family diet.

# Month Eight

THEME: *Exploring New Family Exercise Options.* By now, we hope you have begun to be less sedentary in your daily life and that you are sticking with an individual program of regular exercise. So it's time to branch out a little bit and try some activities that have something new to offer. Does your local Y have classes in tai chi or yoga? Does a nearby pool offer water aerobics or lane swimming? Can you drop into a dojo for martial arts classes? Can you all strap on your helmets and take a bike ride together once or twice a week? How about trying a new stretching tape, or just turning up the music and dancing around the house after dinner one night? Maybe mom and dad can swap the kids a few old moves for some new ones.

The family should continue to try to sneak more physical activity into their day, wash their hands regularly, get enough sleep, eat more whole grains and produce, stick with a regular exercise regimen, and practice a relaxation technique.

ACTIVITY: *Four Animal Exercises*. These are fun to do together, with or without sound effects. Do some gentle warm-up activities first, and then repeat each exercise three times.

*The Cobra:* Lie face down on the floor and relax. Place your palms on the floor next to your upper chest, elbows close to your sides. Slowly raise your head and neck, gently pushing up with the hands so your back curves up while your belly button remains on the floor. Look up without straining your neck. Make a hissing noise like a snake and maybe some snaky tongue movements. Hold the pose for 5 to 10 seconds, breathing easily, and then slowly return to the floor.

*The Flamingo:* Stand straight with feet together. Look at a point on the wall to maintain your balance during the exercise. Lift up one foot and place its heel on the inside of your opposite thigh, as close to your hip as possible. Slowly bring your hands together at chest level. Hold the pose like a sleeping flamingo (bird noises are optional), then slowly return your foot to the floor and repeat with the other foot. If you stretch your arms out over your head in a vee while you hold the pose, this becomes The Tree.

*The Cat:* Get down on your hands and knees with your hands right under your shoulders and your knees right under your hips. Take a deep breath. As you breathe in, slowly arch your back like a cat, curling your head down and tucking in your tailbone. Purr if you like. As you breathe out, slowly raise your head and lift your tailbone, so your spine curves in an easy backbend and your tummy reaches for the ground. Give a few meows. Go gently back and forth between the two poses a few times, slowly and smoothly.

*The Lion:* Sit on your folded legs with your butt resting on the back of your heels. Rest your hands on your knees. Take a deep breath and, keeping your head straight, open your mouth wide and stick your tongue out as far as you can. Look at the tip of your nose. Give a mighty ROAR! Take another deep breath and roar, repeating three times.

# Month Nine

THEME: *Environment.* It's hard to be a healthy kid in an unhealthy physical environment. Do a safety audit of your home looking for such threats to your children's safety as hanging electrical cords and dead batteries in the smoke alarms. Consider what you as a family can do to protect or maintain a healthy environment around you. Institute a family recycling program, or pick up the trash along your street. Join the local Earth Day activities. Explore the natural areas near your house, whether they are city parks or wilderness areas. Discuss with your children the need to respect and care for the wonders of the Earth.

The family should continue to try to sneak more physical activity into their day, wash their hands regularly, get enough sleep, eat more whole grains and produce, stick with a regular exercise regimen, and practice a relaxation technique.

ACTIVITY: *What's in the Garbage Can?* Write down how many cans of garbage you put out for pickup (or take to the dump) each week, and how much you recycle. Brainstorm ways to reduce the amount of waste going to the landfill from your house. The classic strategy for doing this is to follow the 3 Rs: Reduce (buy less or buy fewer things with wasteful packaging), Reuse, and Recycle. Now put the kids in charge of monitoring the household waste stream—with their heightened sense of justice, kids make great cops. At the end of the month compare your weekly garbage and recycling scores with those from the beginning of the month.

# Month Ten

THEME: *Healthy Lunches.* School lunches are frequently abysmal and downright unhealthy, and a lot of the stuff sold in the stores for kids' lunch bags isn't much better. Stand your ground and refuse to buy those plastic containers of "juice drink" anymore, or those prepackaged high-fat lunches, those cute little bags of fried snacks, the mini-candy bars. Resolve not to eat your own lunch out of a vending machine. Obviously this noble attitude won't be enough, and you'll have to come up with five interesting, tasty, and healthy lunch bag menus to get you through a week. Look for help in magazines or books, or ask a creative friend for ideas. Keep a special container for "approved snacks" and allow your children (and your spouse) to pick items from it for their lunches.

The family should continue to try to sneak more physical activity into their day, wash their hands regularly, get enough sleep, eat more whole grains and produce, stick with a regular exercise regimen, practice a relaxation technique, and reduce and recycle their garbage.

ACTIVITY: *Recipes for Healthy Snacks.* We've borrowed some tasty snack ideas from our young friend Julia Schachter, whose mom is a nutritionist.

## Luscious Ladybugs

*2 red organic apples*
*4 tablespoons nut butter (almond, peanut, or cashew)*
*Handful of organic raisins or chocolate chips*

Cut the apples in half and put cut side down. Lay a line of nut butter down the middle of each apple half, and a nut-butter circle at the small end of the apple (this will be the ladybug's head). Put a few dots of nut butter on the ladybug's "skin." Now lay out raisins or chips to make a face on the nut-butter circle, and stick them on the nut-butter dots to darken the ladybug's spots.

## Delicious Crunchers

*8 whole-grain crackers (Julia likes healthy woven-wheat crackers best)*
*4 tablespoons tahini (sesame seed paste)*
*1 tablespoon honey*
*Raisins*

Mix tahini and honey. Spread on crackers and sprinkle with raisins. (*Don't forget that honey should not be given to children under one year.*)

## Red Ants

*Organic cherry tomatoes*
*Stick pretzels*

Thread three cherry tomatoes onto a pretzel stick. Break one pretzel in half and stick both halves into one of the end tomatoes for antennae. (Parents may need to help younger children with the "pre-drilling" of the holes in the tomatoes with a kabob stick or something similar.)

# Month Eleven

THEME: *Social Connection.* People with more social connections seem to live longer, healthier—and certainly richer—lives. These connections can come from religious involvement, social or special-interest clubs, sports teams, and volunteer activities. This month, consider the service your family does in your local community and the world at large. Think about ways you can involve your children in helping others, appropriate for their age. You could encourage them to befriend a child who's new or "different," visit an elderly neighbor, do a chore for a neighbor or friend with no expectation of payment, or raise money for a favorite cause. Perhaps your children can join you in your service work occasionally, or the whole family can volunteer to work together on a service project. Talk with your children about any financial contributions you make to charitable groups as well, and explain why you do it and how it makes you feel.

The family should continue to try to sneak more physical activity into their day, wash their hands regularly, get enough sleep, eat more whole grains and produce, stick with a regular exercise regimen, practice a relaxation technique, reduce and recycle their garbage, and pack healthy lunches.

ACTIVITY: *Helping Others*. Ask your children to make a list of the ways that they help other people. (They may need help with this.) Then ask them if there is anything on the list they would like to do more often. Less often? What issues are important issues for them— the environment, helping the poor, curing a specific disease, kindness to animals? Help them think of ways they could become more involved in areas they care about.

# Month Twelve

THEME: *Alternative Therapies*. In Section II of this book we talked about a number of alternative therapies that we have found to be helpful for our patients and ourselves. This might be a good time to experiment with one or two of them as a preventive or therapeutic tool or to learn a little more about one that intrigues you by checking out some of the resources at the end of the book. You may also find classes offered by alternative practitioners in your community that might give you some feeling for what's involved. You might want to experiment with self-care using homeopathic remedies, massage, or some basic acupressure techniques. Medicine is a field of knowledge that is perpetually in flux, and not the constant and exact science most people mistakenly think it to be. We believe that in the future "conventional medicine" will be much more integrative. In the meanwhile, it is worth trying other therapies that, while not yet "proven," are clearly safe and apparently effective.

The family should continue to try to sneak more physical activity into their day, wash their hands regularly, get enough sleep, eat more whole grains and produce, stick with a regular exercise regimen, practice a relaxation technique, reduce and recycle their garbage, pack a healthy lunch, and volunteer to help others.

ACTIVITY: *Foot Massage.* People of almost any age can learn to massage their own feet or those of a loved one. All you need is five minutes and a little scented oil. Start with self-massage, so you can learn on yourself what does and does not feel good. Sit down and put one foot up on the other thigh. Lube your hands up with a little oil, and, starting with the sole of the foot, rub every part of your foot with your thumbs, applying a good bit of pressure. Pay special attention to any tender spots. Do each toe individually, applying pressure to top, back, and sides. Gently pull toward the end of the toe as you work it. Rub all over the top and sides of the foot to the ankle. When you finish one foot, do the other. Once you get the hang of it, offer to give someone else a foot massage.

the year-long Healthy Child, Healthy Family Program is now over, but we hope that you will continue to guide your children (and yourselves) toward healthy ways of living. By doing so, you not only reduce their risk for the diseases of childhood, but you are building the foundations for a healthy adult life as well. The most serious conditions of adulthood all have their roots in behaviors and attitudes from our early years. By stepping in now, and making sure your children get in the habit of eating well, coping with stress, and staying physically active, you are reducing their risk of cardiovascular disease, diabetes, osteoporosis, and many cancers. You are giving them a gift that lasts a lifetime—good health. We wish you every success.

# References

(Numbers to left of citation indicate page number in book.)

## Introduction

xxii. Visits to alternative practitioners: D. Eisenberg et al., "Trends in Alternative Medicine Use in the United States 1990–1997," *Journal of the American Medical Association* (280) November 21, 1998, 1569–1575.

xxii. Dollars spent on nutritional supplements: Eisenberg, November 1998 *JAMA*, as above.

xxii. Dollars spent on homeopathic remedies: J. Jacobs et al., "Patient Characteristics and Practice Patterns of Physicians Using Homeopathy," *Archives of Family Medicine* (7) November/December 1998, 537–540.

## Chapter 1: Read This First

3. Integrative medicine: D. Eisenberg et al., "Unconventional Medicine in the United States," *New England Journal of Medicine*, (328) January 1993, 246–252. For a greater understanding of integrative medicine, see the books of Dr. Andrew Weil, especially *Natural Health, Natural Medicine* (Houghton Mifflin, 1995) and *Spontaneous Healing* (Alfred A. Knopf, 1995).

11. Varying effects of pharmaceutical drugs: J. Cohen, "Ways to minimize adverse drug reactions," *Postgraduate Medicine* (106) September 1999, 163–174.

13. Money spent on alternative therapies: Eisenberg, November 1998 *JAMA*, as above.

13. Reasons for using alternative medicine: B. Druss and R. Rosenbeck, "Association Between Use of Unconventional Therapies and Conventional Medical Services," *Journal of the American Medical Association*, (282) August 18, 1999, 651–656; and J. Astin, "Why Patients Use Alternative Medicine: Results of a National Study," *Journal of the American Medical Association*, (279) May 20, 1998, 1548–1554.

## Chapter 2: Your Child's Invisible Shield

20. For more on an integrative approach to immunity: Andrew Weil, *Eight Weeks to Optimum Health* (Knopf, 1997).

21. Genetic immunity: L. Oliwenstein, "Dr. Darwin: Darwinian medicine studies the evolutionary purpose of disease," *Discover* (16) October 1995, 111–117.

22. Breast milk and immunity: J. Newman, "How Breast Milk Protects Newborns," *Scientific American* (273) December 1995, 76–79.

25. "Hygiene hypothesis": G. Hamilton, "Let Them Eat Dirt," *New Scientist* July 18, 1998 (accessed online 9/14/99); G. Rook and J. Standford, "Give us this day our daily germs," *Immunology Today* (19) March 9, 1998, 8–11; and S. Carpenter, "Modern Hygiene's Dirty Tricks," *Science News* (156) August 14, 1999, 108–110.

26. Communication between brain, gut, glands, and immune system: Candace Pert, *Molecules of Emotion: Why You Feel the Way You Feel* (Scribner, 1997).

26. Wound-healing under stress: R. Glaser, J. Kiecolt-Glaser, and P. Marucha et al., "Stress-related changes in pro-inflammatory cytokine production in wounds," *Archives of General Psychiatry* (56) May 1999, 450–456; and J. Kiecolt-Glaser, P. Marucha, and W. Malarkey, et al., "Slowing of wound healing by psychological stress," *Lancet* (346) November 4, 1995, 1194–1196.

26. Healing power of humor: Norman Cousins, *Anatomy of an Illness* (Bantam, 1979) and *Head First: The Biology of Hope* (Dutton, 1989).

27. Positive attitude and healing: *"Happy Brains in Healthy Bodies,"* Issue Briefing for Health Reporters from the Center for the Advancement of Health, Washington DC, September 1998.

28. Dangers of tobacco use: J. Wiencke et al., "Early age at smoking

initiation and tobacco carcinogen DNA damage in the lung," *Journal of the National Cancer Institute* (91), 614–19.

## Chapter 3: A Shot in the Arm (or the Leg)

31. Picture of a vaccineless society: "What Would Happen If We Stopped Vaccinations?" National Immunization Program of the Centers for Disease Control and Prevention.

32. MMR, polio, and HiB meningitis statistics: *Epidemiology and Prevention of Vaccine-Preventable Diseases* (Public Health Foundation, 2000).

33. Ear infections and strep: "*Streptococcus pneumoniae*: What the Family Physician Needs to Know," *Family Practice Recertification* (21) November 1999 (supp), 11.

35. Herd immunity: A. Berger, "How does herd immunity work?" *British Medical Journal* (319) December 4, 1999, 1466–7.

35. Diphtheria death: "Six Common Misconceptions About Vaccination," from the National Immunization Program of the Centers for Disease Control and Prevention.

35. Mini-epidemics: "What Would Happen If We Stopped Immunization," above; and T. Sheldon, "Netherlands Faces Measles Epidemic," *British Medical Journal* (320) January 8, 2000, 76.

37. Rotavirus controversy: "Intussusception Among Recipients of Rotavirus Vaccine—United States," CDC Weekly Morbidity and Mortality Report, *Journal of the American Medical Association* (282) August 11, 1999, 520–521; "Rotavirus Vaccination Ends," *Family Practice News* (29) November 15, 1999, 22; "Withdrawal of Rotavirus Vaccine Recommended," CDC Weekly Morbidity and Mortality Report, *Journal of the American Medical Association* (282) December 8, 1999, 2113–2114; and R. Steele, "The Rise and Possible Fall of the Rotavirus Vaccine," Medscape 1999.

38. Heather Whitestone: Barry Glassner, *The Culture of Fear* (Basic Books, 1999), 178.

38. Psychological views of vaccination: L. Ball et al., "Risky Business: Challenges in Vaccine Risk Communication," *Pediatrics* (101), March 1999, 453–458; R. Chen and B. Hibbs, "Vaccine Safety: Current and Future Challenges," *Pediatric Annals* (27) July 1998, 445–454.

39. Overall perspective on vaccine concerns, pro and con: "Six Common Misconceptions About Vaccines," as above; B. Fisher, "Shots in the Dark," from the National Vaccine Information Center.

39. Deaths associated with vaccines: "Six Common Misconceptions About Vaccines" as above.

39. Guillain-Barré and tetanus: J. Tuttle et al., "The risk of Guillain-Barré after tetanus-toxoid-containing vaccine in adults and children in the U.S." *American Journal of Public Health* (87) 1997, 2045–48.

40. Diabetes and vaccines: "Concerns About Diabetes and Vaccines: Questions and Answers," National Immunization Program of the Centers for Disease Control (2/98); and "No Diabetes/Vaccine Link Found," *Family Practice News*, December 15, 1999, 32.

41. MMR and autism/Crohn's disease: A. Wakefield et al., "Ileal-lymphoid-nodular hyperplasia, non-specific colitis, and pervasive developmental disorders in children," *Lancet* (351) February 27, 1998, 637–641; B. Taylor et al., "Autism and measles, mumps, and rubella vaccine: no epidemiological evidence for causal relation," *Lancet* (353) June 12, 1999, 2026–2029; J. Metcalf, "Is measles infection associated with Crohn's disease?" *British Medical Journal* (316) January 17, 1998, 166.

41. Vaccines and mercury: N. Halsey, "Limiting Infant Exposure to Thimerosal in Vaccines and Other Sources of Mercury," *Journal of the American Medical Association* (282) November 10, 1999, 1763–4; "Recommendations Regarding the Use of Vaccines That Contain Thimerosal as a Preservative," CDC Weekly Morbidity and Mortality Report, *Journal of the American Medical Association* (282) December 8, 1999, 2114–2115.

42. Chickenpox complications: T. Jefferson, "Pediatricians Alerted to Five New Vaccines," *Journal of the American Medical Association* (281), June 2, 1999, 1973–1975.

46. Distraction at immunization: B. Felt et al., "Behavioral interventions reduce infant distress at immunization," *Archives of Pediatric and Adolescent Medicine* (154) July 2000, 719–724.

## Chapter 4: Drugs and Bugs

49. Antibiotic statistics: "Antibiotic Resistance: A New Threat to You and Your Family's Health," from the Centers for Disease Control and Prevention accessed from www.cdc.gov/ncidod/dbmd/antibioticresistance/faqs.htm on December 20, 1999; and R. Wenzel and M. Edmond, "Managing Antibiotic Resistance," *New England Journal of Medicine* (343), December 28, 2000, 1961–1963.

49. Resistance in new drug: S. Stapleton, "New antimicrobial raises hope, concern," *American Medical News* (43) May 8, 2000, 1–2.

49. "Technology is losing the arms race with evolution": B. Levin et al., "The Population Genetics of Antibiotic Resistance," *Clinical Infectious Disease* (24 suppl 1) January 1997, S9–S18.

50. Principles of bacterial resistance: S. Levy, "Multi-drug Resistance: A Sign of the Times," *New England Journal of Medicine* (338) May 7, 1998, 1376.

51. Role of day care in promoting resistance: E. Unger, "Daycare Contributes to Antibiotic Resistance," *Medical Tribune* (40) October 1999, 1.

51. Sevenfold increase in ear infections: H. Bauchner et al., "Parents, Physicians, and Antibiotic Use," *Pediatrics* (103) February 1999, 395–401.

52. Antibiotics as societal drugs: S. Levy, "Antibiotic Resistance: An Ecological Imbalance," *Ciba Foundation Symposium* (207) 1997, 9–14.

53. Antibiotics in food and water: S. Levy, "Multi-drug Resistance" as above; and "Why Should You Care About Antimicrobial Resistance?" from the Alliance for the Prudent Use of Antibiotics accessed from www.healthsci.tufts.edu/apua December 20, 1999.

55. Antibiotics as strong medicine: R. Gonzalez and K. Corbett, "The Culture of Antibiotics," *American Journal of Medicine* (107) November 1999, 525–526.

55. Wait-and-see prescribing: C. Cates, "An evidence-based approach to reducing antibiotic use in children with acute otitis media," *British Medical Journal* (318) March 13, 1999, 715–16.

56. Prescriptions for viral illnesses in children: A. Nyquist, R. Gonzalez, J. Steiner, et al., "Antibiotic Prescribing for Children with Colds, Upper Respiratory Infections, and Bronchitis," *Journal of the American Medical Association* (279) March 18, 1998, 875–77.

56. Reasons for delaying antibiotic: N. el-Daher et al., "Immediate vs. delayed treatment of group A beta-hemolytic streptococcal pharyngitis with penicillin," *Pediatric Infectious Disease Journal* (10) February 1991, 126–130; and M. Pichichero et al., "Adverse and beneficial effects of immediate treatment of group A beta-hemolytic streptococcal pharyngitis with penicillin," *Pediatric Infectious Diseases Journal* (6) July 1987, 635–643.

57. Watchful waiting for ear infections: E. Susman, "One in Three Children Seeking Care for Otitis Media Will Be Resistant to Antibiotics," *Emergency Medicine News*, December 1999, 56; A. Walling, "Use of Antibiotics for Acute Otitis Media in Children," *American Family Physician* (57)

March 1, 1998, 1132; and J. Froom'et al., "Antimicrobials for otitis media: A review from the International Primary Care Network," *British Medical Journal* (315) July 12, 1997, 98–102.

58. Probiotics: J. Vanderhoof and R. Young, "Use of Probiotics in Childhood Gastrointestinal Disorders," *Journal of Pediatric Gastroenterology and Nutrition* (27) September 1998, 323–332; T. Arvola, et al., "Prophylactic Lactobacillus GG Reduces Antibiotic-associated Diarrhea in Children with Respiratory Infections: A Randomized Study," *Pediatrics* (104) November 5, 1999, e64; and J. Vanderhoof et al., "*Lactobaccilus GG* in the prevention of antibiotic-associated diarrhea in children," *Journal of Pediatrics* (135), November 1999, 564–568.

59. Antibiotics in milk: S. Begley, "The End of Antibiotics," *Newsweek*, March 28, 1994, 47–52.

59. Day care center study: H. Carabine et al., "Effectiveness of a Training Program in Reducing Infections in Toddlers Attending Daycare Centers," *Epidemiology* (10) May 1999, 219–227.

60. Triclosan resistance: J. Travis, "Popularity of germ fighter raises concern," *Science News* (157) May 27, 2000, 342.

## Chapter 5: The Joy of Eating

61. Family meals: William Doherty, *The Intentional Family: How to Build Family Ties in Our Modern World* (Addison Wesley 1997), 22; and D. A. Gentile and David Walsh, "MediaQuotient: National survey of family media habits, knowledge and attitudes" from the National Institute on Media and the Family, Minneapolis MN, 1999.

61. Outside food: "What We Eat in America food consumption survey," *Food & Nutrition Research Briefs*, April 1996.

61. Fast-food spending: M. Preboth and S. Wright, "Quantum Sufficit: Just Enough," *American Family Physician* (60) October 1, 1999, 1309.

62. What kids eat today: K. Muñoz et al., "Food Intakes of U.S. Children and Adolescents Compared to Recommendations," *Pediatrics* (100) September 1997, 323–329; J. Hampl et al., "The 'age+5' rule: Comparisons of dietary fiber intake among 4- to 10-year-old children," *Journal of the American Dietetic Association* (98) December 1998, 1418–1423; and "Position of the American Dietetic Association: Dietary guidance for healthy children aged 2 to 11," *Journal of the American Dietetic Association* (99), 1999, 93–101.

63. Doubling of obesity: G. Früebeck, "Childhood obesity: time for action, not complacency," *British Medical Journal* (320) February 5, 2000, 328–9.

64. Long-term effects of an unhealthy diet: ADA position paper as above.

64. Food insecurity: ADA position paper, as above.

64. Effect of prenatal nutrition: K. Godfrey, "Maternal regulation of fetal development and health in adult life," *European Journal of Obstetrics and Gynecology and Reproductive Biology* (78) 1998, 141–150.

67. Commercial effects on nursing: C. Howard et al., "Office prenatal formula advertising and its effect on breast-feeding patterns," *Obstetrics & Gynecology* (95) February 2000, 296–303.

67. Benefits of nursing: L. Maher, "Advising parents on feeding healthy babies," *Patient Care* March 15, 1998, 58–74; W. Oddy et al., "Association between breast-feeding and asthma in 6-year-old children," *British Medical Journal* (319) September 25, 1999, 815–19; X. Shu, "Breast-feeding and Risk of Childhood Acute Leukemia," *Journal of the National Cancer Institute* (91) October 20, 1999, 1765–1772; R. Von Kries, "Breast feeding and obesity," *British Medical Journal* (319) July 17, 1999, 147–150; "More Benefit from Breast Milk," *Harvard Women's Health Watch* January 1997, 7; J. Anderson et al., "Breast-feeding and cognitive development: a meta-analysis," *American Journal of Clinical Nutrition* (70) October 1999, 525–35; and P. Newcomb et al., "Lactation in relation to postmenopausal breast cancer," *American Journal of Epidemiology*, (150) July 15, 1999, 174–182.

67. Breast-feeding statistics: K. Springen, "The Bountiful Breast," *Newsweek* June 1, 1998, 71.

69. DHA in formula: E. Birch, et al., "A randomized controlled trial of early dietary supply of long-chain polyunsaturated fatty acids and mental development in term infants," *Developmental Medicine and Child Neurology* (42) March 2000, 174–181.

68. Dark-skinned infants and Vitamin D: M. Shah, et al., "Nutritional rickets still afflict children in north Texas," *Texas Medicine* (96) June 2000, 64–68.

71. Top 10 sources of energy: A. Subar, et al., "Dietary Sources of Nutrients Among US Children 1989–1991," *Pediatrics* (102) October 4, 1998, 913–23.

74. Fiber intake: J. Hempl article cited above.

77. Calcium requirements: NIH Consensus Statement: Optimal Calcium Intake, National Institutes of Health 1994.

81. Recommended fat intake: American Academy of Pediatrics Com-

mittee on Nutrition, "Cholesterol in Childhood," *Pediatrics* (101) January 1998, 141–147.

81. Kids' sugar intake: Subar as above; A. Moshfegh, et al., "Food and Nutrient Intakes by Individuals in the United Sates by Sex and Age 1994–96," USDA 1998; and Lewis, as above.

81. Sugar as a percent of calories: J. Guthrie and J. Morton, "Food sources of added sweeteners in the diets of Americans," *Journal of the American Dietetic Association* (100) January 2000, 43–48, 51.

82. Soda and milk intake: Moshfegh, et al., as above.

83. Salt intake: "The Diets of America's Children," United States Department of Agriculture, 1996.

84. Food additives and behavior: K. S. Rowe and K. J. Rowe, "Synthetic food coloring and behavior: a dose-response effect in a double-blind, placebo-controlled, repeated measures study," *Journal of Pediatrics* (125) November 1994, 691–8.

84. Effects of nitrates: S. Preston-Martin, et al., "Maternal consumption of cured meats and vitamins in relation to pediatric brain tumors," *Cancer Epidemiology, Biomarkers, and Prevention* (5) August 1996, 599–605; and J. Peters, S. Preston-Martin, et al., "Processed meats and risk of childhood leukemia," *Cancer Causes and Control* (5) March 1994, 195–202.

84. Effect of food commercials: ADA position paper as above; and K. Kotz and M. Story, "Food advertisements during children's Saturday morning programming: are they consistent with dietary recommendations?" *Journal of the American Dietetic Association* (94) November 1994, 1296–1300.

86. Effect of family meals: M. Gillman, et al., "Family Dinner and Diet Quality Among Older Children and Adolescents," *Archives of Family Medicine* (9) March 2000, 235–240; B. Bowden and J. Zeisz, "Supper's on!: Adolescent Adjustment and Frequency of Family Mealtimes," presented at the 105th Annual Convention of the American Psychological Association; and M. Resnick, et al., "Protecting Adolescents From Harm," *Journal of the American Medical Association* (278) September 10, 1997, 823–832.

88. Effects of fruit juice: American Academy of Pediatrics Committee on Nutrition, "The Use of Fruit Juice in the Diets of Young Children," *AAP News*, February 1991 (reaffirmed 1994).

89. Artificial sweeteners: H. Roberts, "Aspartame and brain cancer," *Lancet* (349) February 1997, 362; and A. Zehetner and M. McLean, "Aspartame and the internet," *Lancet* (354) July 1999, 78.

90. Vegetarian diet: K. Kolasa, "Is a vegetarian diet healthy for kids?" *Patient Care*, March 15, 2000, 111–128.

## Chapter 6: Don't Just Sit There

93. Obesity and BMI: W. Dietz and M. Bellizi, "Introduction: The use of body mass index to assess obesity in children," *American Journal of Clinical Nutrition* (70), July 1999, 123S–125S.

94. CDC growth charts: "CDC Growth Charts: United States," *Advance Data* (314) May 30, 2000, Vital and Health Statistics of the Centers for Disease Control and Prevention.

94. Extent of childhood obesity: R. Troiano and K. Flegal, "Overweight Children and Adolescents: Description, Epidemiology, and Demographics," *Pediatrics* (101) March 1998, 497–504; Troiano and Flegal, "Overweight Prevalence Among Youth in the United States," *International Journal of Obesity Related Metabolic Disorders* (23), March 1999, S22–27; and J. Hill and F. Trowbridge, "Childhood Obesity: Future Direction and Research Priorities," *Pediatrics* (101) March 1998, 570–574.

95. Genetic influence on obesity epidemic: D. Styne, "Childhood Obesity: Time for Action, Not Complacency," *American Family Physician* (59) February 15, 1999, 758–62, and Troiano and Flegal, *Pediatrics*, as above.

95. Hours of TV watched: A. C. Nielsen, 1988 Report on Television; and policy statement of the American Academy of Pediatrics, "Fitness, Activity, and Sports Participation in the Preschool Child," *Pediatrics* (90) December 1992, 1002–1004.

95. TV and obesity: R. Andersen, et al., "Relationship of Physical Activity and Television Watching with Body Weight and Level of Fatness in Children," *Journal of the American Medical Association* (279) March 25, 1998, 938–959; and S. Gortmaker, et al., "Television viewing as a cause of increasing obesity among children in the United States," *Archives of Pediatric and Adolescent Medicine* (150) April 1996, 356–62.

96. Parental oversight over food: S. Barlow and W. Dietz, "Obesity Evaluation and Treatment: Expert Committee Recommendations," *Pediatrics* (102) September 1998, e29; and Styne, as above.

96. Role of fiber: D. Ludwig, "Dietary Fiber, Weight Gain, and Cardiovascular Disease Factors in Young Adults, *Journal of the American Medical Association* (282) October 27, 1999, 1539–5.

96. Adiposity rebound: A. Dorosty, "Factors associated with early adiposity rebound," *Pediatrics* (105) May 2000, 1115–1118.

97. Impact of obesity: J. Rippe, et al., "Obesity—a chronic disease,"

*Patient Care*, October 15, 1998, 29–32; A. Must, et al., "The Disease Burden Associated with Overweight and Obesity," *Journal of the American Medical Association* (282) October 27, 1999, 1523–29; and A. LaVoie, "Obesity Portends Upswing in Juvenile Diabetes," *Medical Tribune* January 21, 1999, 4.

98. Parental influence: "Pediatric Pearls," *Journal of the American Medical Association* (281) May 26, 1999, 1956; and "Health Check," *Parenting*, June/July 2000, 53.

98. Breast-feeding and obesity: R. von Kries et al., "Breast Feeding and Obesity: Cross Sectional Study," *British Medical Journal* (319) July 17, 1999, 147–150.

98. Behavioral suggestions: B. Baker, "Behavioral Therapy Essential for Childhood Obesity," *Family Practice News* December 1, 1999, 42; and Barlow and Dietz as above.

98. Fidgeting helps maintain normal weight: J. Levine, et al., "Role of nonexercise activity thermogenesis in resistance to fat gain in humans," *Science* (283) January 1999, 212–214.

99. Food ads on TV: Guidelines for School Health Programs to Promote Lifelong Healthy Eating, Centers for Disease Control and Prevention, 1996.

100. Cultural messages about weight: J. Rippe, *Patient Care* as above; and T. Zwillich, "Tally of the Dolls," *Family Practice News* June 15, 1999, 59.

101. Obesity as a family issue: D. Styne, "Childhood Obesity," *American Family Physician* (59) February 15, 1999, 758–62; and M. Golan, A. Weizman, et al., "Parents as the exclusive agents of change in the treatment of childhood obesity," *American Journal of Clinical Nutrition* (67) June 998, 1130–1135.

102. Influence of parents on activity: T. Di Lorenzo, R. Stucky-Roop, et al., "Determinants of exercise among children," *Preventive Medicine* (3) May/June 1998, 470–7; and M. Fogelholm, et al., "Parent-child relationship of physical activity patterns and obesity," *International Journal of Obesity and Related Metabolic Disorders* (23) 1999, 1262–1268.

102. Activity statistics: T. Ganley with T. Sherman, "Exercise and Children's Health," *The Physician and Sports Medicine* (28) February 2000, 85–92; and "Shape of the Nation" survey, National Association for Sport and Physical Education, 1997.

104. Increasing inactivity of girls: CDC's Guidelines for School and Community Programs Promoting Lifelong Physical Activity, from the National Center for Chronic Disease Prevention and Health Promotion of the Centers for Disease Control and Prevention, accessed 2/9/00.

104. University of Michigan study: S. Hofferth and J. Sandberg, "Changes in American Children's Time 1981–1997," research report of the Population Studies Center at the Institute for Social research of the University of Michigan, 1998.

105. Forcing exercise: W. Taylor et al., "The health benefits of physical activity in children and adults: Implications for chronic disease prevention," *European Journal of Pediatrics* (158) 1999, 271–274.

106. Organized sports: AAP position statement as above; and Ganley as above.

108. PE mandates: NASPE report as above.

108. Benefits of PE: G. Payne and the California Governor's Council on Physical Fitness and Sports, "A Powerful Tool," a position paper of the CGCPES; and F. Trudeau, "Daily primary school physical education: effects on physical activity during adult life," *Medical Science of Sports and Exercise* (31) 1999, 111–117.

109. PE goals: "Guidelines for School and Community Programs Promoting Lifelong Physical Activity," Centers for Disease Control and Prevention, 2000; and L. Schnirring, "Can School PE Make Fitter Kids?" *The Physician and Sports Medicine* (27) December 1999, 23–28.

110. Endangered recess: K. Alexander, "Playtime is Cancelled," *Parents*, November 1999, 114–118; and O. Jarrett and D. Maxwell, "Physical Education and Recess: Are Both Necessary?," IPA/USA Newsletter On-Line (55) Spring 1999; and "The Case for Elementary School Recess" fact sheet from the American Association for the Child's Right to Play.

111. Playing and parental weight loss: "Fitting Fitness In," American Heart Association brochure 1996.

112. Late bloomers: H. Clark, "Characteristics of the young athlete: a longitudinal look," *Kinesiology Review* (3) 1968, 33–42.

## Chapter 7: Just Sit There

116. Theory of stress-related pain: See any of the books of Dr. John Sarno, especially *Healing Back Pain* (Warner 1991) and *The Mindbody Prescription* (Warner 1998).

117. Physical effects of stress: Daniel Goleman and Joel Guerin, *Mind/Body Medicine* (Consumer Reports Books, 1993); M. Grey, "Stressors and Children's Health," *Journal of Pediatric Nursing* (8) April 1993, 85–91; J. Turner Cobb et al., "Psychosocial influences on upper respiratory illness

in children," *Journal of Psychosomatic Research* (45) October 1998, 319–330: and M. Small, "Family Matters," *Discover* August 2000, 66–71.

119. Relaxation response: Goleman and Guerin, as above, chapter 14.

123. Use of psychotropic drugs on children: Julie Magno Zito et al., "Trends in the Prescribing of Psychotropic Medications in Preschoolers," *Journal of the American Medical Association* (283) February 23, 2000, 1025–1030, and Joseph Coyle, "Psychotropic Drug Use in Very Young Children," *Journal of the American Medical Association*, as cited, 1059–1060.


## Chapter 8: It's Not Only What They Breathe

129. Pervasiveness of DDT: J. Reigart, "Children's Environmental Health," *The Journal of the South Carolina Medical Association*, August 1997, 286–291.

129. Number and safety of chemicals: Herbert Needleman and Philip Landrigan, *Raising Children Toxic Free* (Farrar Straus & Giroux, 1994) 55; M. Mitka, "Environmental Health Center Aims at Children," *Journal of the American Medical Association* (282) July 21, 1999, 224–225; and P. Landrigan, "Environmental Hazards for Children in the USA," *International Journal of Occupational Medical and Environmental Health* (11) 1998, 189–194.

130. Vulnerability of children: C. Bearer, "Environmental Health Hazards: How Children are Different from Adults," *The Future of Children* (5) Summer/Fall 1995, 11–26.

130. Prenatal effects of solvents: H. Taskinen, "Spontaneous abortions and congenital malformations among the wives of men occupationally exposed to organic solvents," *Scandinavian Journal of Work and Environmental Health* (15) October 1989, 345–352.

130. Prenatal effects of PCBs: J. Jacobson and S. Jacobson, "Intellectual impairment in children exposed to polychlorinated biphenyls in utero," *New England Journal of Medicine* (335) September 1996, 783–789.

130. Pollutants in breast milk: R. Churchill and L. Pickering, "The many pros—and a few cons—of breastfeeding," *Patient Care* (34) April 15, 2000, 177–190; and L. Birnbaum and B. Slezak, "Dietary Exposure to PCBs and Dioxins in Children," *Environmental Health Perspectives* (107), January 1999, 1.

130. Increased exposure of children through diet: Landrigan article as above, and "They Are What They Eat," a report from the Environmental Working Group, Washington DC, February 1999.

131. Increased exposure through inhalation: R. Etzel, "Air pollution hazards to children," *Otolaryngology—Head and Neck Surgery* (114) February 1996, 265–266.

131. Rise in chronic diseases: "An Introduction to Children's Environmental Health," from the Children's Environmental Health Network, www.cehn.org; J. Cushman, "New Toxins Suspected as Cancer Rates Rise in Children," *New York Times* September 29, 1997; and 'Some Facts on Children's Cancers," U.S. Environmental Protection Agency, Office of Children's Protection, June 29, 1998.

132. Landrigan quote: Landrigan article cited above.

132. Lead-poisoning facts: A. Spake and J. Couzin, "In the air that they breathe," *U.S. News and World Report*, December 20, 1999; 54–56, and A. Crochetti, "Determinations of numbers of lead-exposed U.S. children by areas of the U.S.," *Environmental Health Perspectives* (89) 1990, 109–120.

133. Health effects of lead: Needleman and Landrigan, *Raising Children Toxic Free*, 23, 70–76; M. Ellis and K. Kane, "Lightening the Lead Load in Children," *American Family Physician* (62) August 1, 2000, 545–554; Spake and Couzin as above; and personal correspondence with Herbert Needleman.

135. Prenatal effects of mercury: G. J. Myers and P. J. Davidson, "Prenatal methylmercury exposure and children," *Environmental Health Perspectives* (106) June 1998, Supplement 3, 841–847.

135. Mercury in tuna: *In Harm's Way: Toxic Threats to Child Development* (Greater Boston Physicians for Social Responsibility 2000), 63.

136. Prenatal effects of organic solvents: J. Singh and L. Scott, "Threshold for CO-induced fetotoxicity," *Tetrology* (30) October 1984, 253–257; J. Peters, S. Preston-Martin et al., "Childhood tumors and parental occupational exposures," *Teratogenicity, Carcinogenicity, and Mutagenicity* (4) 1984, 137–148; J. Olsen et al., "Parental employment at time of conception and risk of cancer in offspring," *European Journal of Cancer* (27) 1991, 948–965; and J. Fabia and T. Thuy, "Occupation of father at time of birth of children dying of malignant disease," *British Journal of Preventive Social Medicine* (28) May 1974, 98–100.

137. Hormonally active agents: Theo Colburn, Dianne Dumanoski, and John Peterson Myers, *Our Stolen Future* (Plume/Pilgrim 1997); and "Hormone Mimics," *Consumer Reports* June 1998, 52–55.

137. Chlorine exposure in the shower: C. Weisel and W.-K. Jo, "Ingestion, inhalation, and dermal exposures to chloroform and trichloroethylene from tap water," *Environmental Health Perspectives* (104) January 1996, 48–51.

137. Pregnancy and chlorine by-products: D. Vergano, "Tap Water Byproducts Linked to Stillbirths," *Medical Tribune*, May 6, 1999, 20.

139. Effects of passive smoke on children: Needleman and Landrigan, *Raising Children Toxic Free*, as above, 162–165.

139. Drawings of pesticide-exposed children: Judith Raloff, "Picturing pesticides' impacts on kids," *Science News* (153) June 6, 1998, 358.

139. Pesticides and Parkinson's: J. Stephenson, "Exposure to Home Pesticides Linked to Parkinson Disease," *Journal of the American Medical Association* (283) June 21, 2000, 3055–6.

139. NAS report: *Pesticides in the Diets of Infants and Children* (National Academy of the Sciences 1993).

140. Supermarkets offering organic foods: "Organics: Reshaping the Supermarket," *E Magazine*, January/February 2000, 34–35.

140. Percent of two-year-olds getting pesticide residues: "Pesticides in the Diets of Infants and Children," as above.

141. Pesticides on foods: "They Are What They Eat" (as above) and "How 'bout Them Apples?" from the Environmental Working Group, Washington DC, February 1999; and *Regulating Pesticides in Food: The Delaney Paradox* (National Academy of Sciences Press 1987).

141. Pesticides at school: "School Pesticide Use Raises Concerns," Onhealth, www.onhealth.com, January 6, 2000.

141. Pesticide production and use: A. Aspelin, "Pesticide Industry Sales and Usage 1992–1993 Market Estimates," Environmental Protection Agency 1994; and M. Moser, "Designer Poisons," Pesticide Education Center, San Francisco, 1995.

141. Home pesticides and cancer: J. Leiss and D. Savitz, "Home pesticide use and childhood cancer: a case-control study," *American Journal of Public Health* (85) February 1995, 249–252; and R. Lewis, R. Fortmann et al., "Evaluation of methods for monitoring the potential exposure of small children to pesticides in the residential environment," *Archives of Environmental Contamination and Toxicology* (26) January 1994, 37–46.

144. Safety of bottled water: H. Macht, "Bottled hype?" *The Amicus Journal* of the Natural Resources Defense Council, Summer 1999, 7; and J. Lalumandier and L. Ayers, "Fluoride and Bacterial Content of Bottled Water vs. Tap Water," *Archives of Family Medicine* (9) March 2000, 246–250.

145. Percentage of inner-city and suburban kids with high lead levels: M. Friedrich, "Poor Children Subject to 'Environmental Injustice'," *Journal of the American Medical Association* (283) June 21, 2000, 3057.

146. Availability of firearms: M. Schuster et al., "Firearm Storage Pat-

terns in U.S. Homes With Children," *American Journal of Public Health* (90) April 2000, 588–594.

148. Safety of playgrounds: From National Program for Playground Safety, www.uni.edu/playground/home.html.

## Chapter 9: Aliens Are Brainwashing My Kids!

152. TV advertisements seen by children: American Academy of Pediatrics Committee on Communication, "Children, Adolescents, and Advertising," *Pediatrics* (95) February 1995, 295–297.

152. Buying power of kids: "Children and Advertising," Fact sheet from the National Institute for Media and the Family, accessed online April 28, 2000.

152. Developmental inability to recognize advertising: "Children, Adolescents, and Advertising," as above.

153. Viewing of adult shows by children: "Media Violence in Children's Lives," a position paper from the National Association for the Education of Young Children, 1994.

153. Air time for war cartoons: "Media Violence in Children's Lives," as above.

153. Violent acts on TV: "Media Violence in Children's Lives," as above.

156. Poverty in children: "Poverty Rate Lowest in 20 years, Household Income at Record High, Census Bureau Reports," press release, from the U.S. Department of Commerce Bureau of the Census, September 26, 2000.

159. Effects of optimism and pessimism on health: T. Maruta, R. Colligan, et al., "optimists versus pessimists: survival rate among medical patients over a 30-year period," *Mayo Clinic Proceedings* (75) February 2000, 140–143; H. Karpman, "Is Your Life's Wine Bottle Half-Full or Half-Empty?" *Internal Medicine Alert*, June 20, 2000.

159. Girls' self-image: Youth Risk Behavior Study, Centers for Disease Control, 1995.

160. Psychological effects of violent images: "Understanding the Impact of Media on Children and Teens," American Academy of Pediatrics, 2000.

160. Detrimental effects of violent video games: C. Anderson and K. Dill, "Video games and aggressive thoughts, feelings, and behavior in the laboratory and in life" *Journal of Personality and Social Psychology* (78) April

2000, 772–790; and David Walsh, "Video Game Violence: A Research Update," National Institute for Media and the Family, November 23, 1999.

161. Hostility and atherosclerosis: C. Iribarren et al., "Association of Hostility with Coronary Artery Calcification in Young Adults," *Journal of the American Medical Association* (283) May 17, 2000, 2546–2551.

161. Knowledge of tobacco risks: S. Sisley, "Residents help young people understand the truth about tobacco," *Journal of the American Medical Association* (283) May 3, 2000, 2312.

161. Alcohol and tobacco in children's movies: A. Goldstein et al., "Tobacco and Alcohol Use in G-Rated Children's Animated Films," *Journal of the American Medical Association* (281) March 24/31 1999, 1131–1136.

161. Substance use in middle school: "State of Washington's Children," a report from the University of Washington School of Public Health and Community Medicine, Winter 1999; and "High School and Youth Trends," an InfoFax from the National Institute for Drug Addiction, 1999.

162. Dangers of early addiction: "Effect of Advertising on Children's Use of Tobacco," fact sheet from the National Institute for Media and the Family from www.mediaandthefamily.com/tobac.html accessed 4/28/00.

162. Smoking deaths: "Tobacco and kids: Solving the problem before it starts," *AMA Action* May 26, 1999.

163. Sportsmanship classes for parents: Greg Mitchell, "Putting the Play Back in Play Ball," posted at www.youthleagues.com on April 12, 2000.

## Section II Complementary Therapies for Children

166. Use of complementary therapies in pediatric pain management programs: "Alternative Medicine for Kids," *Family Practice News* October 15, 1999, 56.

## Chapter 10: Little Bodies, Big Minds

172. Size of placebo effect: J. Turner, "The importance of placebo effects in pain treatment and research," *Journal of the American Medical Association* (271) May 25, 1994, 1609–1614.

172. Placebo and asthma study: T. Luparello, et al., "Influences of suggestion on airway reactivity in asthmatic subjects," *Psychosomatic Medi-*

*cine* (30) 1968, 819; and W. Brown, "Harnessing the Placebo Effect," *Hospital Practice*, July 15, 1998, 107–116.

173. Psychoneuroimmmunology: Candace Pert, *Molecules of Emotion: Why You Feel the Way You Feel* (Scribner 1997); and R. Ader, D. Felten, et al., "Interactions between the brain and the immune system," *Annual Review of Pharmacology and Toxicology* (30) 1990, 561–602.

175. Psycho-physiologic influences on pediatric illness: Figures presented at the first annual Conference on Pediatric Integrated Medicine, Tucson, Arizona February 18, 2000; and S. Vollmer, "How to detect and treat pediatric somatization," *Family Practice Recertification* (22) March 2000, 47–66.

179. Iyenegar quote: Mirka Knaster, *Discovering the Body's Wisdom* (Bantam 1996), 346.

180. Relaxation response and progressive muscular relaxation: Herbert Benson and Miriam Klipper, *The Relaxation Response* (Avon 1976).

182. Benefits of social connection: S. Kohen, et al., "Social Ties and Susceptibility to the Common Cold," *Journal of the American Medical Association* (277) June 25, 1997, 1940–1944; R. Hagerty, "Life stress, illness and social support," *Developmental Medicine and Child Neurology* (22) June 1980, 391–400; T. Glass, et al., "Population based study of social and productive activities as predictors of survival among elderly Americans," *British Medical Journal* (319) August 21, 1999, 478–483; and John Rowe and Robert Kahn, *Successful Aging* (Pantheon 1998), 152–166.

182. Health benefits of yoga: H. Nagendra and R. Nagarathna, "An integrated approach of yoga for bronchial asthma: a 3–54 month integrated study," *Journal of Asthma* (23) 1986, 123–137; M. Garfinkel, A. Singhal, et al., "Yoga-Based Intervention for Carpal Tunnel Syndrome," *Journal of the American Medical Association* (280) November 11, 1998, 1601–1603; and K. Uma, et al., "The integrated approach of yoga: a therapeutic tool for mentally retarded children: a one-year controlled study," *Journal of Mental Deficiency Research* (33) 1989, 415–421.

183. Health benefits of meditation: H. Benson, C. Edwards, et al., "Using mind-body therapies in primary care," *Patient Care* (33) July 15, 1999, 108–129; and N. Waring, "Mindfulness Meditation," *Hippocrates*, July 2000, 19–21.

184. Mindfulness Meditation: Jon Kabat-Zinn, *Full Catastrophe Living: Using the Wisdom of Your Body and Mind to Face Stress, Pain and Illness* (Dell 1990).

186. Video-game analogy: Melvin Levine, William Carey, and Allen

Crocker, *Developmental-Behavioral Pediatrics*, 3rd Edition (W. B. Saunders 1999), 847.

186. Health benefits of biofeedback: T. Culbert, R. Kajander, et al., "Biofeedback with Children and Adolescents: Clinical Observations and Patient Perspectives," *Developmental and Behavioral Pediatrics* (17) October 1996, 342–350.

189. Health benefits of hypnosis/imagery: L. Sugarman, "Hypnosis in a primary care practice: Developing Skills for the 'New Morbidities'," *Developmental and Behavioral Pediatrics* (17) October 1996, 300–305; and K. Olness and D. Kohen, *Hypnosis and Hypnotherapy with Children* (Guilford 1996).

## Chapter 11: The Healing Touch

195. Craniosacral manipulation: Andrew Weil, *Spontaneous Healing* (Knopf 1995), 25–39.

197. Divisions of chiropractors: Kenneth Pelletier, *The Best Alternative Medicine: What Works? What Does Not?* (Simon & Schuster 2000).

198. Chiropractic manipulation for acute low back pain: S. Bigos, O. Bowyer, et al., "Clinical Practice Guideline Number 14: Acute Low Back Pain Problems in Adults," U.S. Agency for Healthcare Policy and Research, 1994.

198. Chiropractors and primary care: S. Benjamin, "Chiropractic: Defining its role," *Patient Care* (33) June 15, 1999, 23–30; P. Shekelle, "What Role for Chiropractic in Health Care?" *New England Journal of Medicine* (339) October 8, 1998, 1074–5 and A. Mainous, J. Gill, et al., "Fragmentation of Patient Care Between Chiropractors and Family Physicians," *Archives of Family Medicine* (9) May 2000, 446–450.

199. Benefits of therapeutic massage: T. Field, "Massage therapy effects," *American Psychology* (53) 1998, 1270–1281. Other massage studies can be found at the Touch Research Institute Web site www.miami.edu/touch-research/

## Chapter 12: "Herbs and Spices"

205. Prescription drugs originally derived from plants: Michael Murray, *The Healing Power of Herbs,* 2nd edition (Prima 1995), xi.

206. Spending on botanical medicines: E. Ernst, "Herbal medicines: where is the evidence?" *British Medical Journal* (321) August 12, 2000, 395–396.

212. Dosage for children: Personal correspondence from Francis Brinker, N.D.

213. Herbs that increase bleeding: Frances Brinker, *Herbal Contraindications and Drug Reactions* (Eclectic Institute 1997).

214. Echinacea studies: D. Melchart, K. Linde, et al., "Echinacea for preventing and treating the common cold," Cochrane Database System Review (2) 2000; and D. Melchart, "Echinacea root extracts for the prevention of upper respiratory tract infections," *Archives of Family Medicine* (7) November/December 1998, 741.

214. Actions of astragalus: Michael Murray and Joseph Pizzorno, Jr. *An Encyclopedia of Natural Medicine* (Prima 1990), 230.

215. Ginger studies: T. Mustapha, et al., "Ginger (Zingiber officinale) in migraine headache," *Journal of Ethnopharmacology* (29) July/August 1988, 267–273; K. Srivastava, et al., "Ginger (Zingiber officinale) in rheumatism and musculoskeletal disorders," *Medical Hypotheses* (39) December 1992, 342–348; and A. Grontved, "Ginger root against seasickness: A controlled trial on the open sea," *Acta Otolaryngology* (105) January/February 1988, 45–9.

215. Garlic studies: James Robbers and Varro Tyler, *Tyler's Herbs of Choice: The Therapeutic Use of Phytomedicinals* (Haworth 1999).

216. Elderberry and flu: Z. Zakay-Rones, et al., "Inhibition of several strains of influenza virus in vitro and reduction of symptoms by an elderberry extract (Sambucus nigra L.) during an outbreak of influenza B Panama," *Journal of Alternative and Complementary Medicine* (1) Winter 1995, 361–369.

216. Chamomile and diarrhea: S. de la Motte, et al., "Double-blind comparison of a preparation of pectin/chamomile extract and placebo in children with diarrhea," *Arzneimittel Forschung* (47) November 1997, 1247–9.

217. Green tea and health: Lester Mitscher and Victoria Dolby, *The Green Tea Book: China's Fountain of Youth* (Avery 1998).

218. Comparative caffeine content of green tea: D. Schardt and S. Schmidt, "Caffeine: The Inside Scoop," *Nutrition Action* health letter, December 1996.

218. Infants and green tea: "Medicinal Foods," *Alternative Medicine Alert: Clinician Alert,* May 2000.

219. Medicinal mushrooms: Paul Stamets, *Growing Gourmet and Med-*

*icinal Mushrooms* (Ten Speed Press 1993); Kenneth Jones, *Shiitake: The Healing Mushroom* (Healing Arts 1995); and "Miraculous Mushrooms," *Dr. Andrew Weil's Self Healing* newsletter, May 1997.

220. Use of essential oils: Robert Tisserand and Tony Balacs, *Essential Oil Safety: A Guide for Health Care Professionals* (Churchill Livingstone 1995).

## Chapter 13: Like Cures Like

225. Homeopathic studies: K. Linde, S. Clausius, et al., "Are the clinical effects of homeopathy placebo effects?: A meta-analysis of placebo-controlled trials" *Lancet* (350) September 20, 1997, 834–843; E. Ernst and T. Kaptchuk, "Homeopathy Revisited," *Archives of Internal Medicine* (156) October 28, 1996, 2162–2164; and Wayne Jonas and Jennifer Jacobs, *Healing with Homeopathy: The Doctor's Guide* (Warner 1996).

225. Sales of homeopathic remedies in 1996: S. Benjamin, "Can like cure like?" *Patient Care* (33) December 15, 1999, 16–27.

230. Choosing homeopathic remedies: Robert Ullman and Judyth Reichenberg-Ullman, *Homeopathic Self-Care* (Prima 1997); Andrew Lockie and Nicola Geddes, *The Complete Guide to Homeopathy* (Dorling Kindersley 1995); Dana Ullman, *A Consumer's Guide to Homeopathy* (J. P. Tarcher 1995); and Maesimund Panos and Jane Heimlich, *Homeopathic Medicine at Home: Natural Remedies for Everyday Ailments and Minor Injuries* (J. P. Tarcher 1980).

## Chapter 14: A Billion People Can't Be Wrong

234. Western studies of Chinese medicine: A. Bensoussan, N. Talley, et al., "Treatment of Irritable Bowel Syndrome with Chinese Herbal Medicine: A Randomized Controlled Trial," *Journal of the American Medical Association* (280) November 11, 1998, 1585–1589; "Acupuncture," consensus statement from the National Institutes of Health, November 1997; W.-J. Xu, et al., "Modulation by Chinese herbal therapies of immune mechanisms in the skin of patients with atopic dermatitis," *British Journal of Dermatology* (136) January 1997, 54–59; D. Young, et al., "The Effects of Aerobic Exercise and Tai Chi on Blood Pressure in Older People: Results of a Randomized Trial," *American Journal of Geriatrics* (47) March 1999; S.

Wolf, et al., "Reducing frailty and falls in older persons: an investigation of tai chi and computerized balance training," *Journal of the American Geriatric Society* (44) May 1996, 489–497; and I. Chen, "Finding the Right Balance," *Hippocrates,* March 1999, 28–9.

235. Philosophy of Chinese medicine: Harriet Beinfield and Efrem Korngold, *Between Heaven and Earth: A Guide to Chinese Medicine* (Random House 1991); Ted Kaptchuk, *The Web That Has No Weaver: Understanding Chinese Medicine* (NTC/Contemporary 2000); Marc Micozzi, ed., *Fundamentals of Complementary and Alternative Medicine* (Churchill Livingstone 1996), 185–223 (written by Kevin Ergil); and Tom Williams, *The Complete Illustrated Guide to Chinese Medicine* (Element 1996).

237. James Reston: *New York Times* July 26, 1971 (1,6).

237. Acupuncture training: D. Grandinetti, "Acupuncture in 2000: Working its way into mainstream medicine," *Medical Economics,* August 7, 2000, 99–110.

238. "If Yin is a noun . . .": Korngold and Beinfield as above, 52.

242. Effects of acupuncture: "Proof that acupuncture alleviates pain." *Modern Medicine* (68) January 2000, 13; J. Helms, "An overview of medical acupuncture," *Alternative Therapies in Health and Medicine* (4) May 1998, 35–45; and NIH consensus statement on acupuncture, as above.

## Chapter 15: *Good Vibrations*

250. Heart-brain connection study: L. Russek and G. Schwartz, "Interpersonal Heart-Brain Registration and Perception of Parental Love," *Subtle Energies* (5) 1994, 195–208.

250. Religious participation studies: B. Bower, "Religious commitment linked to longer life," *Science News* (157) June 3, 2000, 359; D. Mathews, M. McCullough, et al., "Religious Commitment and Health Status," *Archives of Family Medicine* (7) March/April 1998, 118-124.

250. Intercessory prayer studies: Harold Koenig, *The Healing Power of Faith* (Simon & Schuster 1999); J. Astin, "The efficacy of 'distant healing': a systematic review of randomized trials," *Annals of Internal Medicine* (132) June 6, 2000, 903–910; W. Harris, M. Gowda, et al., "A randomized controlled trial of the effects of remote intercessory prayer on outcomes in patients admitted to the coronary care unit," *Archives of Internal Medicine* (159) October 25, 1999, 2273–8; F. Sicher, et al., "A randomized double-blind study of the effect of distant healing in a population with advanced

AIDS: report of a small-scale study," *Western Journal of Medicine* (169) December 1998, 356–363; and R. Byrd, "Positive therapeutic effects of intercessory prayer in a coronary care unit population," *Southern Medical Journal* (81) July 1988, 826–829.

255. American belief in the power of prayer: J. Levin, D. Larson, et al., "Religion and Spirituality in Medicine: Research and Education," *Journal of the American Medical Association* (278) September 3, 1997, 792–793.

256. Desire for doctors to address spiritual needs: "Vital Statistics," *Health*, October 1999, 20.

256. Herbert Benson: M. Moran, "What is the role of spirituality in medicine?" *American Medical News*, April 12, 1999, 1, 52–53.

## Chapter 16: Cold and Flu Defense

263. Colds per year: T. Nordenberg, "Colds and Flu: Time is the Only Sure Cure," *FDA Consumer*, May 1999 (revised).

263. Antibiotics for viral URIs: S. Dosh, et al., "Predictors of Antibiotic Prescribing for Non-Specific Upper Respiratory Infections, Acute Bronchitis and Acute Sinusitis," *The Journal of Family Practice* (49) May 1999, 407–414.

265. Sales of OTC cold medicines: Nordenberg, as above.

266. Handwashing studies: J. Niffenegger, "Proper handwashing promotes wellness in child care," *Journal of Pediatric Health Care* (11) January/February 1997, 26–31; and J. Green, "Quantum Sufficit," *American Family Physician* (61) January 15, 2000, 295.

267. Day care and colds: C. Ryan and E. Bean, "Management of Upper Respiratory Syndromes in Children," *Family Practice Recertification* (22) March 15, 2000, 41–55.

267. Vitamin C and colds: H. Hemila, "Vitamin C and the Common Cold," *British Journal of Nutrition* (67) January 1992, 3–16.

267. Echinacea and colds: B. Barret, et al., "Echinacea for Upper Respiratory Infection," *The Journal of Family Practice* (48) August 1999, 628–634; and studies listed above in the note for page 266.

268. Zinc and colds: A. Prasad, et al., "Duration of symptoms and plasma cytokine levels in patients with the common cold treated with zinc acetate," *Annals of Internal Medicine* (133) August 15, 2000, 245–252; M. Macknin, et al., "Zinc Gluconate Lozenges for Treating the Common Cold in Children," *Journal of the American Medical Association* (279) June 24,

1999, 1962–1967; and A. Gadomski, "A Cure for the Common Cold? Zinc Again," *Journal of the American Medical Association* (279) June 24, 1998, 1999–2000.

270. Chicken soup study: B. Rennard, "Chicken soup inhibits neutrophil chemotaxis in vitro," *Chest* (118) October 2000, 1150–1157.

275. Incidence of viral vs bacterial sinusitis: K. O'Brien, et al., "Acute Sinusitis: Principles of Judicious Use of Antimicrobial Agents," *Pediatrics* (101) January 1998, 174–177.

280. Sambucol studies: Z. Zackay-Rones, et al., "Inhibition of several strains of influenza virus in vitro and reduction of symptoms by an elderberry extract (Sambuccus nigra L.) during an outbreak of influenza B Panama," *Journal of Alternative and Complementary Medicine* (1) Winter 1995, 361–369.

280. Side effects of zanamivir: G. Yamey, "Drug company issues warning about flu drug," *British Medical Journal* (320) February 5, 2000, 334.

## Chapter 17: Is It Strep?

283. Incidence of strep throat: M. Pichichero, "Pharyngitis: When to Treat," *Consultant* (40 ) August 2000, 1669–1674; and M. Tucker, "Testing for Strep Throat Before Using Antibiotics," *Family Practice News,* May 15, 2000, 14.

284. Effectiveness of throat cultures: J. Tsevat and U. Kotagal, "Management of Sore Throats in Children: A Cost-Effectiveness Analysis," *Archives of Pediatric and Adolescent Medicine* (153) June 1999, 681–688.

285. Desirability of time to build potential immune response: R. Pitetti and E. Wald, "Strep throat: Considering the diagnostic options," *Patient Care* (33) April 30, 1999, 119–145; and see page 74 above.

## Chapter 18: Listen Up!

288. Incidence of ear infections: V. Howie, "Natural history of otitis media," *Annals of Otology, Rhinology, and Laryngology* (84) 1975, 67.

288. Office visits for: G. Bosker and S. Winograd, "Acute Otitis Media (AOM) Year 2000 Update: A Rational and Evidence-Based Analysis of Current Controversies in Antibiotic Therapy and Drug Selection for AOM," *Emergency Medicine Reports* (21) March 27, 2000.

288. Prescriptions for: H. Baucher and B. Phillip, "Reducing Inappropriate Oral Antibiotic Use: A Prescription for Change," *Pediatrics* (102) July 1998, 142–4.

288. Increased risk from day care: "Acute Otitis Media in Children: Challenging the Guidelines and Course of Antibiotic Therapy," *Medical Crossfire* (1) June 1999, 37–68; and S. Chartrand, "Acute otitis media: Management in an era of antibiotic resistance," *Family Practice Recertification* (21) April 15, 1999, 49–64.

289. Unnecessary prescriptions for: Bauscher and Phillip, as above.

292. Amount caused by viruses: T. Heikkinen, et al., "Serum Interleukin-6 in Bacterial and Nonbacterial Acute Otitis Media," *Pediatrics* (102) August 1998, 296–9.

292. Percent resolving on their own: "Acute Otitis Media in Children," as above.

293. Percent of resistant bacteria: E. Susman, "One in Three Children Seeking Care for Otitis Media Will Be Resistant to Antibiotics," *Emergency Medicine News*, December 1999, 56.

293. Watchful waiting studies: R. Damoiseux, et al., "Primary-care-based, randomized double-blind trial of amoxicillin versus placebo for acute otitis media in children aged under two years," *British Medical Journal* (320) February 5, 2000, 350–354; J. Froom, et al., "Antimicrobials for otitis media: A review from the International Primary Care Network," *British Medical Journal* (315) July 12, 1997, 98–102.

294. Doctor visits for AOM: "Recurrent Acute Otitis Media: Medical Versus Surgical Options," *Medical Crossfire* (2) March 2000, 45–55.

294. Risk factors for AOM: Bosker and Winograd, as above; G. Ehrlich and J. Post, "Susceptibility to Otitis Media," *Journal of the American Medical Association* (282) December 8, 1999, 2167–9; and G. Gates, "Otitis Media—The Pharyngeal Connection," *Journal of the American Medical Association* (282) September 8, 1999, 987–9.

295. Incidence of S. pneumoniae: Chartrand, as above.

295. Efficacy of nasal flu vaccine: R. Belshe, "The efficacy of live attenuated, cold-adapted, trivalent, intranasal influenza virus vaccine in children," *New England Journal of Medicine* (338) May 14, 1998, 1405–1412.

296. Risk from passive smoke: Chartrand, as above.

296. Risk reduction from breastfeeding: Chartrand, as above.

297. Homeopathy: K. Friese, et al., "The homeopathic treatment of otitis media in children—comparisons with conventional therapy,"

*International Journal of Clinical Pharmacology Therapy* (35) July 1997, 296–301.

## Chapter 19: Cry Babies, Cry Parents

298. Incidence of colic: D. Fleisher, "Coping with colic," *Patient Care* (33) April 15, 1999, 125–140.
299. Cause of colic: Fleisher, as above.
300. Chamomile for colic: Z. Weizman, et al., "Efficacy of herbal tea preparation in infantile colic," *Journal of Pediatrics* (122) April 1993, 650–652.
304. Tobacco smoke and reflux: S. Shahib, et al., "Passive smoking is a risk factor for esophagitis in children," *Journal of Pediatrics* (127) 1995, 435–437.

## Chapter 20: Tummy Troubles

307. Benefit of probiotics for constipation: K. Niedzielin and H. Kordecki, "Therapeutic usefulness of "Pro-Viva" solution in the treatment of irritable bowel syndrome and hemorrhoids," presented at the Symposium of Gastroenterology in Heiligenstadt (Germany), May 3–5, 1996.
308. Fruit juice and diarrhea: F. Lifshitz, "Role of Juice Carbohydrate Malabsorption in Chronic Non-specific Diarrhea in Children," *Journal of Pediatrics* (82) 1992, 64–68.
309. *Lactobacillus GG* for diarrhea: T. Arvola, et al., "Prophylactic Lactobacillus GG Reduces Antibiotic-Associated Diarrhea in Children with Respiratory Infections: A Randomized Study," *Pediatrics* (104) November 5, 1999, e64; and J. Vanderhoof and R. Young, "Use of Probiotics in Childhood Gastrointestinal Disorders," *Journal of Pediatric Gastroenterology and Nutrition* (27) September 1998, 323–332.
313. Treatment of *H. pylori*: C. Maltz, "14 commonly asked questions about *Helicobacter pylori* infection," *Emergency Medicine* (32) August 2000, 21–23.
313. Ginger and ulcer: James Duke, *The Green Pharmacy* (Rodale 1997), 435–6; and J. Yamahara et al., "The anti-ulcer effect in rats of ginger constituents," *Journal of Ethnopharmacology* (23) July/August 1988, 299–304.

# Chapter 21: It's Not All in Your Head

314. Incidence of headache: S. Diamond, "Migraine in Children: How to Recognize—How to Treat," *Consultant* (39) July 1999, 2045–2054.

319. Genetic component of migraine: R. Cady and K. Farmer-Cady, "Migraine: Changing Perspectives on Pathophysiology and Treatment," *Consultant* (40) September 15, 2000, S13–19.

320. Missing a meal: T. Rozen, et al., "Food for Thought About Dieting and Migraine," *Consultant* (39) May 2000, 968.

320. Efficacy of hypnosis: K. Olness, et al., "Prospective study comparing propranodol, placebo, and hypnosis in the treatment of juvenile migraine," *Pediatrics* (79) April 1987, 593–7.

322. Feverfew: S. Foster, "Feverfew: When the Head Hurts," *Alternative and Complementary Therapies*, September/October 1995, 335–337.

# Chapter 22: Sneezes and Wheezes

323. Increase in childhood asthma: P. Newacheck and N. Halpfon, "Prevalence, impact, and trends in childhood disability due to asthma," *Archives of Pediatric and Adolescent Medicine* (154) March 2000, 287–293.

323. Missed school days: The American Academy of Allergy, Asthma, and Immunology Task Force on Allergic Disorders, "Promoting Best Practice. Raising the Standard of Care for Patients with Allergic Disorders," (Executive Summary Report). Milwaukee, WI: AAAAI, November 1998; and E. Mechcatie, "User-friendly pediatric asthma guide posted on the Internet," *Family Practice News*, January 2000, 24.

324. Asthma and hospitalization: J. Horstman, "Living with asthma and allergies," *Hippocrates* (supplement), Spring 1998, 3–24).

324. Air pollution and asthma: H. Pikhart, et al., "Outdoor air concentrations of nitrogen dioxide and sulfur dioxide and prevalence of wheezing in children," *Epidemiology* (11) March 2000, 153–160; H. Anderson, et al., "Air pollution, pollens, and daily admissions for asthma in London 1987–92," *Thorax* (53) 1998, 842–848; J. Devalia, et al., "Allergen/irritant interaction: its role in sensitization and allergic disease," *Allergy* (53) April 1998, 335–345; and C. Meza and M. E. Gershwin, "Why is asthma becoming more of a problem?" *Current Opinions in Pulmonary Medicine* (3) January 1997, 6–9.

325. Hygiene hypothesis studies: P. Steerenberg, "Environmental and lifestyle factors may act in concert to increase the prevalence of respiratory allergy including asthma," *Clinical and Experimental Allergy* (29) October 1999, 1303–8; J. Celedon, et al., "Day care attendance in the first year of life and illnesses of the upper and lower respiratory tract in children with a family history of atopy," *Pediatrics* (104) September 1999, 495–500; U. Kramer, et al., "Age of entry to day nursery and allergy in later childhood," *Lancet* (353) February 1999, 450–454; and Sandra Christianson, "Please, sneeze on my child," *New England Journal of Medicine* (343) August 24, 2000, 574–575.

326. Breast-feeding and allergy: U. Hoppu, et al., "Maternal diet rich in saturated fat during breastfeeding is associated with atopic sensitization of the infant," *European Journal of Clinical Nutrition* (54) September 2000, 702–5.

327. Smoking exposure: S. Sarpong and J. Corey, "Assessment of the indoor environment in respiratory allergy," *Nose and Throat Journal* (77) December 1998, 960–964; 397.

327. Incidence of food allergy: National Center for Nutrition and Dietetics 1996 Fact Sheet; and H. A. Sampson, "Food allergy: from biology toward therapy," *Hospital Practice* (35) May 15, 2000, 67–76.

329. Peanut allergies: J. Raloff, "Family allergies? Keep nuts away from babies," *Science News* (149) May 4, 1996, 279.

330. Effects of smoking: J. Schwartz, et al., "Respiratory effects of environmental tobacco smoking a panel study of asthmatic and symptomatic children," *American Journal of Respiratory Critical Care Medicine* (161) March 2000, 802–806.

331. Value of fruits and vegetables: A. Soutar, et al., "Bronchial reactivity and dietary antioxidants. A lack of sufficient dietary antioxidants may promote bronchial reactivity," *Thorax* (52) February 1997, 166–170; J. Britton, et al., "The effects of dietary antioxidants on lung function in the general population," *American Review of Respiratory Disease* (147) 1993, A369; and J. Schwartz and S. Weiss, "Relationship between dietary vitamin C intake and pulmonary function: the first National Health and Nutrition Examination Survey (NHANES 1)," *American Journal of Clinical Nutrition* (59) January 1994, 110–114.

331. Vitamin C and asthma: C. Monteleone and A. Sherman, "Nutrition and asthma," *Archives of Internal Medicine* (157) January 1997, 23–34; and F. Forestiere, et al., "Consumption of fresh fruit rich in Vitamin C and wheezing symptoms in children," *Thorax* (55) April 2000, 283–8.

332. Hay fever statistics: P. Newacheck and J. Stoddard, "Prevalence and impact of multiple childhood chronic illnesses," *Journal of Pediatrics* (124) January 1994, 40–48; American Academy of Allergy, Asthma, and Immunology, The Task Force on Allergic Disorders: Promoting Best Practice. Raising the Standard of Care for Patients with Allergic Disorders. Executive Summary Report. Milwaukee, WI: AAAAI; November 1998.

332. Incidence of allergic rhinitis in children and number of school days missed: "Allergic Rhinitis: Impact and Diagnosis in the Primary Care Setting," white paper of University of Wisconsin-Madison Medical School Office of Continuing Medical Education, December 1999.

333. Dangers of ozone generators: "Ozone Generators That Are Sold as Air Cleaners: An Assessment of Effectiveness and Health Consequences," a report of the U.S. Environmental Protection Agency, April 16, 1998, accessed at www.epa.gov/iaq/pubs/ozonegen.html October 2, 2000.

334. Side effects of antihistamines: D. Aaronson, "Side effects of rhinitis medications," *Journal of Allergy and Clinical Immunology* (101 suppl) February 1998, S379–S382; and E. Vuurman, et al., "Seasonal allergic rhinitis and antihistamine effects on children's learning," *Annals of Allergy* (71) August 1993, 121–126.

335. Steroid growth suppression: L. Agertoft and S. Petersen, "Effect of long-term treatment with inhaled budesonide on adult height in children with asthma," *New England Journal of Medicine* (343) October 2000, 1064–1069.

335. Allergy component in all childhood asthma: S. Weiss, et al., "The inter-relationship among allergy, airways responsiveness and asthma," *Journal of Asthma* (30) 1993, 329–349; and B. Burrows, et al., "Association of asthma with serum IgE levels and skin-test reactivity to allergens," *New England Journal of Medicine* (320) February 2, 1989, 271–277.

336. Number of kids with asthma: D. Flapan, "Children with Asthma and Allergies Should Take Precautions at School," American Academy of Allergy and Immunology/Medscape Wire, August 24, 2000.

336. Asthma and diet: N. Hijazi et al., "Diet and childhood asthma in a society in transition: a study in urban and rural Saudi Arabia," *Thorax* (55) September 2000, 775–779.

338. Mind/body techniques: R. Greenfield, "Yoga as an adjunctive therapy in the treatment of asthma," *Alternative Medicine Alert* (1) November 1998, 127–130; R. Hackman, et al., "Hypnosis and asthma: a critical review," *Journal of Asthma* (37) February 2000, 1–15; D. Kohen, et al.,

"The use of relaxation-mental imagery (self-hypnosis) in the management of 505 pediatric behavioral encounters," *Journal of Developmental and Behavioral Pediatrics* (5) February 1984, 21–25; and J. Smyth, et al., "Effects of Writing About Stressful Experiences on Symptom Reduction in Patients with Asthma or Rheumatoid Arthritis: A Randomized Trial," *Journal of the American Medical Association* (281) April 14, 1999, 1304–9.

339. Obesity and asthma: "Obesity Found to Raise Kids' Asthma Risk," *Medical Tribune*, May 20, 1999; and B. Baker, "Obesity Tied to New-Onset Asthma in Ages 9–14," *Family Practice News*, June 15, 1999, 26.

339. Exercise and asthma: E. McFadden, "Exercise-induced airway obstruction," *Clinical Chest Medicine* (16) December 1995, 671–682.

341. Effects of steroid drugs: S. Kannisto, et al., "Adrenal suppression evaluated by a low-dose adrenocorticotropin test, and growth in asthmatic children treated with inhaled steroids," *Journal of Clinical Endocrinology and Metabolism* (85) February 2000, 652–7; and G. Sampraj and L. Kuritzky, "Inhaled Corticosteroids: Systemic Toxicity," *Hospital Practice* (35) June 15, 2000, 35–8.

## Chapter 23: A Rash of Complaints

346. Incidence of eczema: C. Correale, et al., "Atopic Dermatitis: A Review of Diagnosis and Treatment," *American Family Physician* (60) September 15, 1999, 1191–1198.

348. Probiotics and eczema: T. Kirn, "Probiotics Reduced Atopic Dermatitis," *Family Practice News*, June 1, 2000, 40.

## Chapter 24: "What Did You Say?"

353. Connection with other conditions: D. Phillips, et al., "School Problems and the Family Physician," *American Family Physician* (59) May 15, 1999, 2816–2824.

353. Smoking in pregnancy: S. Milberger, J. Biederman, et al., "Is Maternal Smoking During Pregnancy a Risk Factor for Attention Deficit Disorder in Children?" *American Journal of Psychiatry* (153) September 1996, 1138–1142.

353. Incidence of ADD/ADHD: "Managing Attention Deficit Hyperactivity Disorder: What Works?" *Consultant* (39) May 1999,

1507–1511; and "Attention-Deficit/Hyperactivity Disorder: Latest Guidelines for Diagnosis," *Consultant* (40) June 2000, 1265–1268.

354. Misdiagnosis: S. Stapleton, "Pediatricians add rigor to ADHD diagnosis," *American Medical News*, May 22/29, 2000, 35 and 39; B. Bower, "Study of stimulant therapy raises concerns," *Science News* (158) July 29, 2000, 69; and E. Littman, "ADHD Under-diagnosed in Girls," *Family Practice News*, April 1, 2000, 8.

354. Ritalin prescriptions: J. Zito, et al., "Trends in the Prescribing of Psychotropic Medications to Preschoolers," *Journal of the American Medical Association* (283) February 23, 2000, 1025–1030; and J. Coyle, "Psychotropic Drug Use in Very Young Children," *Journal of the American Medical Association* (283) February 23, 2000, 1059–1060.

356. Academic effects of Ritalin use: "Managing Attention Deficit Hyperactivity Disorder: What Works?" *Consultant* (39) May 1999, 1507–1511.

358. Essential fatty acids: J. Burgess, et al., "Long-chain polyunsaturated fatty acids in children with attention-deficit hyperactivity disorder," *American Journal of Clinical Nutrition* (71) January 2000 (Suppl), 327S–330S; and L. Stevens, et al., "Essential fatty acid metabolism in boys with attention-deficit hyperactivity disorder," *American Journal of Clinical Nutrition* (62) October 1995, 761–8.

# Resources

Here are some books, newsletters, videos, cassettes, organizations, web sites, and other sources of additional information on the topics covered in this book. Web sites come and go, so take the Internet addresses listed here with a grain of salt, and be prepared to use a search engine to locate an organization's new site.

## General Information on Integrative Medicine

*Natural Health, Natural Medicine: A Comprehensive Manual for Wellness and Self-Care,* by Andrew Weil, M.D. (Houghton Mifflin, 1998)

*Eight Weeks to Optimum Health,* by Andrew Weil, M.D. (Knopf, 1997)

*Spontaneous Healing,* by Andrew Weil, M.D. (Knopf, 1995)

*The Complete Illustrated Encyclopedia of Alternative Health Therapies,* C. Norman Shealy, M.D., consultant editor (Element, 1999)

*The Best Alternative Medicine: What Works? What Does Not?,* by Kenneth Pelletier, M.D. (Simon & Schuster, 2000)

*Medicine and Culture,* Lynn Payer (Henry Holt, 1996)

*Dr. Andrew Weil's Self Healing* newsletter, 42 Pleasant Street, Watertown MA 02172; (800) 523-3296; www.drweilselfhealing.com

National Center for Complementary and Alternative Medicine Clearinghouse, National Institutes of Health, P.O. Box 8218, Silver Spring MD 20907; (888) 644-6226; www.nccam.nih.gov

American Holistic Medical Association, 6728 Old McLean Village Drive, McLean VA 22101; (703) 556-9245; www.holisticmedicine.org

The Alternative Medicine Home Page at the University of Pittsburgh www.pitt.edu/~cbw/altm.html

Dr. Andrew Weil's Web site: www.drweil.com

## General Information on Pediatrics

*Caring for Your Baby and Young Child: Birth to Age 5,* by The American Academy of Pediatrics, Steven Shelov, M.D., editor (Bantam Doubleday, 1998)

*Caring for Your School-Age Child: Ages 5 to 12,* by The American Academy of Pediatrics, Edward Schur, M.D., editor (Broadway, 1999)

*The Natural Nursery: The Parent's Guide to Ecologically Sound, Non-Toxic, Safe, and Healthy Baby Care,* by Louis Pottkotter, M.D. (Contemporary Books, 1994)

*What to Expect When You're Expecting (1996), What to Expect the First Year (1996),* and *What to Expect the Toddler Years (1996),* by Arlene Eisenberg, Heidi Murkoff, and Sandra Hathaway, B.S.N. (all Workman)

*Everyday Blessings: The Inner Work of Mindful Parenting,* by Myla Kabat-Zinn and Jon Kabat-Zinn (Hyperion, 1997)

The Nemours Center for Children's Health Media Web site: www. Kidshealth.org

American Academy of Pediatrics You and Your Family Web site: www.aap.org/family/

American Academy of Family Physicians Web site: http://familydoctor.org

PubMed, the National Institutes of Health database on research: www.ncbi.nlm.nih.gov/PubMed/

## Immunity

*Health and Healing,* by Andrew Weil, M.D. (Houghton Mifflin, 1995)

*Molecules of Emotion: Why You Feel the Way You Feel,* by Candace Pert, Ph.D. (Scribner, 1997)

How Your Immune System Works: www.howstuffworks.com/immune-system.htm

## Vaccinations

*Vaccinating Your Child: Questions and Answers for the Concerned Parent,* by Sharon Humiston, M.D., and Cynthia Good (Peachtree, 2000)

National Immunization Program, Centers for Disease Control and Prevention, 1600 Clifton Road, Mailstop E-05, Atlanta GA 30333; (800) CDC-SHOT; www.cdc.gov/nip

Facing Parents' Concerns About Vaccines: www.medscape.com/ pediatrics/features/newsbeat/2000/0400/ID-Vaccines.html

Immunization Action Coalition, 1573 Selby Avenue, St. Paul MN 55104; (651) 647-9009; www.immunize.org

*Vaccines—Ask the Experts,* by William L. Atkinson, M.D., M.P.H., Harold Margolis, M.D., and Linda Moyer, R.N. [*NEEDLE TIPS* 9(2): 1999. © 1999 Immunization Action Coalition]

## Antibiotics

*The Antibiotic Paradox: How Miracle Drugs Are Destroying the Miracle,* by Stuart Levy, M.D. (Perseus, 1992)

*Breaking the Antibiotic Habit: A Parent's Guide to Coughs, Colds, Ear Infections, and Sore Throats,* by Paul Offit, M.D., and Louis Bell, M.D. (John Wiley, 1999)

Alliance for the Prudent Use of Antibiotics, 75 Kneeland Street, Boston MA 02111; (617) 636-0966; www.healthsci.tufts.edu/apua/

Fact sheets from the National Institute of Allergies and Infectious Diseases, Building 31, Room 7A50, 31 Center Drive, Bethesda MD 20892; www.niaid.nih.gov

Centers for Disease Control and Prevention, National Center for Infectious Disease, Division of Bacterial and Mycotic Diseases, 1600 Clifton Road, MSC23, Atlanta GA 30333; www.cdc.gov/ncidod/dbmd/ antibioticresistance/faqs.htm

Pamphlets from National Consumers' League, 1701 K Street NW, Suite 1200, Washington DC 20006; (202) 835-3323; www.nclnet.org

## Nutrition

*Eating Well for Optimum Health: The Essential Guide to Food, Diet, and Nutrition,* by Andrew Weil, M.D. (Knopf, 2000)

*How to Get Your Child to Eat . . . But Not Too Much* (1987) and *Child of Mine: Feeding with Love and Good Sense* (2000), by Ellyn Satter (Bull Publishing)

*Safe Eating,* by David W. K. Acheson, M.D., and Robin K. Levinson (Dell, 1998)

*The PDR Family Guide to Nutrition and Health* (Medical Economics, 1995)

*Feeding Your Child for Lifelong Health,* by Susan B. Roberts, Ph.D., and Melvin B. Heyman, M.D. with Lisa Tracy (Bantam, 1999)

*The Yale Guide to Children's Nutrition,* William Tamborlane, M.D., editor (Yale University Press, 1997)

*Breastfeeding Your Baby,* by Sheila Kitzinger (Knopf, 1998)

*The Nursing Mother's Companion,* by Kathleen Huggins (Harvard Common Press, 1995)

*The Crazy Makers: How the Food Industry Is Destroying Our Minds and Harming Our Children,* by Carol Simontacchi (Putnam, 2000)

*The Mash and Smash Cookbook: Fun and Yummy Recipes Every Kid Can Make!,* by Marion Buck-Murray (John Wiley, 1997)

Free materials on healthy foods for adults and children from the American Institute for Cancer Research, 1759 R Street NW, Washington DC 20009; (800) 843-8114; www.aicr.org

*Nutrition and Your Child* newsletter, Children's Nutrition Research Center at Baylor College of Medicine, 1100 Bates Street, Houston TX 77030; (713) 798-7000; www.bcm.tmc.edu/cnrc/

Food and Drug Administration Center for Food Safety and Applied Nutrition, (800) 332-4010; www.foodsafety.gov

*Nutrition Action,* newsletter of the Center for Science in the Public Interest, Suite 300, 1875 Connecticut Avenue NW, Washington DC 20009; (202) 332-9110; www.cspinet.org

Farmers' markets are listed at www.ams.usda.gov/farmersmarkets

USDA Healthy School Meals Resource Program: http://schoolmeals.nal.usda.gov:8001/Resource/

American Academy of Pediatrics, *American Academy of Pediatrics Guide to Your Child's Nutrition: Making Peace at the Table and Building Healthy Eating Habits for Life,* W. H. Dietz and L. Stern, American Academy of Pediatrics, editors (Villard Books, 1999)

Notes about super-sizing meals, etc. American Institute of Cancer Research Website: http://www.aicr.org/

## Physical Fitness/Obesity

*Save Your Child from the Fat Epidemic,* by Gayle Povis Alleman, M.S., R.D. (Prima, 1999)

*The Case for Elementary School Recess,* by Rhonda Clements (American Press, 1999)

*Promoting Physical Activity: A Guide for Community Action* (Centers for Disease Control, 1999)

*Moving With a Purpose: Developing Programs for Preschoolers of All Abilities,* by Renee McCall and Diane Craft (Human Kinetics, 2000)

National Association for Sport and Physical Education, 1900 Association Road, Reston VA 22091; (703) 476-3410; www.aahperd.org/naspe

American Association for the Child's Right to Play: www.ipausa.org

TV-Free America, 1611 Connecticut Avenue NW, Suite 3A, Washington DC 20009; (202) 887-0436; www.tvfa.org

BodyWise, an area on the Girl Power! Web site at www.health.org/gpower/girlarea/Bodywise/ from the National Clearinghouse for Alcohol and Drug Information (800-729-6686)

Human Kinetics Web site: www.humankinetics.com

Growth charts for Children from the Centers for Disease Control and Prevention: www.cdc.gov/nccdphp/dnpa/bmi/bmi-for-age.htm

You can find growth charts and other tools for assessing children's health at a site in which Dr. Stu holds an interest: www.MyFamilyMD.com

*Dynamic Physical Education for Elementary School Children,* by R. P. Pangrazi (Allyn and Bacon, 1998)

Better Health and Fitness Through Physical Activity: www.aap.org/family/fitness.htm

*Outcomes of Quality Physical Education Programs;* American Alliance for Health, Physical Education, Recreation and Dance, 1900 Association Drive, Reston, VA 22091

## Stress Management

*Stress-Proofing Your Child: Mind-Body Exercises to Enhance Your Child's Health,* by Sheldon Lewis and Sheila Kay Lewis (Bantam, 1996)

*Seven Times the Sun: Guiding Your Child Through the Rhythms of the Day,* by Shea Darian (LuraMedia, 1994)

*Conscious Breathing: Breathwork for Health, Stress Release, and Personal Mastery,* by Gay Hendricks, Ph.D. (Bantam, 1995)

*The Wellness Book: The Comprehensive Guide to Maintaining Health and Treating Stress-Related Illness,* by Herbert Benson, M.D., and Eileen Stuart, R.N., M.S. (Fireside, 1993)

*Relax,* by Catherine O'Neill Grace (1993)

*Cool Cats, Calm Kids: Relaxation and Stress Management for Young Kids,* by Mary L. Williams (Impact, 1996)

*Full Catastrophe Living: Using the Wisdom of the Body and Mind to Face Stress, Pain, and Illness,* by Jon Kabat-Zinn (Delacorte, 1990)

*Aromatherapy for Babies and Children: Gentle Treatments for Health and Well-Being,* by Shirley Price and Penny Price Parr (Thorsons/Harper, 1996)

*Breathing, the Master Key to Self Healing,* cassette or CD by Andrew Weil, M.D. (Sounds True, 1999)

## Environmental Issues

*In Harm's Way: Toxic Threats to Child Development* (Greater Boston Physicians for Social Responsibility, 2000)

*Raising Children Toxic Free,* by Herbert Needleman, M.D., and Philip Landrigan, M.D. (Farrar Straus and Giroux, 1994)

*Mothers and Others Guide to Natural Baby Care,* by Mindy Pennypacker and Aisha Ikramuddin (John Wiley & Sons, 1999)

*Our Stolen Future,* by Theo Colburn, Dianne Dumanoski, and John Peterson Myers (Plume/Penguin, 1997)

*Generations at Risk: Reproductive Health and the Environment,* by Ted Schettler, M.D., Gina Solomon, M.D., Maria Valenti, and Annette Huddle (MIT Press, 2000)

*Home Safe Home: Protecting Yourself and Your Family from Everyday Toxics and Harmful Household Products,* by Debra Lynn Dadd (Jeremy Tarcher/Putnam, 1997)

*Now I Know Better* and *Now I Know Better, Too,* (kids' own safety stories) from Yale New Haven Health (800) 925-3606

*The Geography of Childhood: Why Children Need Wild Places,* by Gary Paul Nabhan and Stephen Trimble (Beacon, 1994)

*Our Children's Toxic Legacy:How Science and Law Fail to Protect Us From Pesticides,* by John Wargo (Yale University Press, 1998)

Office of Children's Health Protection, Environmental Protection Agency, 1200 Pennsylvania Avenue NW, Mail Code 1107A, Room 2512 Ariel Rios North, Washington DC 20004; (202) 564-2188; www.epa.gov/children

Children's Environmental Health Network, 110 Maryland Avenue NE, Suite 511, Washington DC 20002; (202-543-4033); www.cehn.org

Mothers and Others for a Livable Planet, 40 W. 20th Street, New York NY 10011; (888) ECO-INFO; www.mothers.org

Childproofing Our Communities campaign of the Center for Health, Environment and Justice, P.O. Box 6806, Falls Church VA 22040; (703-237-2249); www.childproofing.org

Environmental Concepts Made Easy, from Tulane University School of Medicine; www.som.tulane.edu/ecme

Alliance to End Childhood Lead Poisoning, 227 Massachusetts Avenue NE, Suite 200, Washington DC 20002; (202) 543-1147; www.aeclp.org

National Lead Information Center, (800) 424-LEAD

The National SAFE KIDS Campaign 1301 Pennsylvania Avenue NW, Suite 1000, Washington DC 20004; (202) 662-0600; www.safekids.org

Environmental Defense, 257 Park Avenue South, New York NY 10010; (212) 505-2100; www.environmentaldefense.org

Environmental Working Group, 1718 Connecticut Avenue NW, Washington DC 20009; (202-667-6982); www.ewg.org

Environmental Protection Agency Safe Drinking Water Hot Line (800) 426-4791; www.epa.gov/safewater/dwinfo.htm

Defenders of Wildlife's Kids' Planet: www.kidsplanet.org

Books for Young People on Environmental Issues (grades K-6 and 7-12): www.epa.state.il.us/kids/teachers/books.html

EPA Office of Water: http://www.epa.gov/safewater/dwinfo.htm

EPA – The Children's Healthline Issue: Your child asks for a drink of water . . . http://www.epa.gov/reg3esd1/childhealth/ch3.pdf

EPA's Safe Water Hotline at 1-800-426-4791

## Cultural Issues

*Raising Children in a Socially Toxic Environment,* by James Garbarino (Jossey-Bass, 1999)

*Bringing Up a Moral Child,* by Michael Schulman and Eva Mekler (Addison Wesley, 1985)

*Raising Spiritual Children in a Material World,* by Phil Calalfo (Berkley, 1997)

*Put Your Heart on Paper: Staying Connected in a Loose-Ends World,* by Henriette Anne Klauser (Bantam, 1995)

*The Whole Parenting Guide,* by Alan Reder, Phil Catalfo, and Stephanie Renfrow Hamilton (Broadway, 1999)

*The Smart Parents' Guide to Kids TV,* by Milton Chen and Andy Bricky (Bay Books, 1994)

*Raising Peaceful Children in a Violent World,* by Nancy Lee Cecil and Patricia Roberts (LuraMedia, 1995)

National Institute for Media and the Family, 606 24th Avenue South, Suite 606, Minneapolis MN 55454; (888-672-5437); www.mediaandthefamily.com

The Media Literacy Online Project of the University of Oregon College of Education: http://interact.uoregon.edu/MediaLit/HomePage

The Center for Media Literacy, 4727 Wilshire Boulevard, #403, Los Angeles CA 90010; (800) 226-9454; www.medialit.org

Media Awareness Network: www.media-awareness.ca

Movie ratings: www.filmratings.com

Entertainment Software Rating Board, 845 Third Avenue, New York NY 10022; (800) 771-3772; www.esrb.org

The Lions & Lambs Project, 4300 Montgomery Avenue, Suite 104, Bethesda MD 20814; (301) 654-3091; www.lionlamb.org

Chinaberry Books, 2780 Via Orange Way, Suite B, Spring Valley CA 91978; (800) 776-2242; www.chinaberry.com

## Mind/Body Medicine

*Timeless Healing: The Power and Biology of Belief,* by Herbert Benson, M.D. with Marg Stark (Scribner, 1996)

*Mind/Body Medicine: How to Use Your Mind for Better Health,* by Daniel Goleman and Joel Guerin (Consumer Reports Books, 1993)

*Healing and the Mind,* by Bill Moyers (Doubleday, 1993)

*Anatomy of an Illness* (Bantam, 1979) and *Head First: The Biology of Hope* (E. P. Dutton, 1989), by Norman Cousins

*Guided Imagery for Self Healing,* by Martin Rossman, M.D. (H.J. Kramer, 2000)

*Meditating with Children: The Art of Concentration and Centering,* by Deborah Rozman (Planetary, 1994)

*Teaching Meditation to Children: A Practical Guide to the Use and Benefits of Modern Meditation Techniques,* by David Fontana and Ingrid Slack (Element, 1998)

*Moonbeam: A Book of Meditations for Children* (1999) and *Earthlight: New Meditations for Children* (1997), by Maureen Garth (HarperCollins, Australia)

Academy for Guided Imagery, P.O. Box 2070, Mill Valley CA 94942; (800) 726-2070; www.healthy.net/agi

*Imaginative Medicine: Hypnosis in Pediatric Practice*, video from Dr. Lawrence Sugarman, 880 Westfall Rd., Rochester, NY 14618-3906.

Guided Imagery Resource Center: www.healthjourneys.com

Center for Mind-Body Medicine, 5225 Connecticut Avenue NW, Suite 414, Washington DC 20015; (202) 966-2589; www.cmbm.org

Biofeedback Certification Institute of America, 10200 West 44th Avenue, Suite 304, Wheat Ridge CO 80033; (303) 420-2902

American Society of Clinical Hypnosis, 2200 East Devon Avenue, Suite 291, Des Plaines IL 60018; www.asch.net

American Music Therapy Association, 8455 Colesville Road, Silver Springs, MD 20910

Certification Board for Music Therapists, 589 Southlake Boulevard, Richmond, VA 23236; (800) 765-CBMT or (804) 379-9397

Association for Applied Psychotherapy and Biofeedback (AAPB), 10200 West 44th Ave., Suite 304, Wheatridge CO 80033; (303) 422-8436

## Manual Medicine

*Discovering the Body's Wisdom*, by Mirka Knaster (Bantam, 1996)

*Acupressure's Potent Points: A Guide to Self-care for Common Ailments*, by Michael Reed Gach (Bantam, 1990)

*The Complete Illustrated Guide to Massage: A Step-by-Step Approach to the Healing Art of Touch*, by Stewart Mitchell (Element Books, 1997)

*Infant Massage: A Handbook for Loving Parents*, by Vimala McClure (Bantam, 1989)

*The Reflexology Manual: An Easy-to-Use Illustrated Guide to the Healing Zones of the Hands and Feet*, by Pauline Wills (Healing Arts Press, 1995)

*In Your Hands: Baby Massage Therapy Techniques,* video at www.trusttouch.com

*Principles of Manual Medicine*, 2nd edition, by Philip E. Greenman, D.O., F.A.A.O., (Wiliams and Wilkins, 1996)

American Massage Therapy Association, 820 Davis Street S-100, Evanston IL 60201; (847) 864-0123; www.amtamassage.org

Acupressure Institute, 1533 Shattuck Avenue, Berkeley CA 94709; (510) 845-1059; www.acupressure.com

American Osteopathic Association, 142 East Ontario Street, Chicago IL 60611; (800) 621-1773; www.am-osteo-assn.org

The Cranial Academy, 8202 Clearvista Parkway, Building 9, Suite D, Indianapolis IN 46256; (317) 594-0411

The Osteopathic Center for Children : www.osteopathic-ctr-4child.org

Living Arts (massage video series including infant massage, acupressure, and reflexology); (800) 254-8464; www.gaiam.com

## Botanical Medicine

*Kids, Herbs, and Health: A Parent's Guide to Natural Remedies*, by Linda B. White, M.D., and Sunny Mavor A.H.G. (Interweave Press, 1998)

*The Healing Power of Herbs*, by Michael Murray, N.D. (Prima, 1995)

*The Encyclopedia of Natural Medicine*, Joseph Pizzorno, N.D., and Michael Murray, N.D. (Prima, 1998)

*Herbal Prescriptions for Better Health*, by Donald Brown (Prima, 1995)

*Herbs of Choice: The Therapeutic Use of Phytomedicinals*, by James Robbers, Ph.D., and Varro Tyler, Ph.D., Sc.D. (Haworth, 1999)

American Herbalists Guild, 1931 Gaddis Road, Canton GA 30115; (770) 751-6021; www.healthy.net/herbalists

American Botanical Council, P.O. Box 144345, Austin TX 78714; www.herbalgram.org

HerbMed of the Alternative Medicine Foundation: www.herbmed.org

Longwood Herbal Task Force Web site: www.mcp.edu/herbal

Institute for Natural Products Research Web site: www.naturalproducts.org

Rx List, the Internet Drug Index: www.rxlist.com/westherb.htm

## Homeopathic Medicine

*Homeopathic Self-Care: The Quick and Easy Guide for the Whole Family*, by Robert Ullman, N.D., and Judyth Reichenberg-Ullman, N.D. (Prima, 1997)

*Homeopathic Medicine for Children and Infants*, by Dana Ullmann (Jeremy Tarcher, 1992)

*Healing with Homeopathy*, by Wayne Jonas, M.D., and Jennifer Jacobs, M.D. (Warner, 1996)

Homeopathic Education Services, 2124 Kittredge Street, #71-Q, Berkeley CA 94704; (510) 649-0294

National Center for Homeopathy, 801 N Fairfax Street, Suite 306, Alexandria VA 22314; (703) 246-7790; www.homeopathic.org

# Chinese Medicine

*Between Heaven and Earth: A Guide to Chinese Medicine*, by Harriet Beinfield Lac and Efrem Korngold Lac, O.M.D. (Ballantine, 1991)

*The Web That Has No Weaver: Understanding Chinese Medicine*, by Ted Kaptchuk, O.M.D. (NTC/Contemporary, 2000)

*The Complete Illustrated Guide to Chinese Medicine: A Comprehensive System for Health and Fitness*, by Tom Williams (Element, 1996)

*Encounters with Qi: Exploring Chinese Medicine*, by David Eisenberg and Thomas Lee Wright (W. W. Norton, 1995)

*The Natural Healer's Acupressure Handbook: G-Jo Fingertip Technique*, by James Blate (Henry Holt, 1976)

National Commission for the Certification of Acupuncturists, 1424 16th Street NW, Suite 601, Washington DC 20036; (202) 232-1404

American Association of Oriental Medicine, 433 Front Street, Catasauqua PA 18032; (888) 500-7999; www.aaom.org

American Academy of Medical Acupuncture, 5820 Wilshire Boulevard, Suite 500, Los Angeles CA 90036; (213) 937-5514; www.medical acupuncture.org

National Acupuncture and Oriental Medicine Alliance Web site: www.acuall.org

# Energy Medicine

*The Living Energy Universe: A Fundamental Discovery that Transforms Science and Medicine*, by Gary Schwartz and Linda Russek (Hampton Roads, 1999)

*Infinite Grace: Where the Worlds of Science and Spiritual Healing Meet*, by Diane Goldner (Hampton Roads, 1999)

*Accepting Your Power to Heal: Personal Practice Therapeutic Touch*, by Dolores Kreiger, Ph.D., R.N. (Bear and Company, 1993)

*The Touch of Healing: Energizing the Body, Mind, and Spirit with Jin Shin Jyutsu*, by Alice Burmeister and Tom Monte (Bantam, 1997)

*The Spiritual Life of Children*, by Robert Coles (Houghton Mifflin, 1991)

*Prayer Is Good Medicine,* by Larry Dossey, M.D. (HarperSan Francisco, 1996)

International Center for Reiki Training, 29209 Northwestern Highway, #592, Southfield MI 48034; (800) 332-8112; www.reiki.org

Reiki Alliance, P.O. Box 41, Cataldo ID 83810

Healing Touch International, 12477 W Cedar Drive, Suite 202, Lakewood CO 80228; (303) 989-7982; www.healingtouch.net

Jin Shin Jyutsu, 8719 E San Alberto, Scottsdale AZ 85258; (480) 998-9331

## Otitis Media

*Management of Acute Otitis Media* is available in summary on the AHRQ Web site: *http://www.ahrq.gov/clinic/otitisum.htm*

## Allergy and Asthma

*American Academy of Pediatrics Guide to Your Child's Allergies and Asthma: Breathing Easy and Bringing Up Healthy Active Children*, by Michael Welch (Random House, 2000)

*The American Lung Association's Family Guide to Asthma and Allergy*, by Norman Edelman (Little, Brown, 1997)

*What You Really Need to Know About Caring for a Child with Asthma*, by Robert Buckman (Lebhar-Friedman Books, 1999)

The Food Allergy Network, 10400 Eaton Place, Suite 107, Fairfax VA (800) 929-4040; www.foodallergy.org or their site for kids www.fan kids.org

Allergy and Asthma Network-Mothers of Asthmatics, 2751 Prosperity Avenue, Suite 150, Fairfax VA 22031; (800) 878-4403; www.aanma.org

American Lung Association Web site: www.lungusa.org

National Jewish Research Center Web site: www.njc.org

Allergy, Asthma, and Immunology Online: www.allergy.mcg.edu

## IBD

*Breaking the Vicious Cycle: Intestinal Health Through Diet*, by Elaine Gottschall (Kirkton Press, 1994)

## ADHD

*Power Parenting for Children with ADD/ADHD: A Practical Parent's Guide for Managing Difficult Behavior* (1996), and *ADD/ADHD Behavior-Change Resource Kit* (1998), by Grad Flick, Ph.D. (The Center for Applied Research in Education)

*Living with ADHD: A Practical Guide to Coping with Attention Deficit Hyper-*

*activity Disorder*, by Rebecca Kajander, B.S.N., R.N., M.P.H. (Park Nicollet Medical Foundation, 1999)

*Ritalin-Free Kids*, by Judyth Reichenberg-Ullman, N.D., M.S.W., and Robert Ullman, N.D. (Prima, 2000)

Agency for Health Care Policy and Research (AHCPR): http://www.ahrq.gov/clinic/adhdsum.htm

## *Yoga*

Living Arts, (800) 254-8464, carries excellent instructional videotapes, including *YogaKids*, by Marsha Wenig

*A Yoga Parade of Animals: A first fun picture book of yoga*, by Pauline Mainland (Element, 1998)

*Children's Book of Yoga*, by Thia Luby (Clear Light, 1998)

*The Complete Idiot's Guide to Yoga with Kids*, by Jodi Komitor and Eve Adamson (Alpha, 2000)

# Index

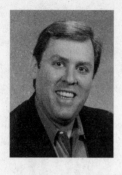

STUART H. DITCHEK, M.D., is a practicing pediatrician, a diplomat of the American Board of Pediatrics, a fellow of the American Academy of Pediatrics, and a clinical assistant professor of pediatrics at New York University School of Medicine. He lives in Brooklyn, New York, with his wife and five children. (PHOTO: ©2001 ZELMAN STUDIOS)

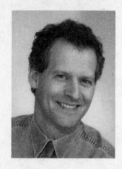

RUSSEL H. GREENFIELD, M.D., was one of the first four physicians nationwide to be admitted to Doctor Andrew Weil's program in integrative medicine at the University of Arizona Health Sciences Center. He is the director of Carolinas Integrative Health (CIH) in Charlotte, North Carolina, and speaks around the globe on topics related to integrated medicine. He lives in Charlotte with his wife and two children. (PHOTO: ©2001 LANCE FAIRCHILD PHOTOGRAPHY STUDIO)

LYNN MURRAY WILLEFORD is a freelance writer specializing in health, associate editor of the newsletter *Dr. Andrew Weil's Self Healing,* and a contributing editor of *New Age Journal.* She lives on Whidbey Island, Washington, with her husband and son.